TWIN BLOCK FUNCTIONAL THERAPY

Applications in Dentofacial Orthopaedics

William J Clark BDS, DDO

Orthodontist,
Fife, Scotland

Foreword by Professor T M Graber

Clinical Professor of Orthodontics,
University of Illinois at Chicago

Mosby-Wolfe

London Baltimore Bogotá Boston Buenos Aires Caracas Carlsbad, CA Chicago Madrid Mexico City
Milan Naples, FL New York Philadelphia St. Louis Sydney Tokyo Toronto Wiesbaden

Project Manager:	Dave Burin
Developmental Editors:	Lucy Hamilton, Claire Hooper
Designer:	Ian Spick
Cover Design:	Ian Spick
Illustration/Layout:	Frank Dingwall
Production:	Mike Heath
Publisher:	Geoff Greenwood

Copyright © 1995 Times Mirror International Publishers Limited

Published in 1995 by Mosby–Wolfe, an imprint of Times Mirror International Publishers Limited

Printed in Italy by G. Canale & C. S.p.A. - Borgaro T.se - TURIN

ISBN 0 7234 2120 X

For full details of all Times Mirror International Publishers Limited titles, please write to Times Mirror International Publishers Limited, Lynton House, 7–12 Tavistock Square, London WC1H 9LB, England.

A CIP catalogue record for this book is available from the British Library.

Library of Congress Cataloging-in-Publication Data has been applied for.

FOREWORD

If I have seen further it is by standing on the shoulders of giants

This quote from that eminent English scientist Sir Isaac Newton (1642–1727) should have been used by the author to introduce this valuable volume on functional orthopaedics. As a mature, experienced clinician who has faced and solved multiple orthodontic and orthopaedic problems, and as a frequent lecturer to orthodontic societies around the world, he has amassed an enormous amount of clinical material. This book is the culmination of a career dedicated to excellence and is a valuable addition to our compendium of knowledge.

In Chapter 1, Bill Clark wisely recognises the **art** of orthodontics. Quoting Edward H. Angle, he stresses that the philosophical challenges of our field were recognised at the turn of the century.

The study of orthodontia is indissolubly connected with that of art as related to the human face. The mouth is a most potent factor in making or marring the beauty and character of the face, and the form and beauty of the mouth largely depend on the occlusal relations of the teeth.

Truly a biological, as well as a mechanical artist, the author stresses that to achieve the optimal therapeutic results, in line with Angle's concepts (and those of his artistic mentor, Edmund Wuerpel), modern therapy is more than occlusion of the teeth. By virtue of whatever therapeutic means possible, it is our duty as orthodontists to effect changes that transcend occlusal relationships and encompass the total dentofacial complex. We must satisfy the wider aesthetic and holistic aims of our specialty. Excellent discussions of the aims and objectives of treatment, the analogy of 'dental chess', differentiation between orthodontics and orthopaedics, the philosophical divide and the genetic paradigm prepare the reader for the Twin Block technique.

Chapter 2 is a very complete description of the construction and use of the Twin Block orthopedic appliances, with appliance design and variations, stages and timetable of treatment, and response to treatment, with ample case reports. After briefly discussing the evolution of fixed appliance principles and techniques, to better understand orthodontic versus orthopaedic aspects of therapy. Chapter 3 then proceeds with a beautiful in-depth analysis of form and function, including the temporomandibular joint, objectives of functional treatment, the precursor to the Twin Block appliance (the Schwarz double plate), bite registration and control of the vertical dimension. This succinct but incisive discussion clearly delineates the challenges of orthopaedic treatment.

Chapter 4 provides more background and understanding of the growth guidance potential of functional appliances, elaborating on experimental animal studies. The clinician will appreciate especially the discussion of neuromuscular and skeletal adaptations and the paradigm of genetic control. The Twin Block response is compared with that of animal studies. This is again discussed in Chapter 13.

By the time the reader gets to that all important Chapter 5 on diagnosis and treatment planning, he has an excellent understanding of the challenges and potentials of functional appliance treatment. Although most clinicians already know how to take and interpret orthodontic records, excellent discussions of clinical guidelines and the means of assessment of records, for example, stress the most salient features of a proper diagnostic approach.

Chapter 6 is devoted to a comprehensive discussion of cephalometric analyses. Interestingly, Bill Clark cites the research of Eugene Coben and his means of superimposition. Incorporating elements from Ricketts, McNamara and Bimler, and the role of posture, the resultant cephalometric analysis is a melding of the latest concepts and provides a superb tool for the clinician, regardless of the appliance being used. This chapter alone justifies ownership of the book. Case studies elucidate the cephalometric approach and analyse treatment responses, particularly the section on facial changes with Twin Block treatment.

Chapter 7 is a comprehensive presentation on appliance design and construction that is well illustrated to prevent any misunderstanding. Clinical management of Class II, Division 1, deep bite cases are covered in Chapter 8, which considers all facets of appliance manipulation and uses case reports to illustrate the salient features. Initial adjustment, the support phase and retention are described.

Chapter 9 discusses one of the most rapidly developing orthodontic treatment areas – mixed dentition treatment. Growth guidance, functional control, treatment steps, duration, etc., are illustrated with case reports – again the hallmark of the book—clinical orientation for the average practitioner, without esoteric discussions of satellite considerations. Two-phase treatment mixed and permanent dentition are discussed and profusely illustrated by actual cases.

Chapter 10 covers combination therapy in the permanent dentition, utilising case reports, while Chapter 11 describes the use of extraoral traction in selected cases, in conjunction with the Twin Block. Chapter 12 discusses anterior open bite treatment, again with suitable appliance modifications, and uses case reports to show the correct Twin Block treatment. Orthopaedic control of vertical growth is described and illustrated. Intraoral traction to close the bite is also discussed fully.

Chapter 13 again has a detailed discussion of therapy—this time, for Class II, Division 2 malocclusions. Differences from Class II, Division I therapy are described and illustrated. Class III malocclusions are treated with reverse Twin Blocks in Chapter 14. All treatment aspects are covered, with case reports showing varying responses to appliance guidance.

Chapter 15 is a broader discussion of differential diagnosis that examines extraction therapy and arch length discrepancy. A logical follow up is the management of crowding cases. The excellent case reports provide a broad understanding of diagnostic and therapeutic principles. Crowding is discussed in Chapter 16, while extraction therapy is again discussed in Chapter 17. Facial asymmetry problems are described and sample treated cases are shown in Chapter 18. The latest modification to enhance the functional aspects of Twin Block therapy, the use of magnets with Twin Blocks, are described in Chapter 19. Though more limited in potential, Chapter 20 illustrates the Twin Block appliance use for adults. A logical following chapter is Twin Block use in temporomandibular joint problems. It is well known that forward posturing of the mandible has a beneficial effect in most TMD patients. The author describes the effective use of the appliances, along with a discussion of various aspects of TMJ derangement.

Some clinicians enhance functional appliance results by bonding them in place – i.e. using the Hamilton expansion-activator and the Herbst appliance. That this can be done with the Twin Block appliance, reducing patient compliance demands, is shown in the penultimate chapter. Here, again, the broad potential of this most versatile appliance is evident.

The last chapter is, in a way, a postscript to the book: a discussion of the growth responses to Twin Block treatment. Various studies are cited to illustrate the potential of the appliance. The final quote from the great Scottish poet, Robert Burns, is a fitting commentary on the challenge of growth guidance.

T. M. GRABER

To catch Dame Fortune's Golden smile,
Assiduous wait upon her,
And gather gear by ev'ry wile,
That's justified by honour.

Epistle to a Young Friend,
Robert Burns, 1759–1796

DEDICATION

To Sheila, Fiona and Alastair for their love, support and understanding over the years during the

development of the Twin Block technique and the preparation of this book.

PREFACE

The opinions expressed in this book are based on the author's experience over 34 years in orthodontic practice. This is not intended to be a circumscribed view; the author acknowledges that other practitioners may differ in some respects but hopes that the material presented may help to integrate the orthodontic and orthopaedic objectives of our profession.

Abnormal musculoskeletal development is frequently the fundamental cause of dental malocclusion. The treatment objective in the growing child with a resultant skeletal discrepancy changes from an orthodontic approach, aiming to correct the dental irregularity, to an orthopaedic approach, where the objective is to correct the underlying skeletal abnormality. This difference in emphasis reflects the existence of two distinct schools of thought in evaluating the aims of orthodontic and dental orthopaedic treatment.

The purpose of this book is to advance the recognition of dentofacial orthopaedics as the treatment of choice for correction of malocclusion that results from abnormal skeletal development. The present philosophical basis of orthodontic and orthopaedic technique is examined with reference to current practice and research.

This book extends the armamentarium of dental orthopaedic treatment by introducing the Twin Block appliance system. Twin Blocks are designed for full-time wear in order to overcome problems associated with conventional functional appliances that were designed in one piece to fit the teeth in upper and lower dental arches. Twin Blocks are more comfortable, more aesthetic and more efficient than alternative functional appliances. The emphasis in this book is to provide practical advice and instruction that is of direct value to the teacher, practitioner and student of orthodontics.

The Twin Block technique is demonstrated in case reports to give guidance on diagnosis, treatment planning, and clinical management of the various types of appliances involved in the system. The clinical approach to treatment is supported by scientific investigation and analysis of patients treated consecutively, which evaluates the dentofacial changes that result from treatment with the Twin Block technique.

The purpose in presenting the material in this fashion is to provide both comprehensive analysis and instruction in a well-illustrated format that is easy to understand. Then the principles of diagnosis and therapy will in turn more readily provide a sound basis for clinical application of the techniques described.

WILLIAM J. CLARK

ACKNOWLEDGEMENTS

This book is based on the development of a new approach to functional orthopaedics in clinical orthodontic practice. I wish to acknowledge first the cooperation of many excellent patients and their primary role in the development of the Twin Block technique, not least Colin Gove, the first patient I treated with Twin Blocks in 1977.

My dental technician, Jim Watt, has made my appliances for the past 29 years, and still does. He made the first Twin Blocks and I should like to acknowledge his invaluable contribution and support in providing the expert technical help I needed to develop the Twin Block technique.

It has been interesting and challenging to travel and teach throughout the world, and to all the people who have offered their support and encouragement over the years, I offer my sincere thanks. There are too many to mention in this short acknowledgement. My former partners in orthodontic practice, Duncan McCallum and Ken Lumsden, were among the first to adopt the technique, and were always unfailing in their support.

I should like to acknowledge those who offered support in the early days and helped to champion the cause of Twin Block therapy. Hans Eirew, former president of the British Association of Orthodontists and a leader in the cause of dentofacial orthopaedics, has been a great friend, who offered unstinting and eloquent support over the years. He came to the first ever Twin Block course with Peter Cousins, another past president and friend, who offered me my first position as assistant in his orthodontic practice in 1961. Philip Adams also attended an early course and displayed an academic mind, completely open to new ideas.

Distinguished orthodontic teachers of functional therapy who recognised the potential of Twin Blocks were Harry Orton, Jim McNamara, Tom Graber and Jim Broadbent. My decision to travel abroad and teach Twin Block courses was first supported by Jim McNamara, when he organised a lecture tour of American Universities in 1983. I also thank Bill Profitt and Ram Nanda for their interest and support.

In preparing the text of this book I am especially indebted to Tom Graber, Jim McNamara, Hans Eirew and Terry Spahl for their constructive criticism of the text and for their help and support over the years in the teaching of Twin Block technique.

For assistance with my statistical analysis of Twin Block therapy I am greatly indebted to Peter Baker for programming data and generating the results. I am grateful also to Professors Jimmy McEwen, Derek Chisholm and David Stirrups of the University of Dundee for advice on presentation of the statistical results.

Gordon Kluzak is a good friend and pioneer of Twin Block technique in Canada who offered research facilities to investigate the results of treatment. Christine Mills carried out a detailed statistical investigation in her orthodontic practice in Vancouver. Mel Taskey offered advice on the management of temporomandibular disorders with Twin Blocks.

Illustrations

The computerised diagrams and tracings were prepared by Frank Dingwall, whose skill and dedication I wish to acknowledge in recognition of his patience and expertise. Thanks are due also for the additional drawings in Chapter 2 provided by William Bruden under the direction of Jim McNamara in the University of Michigan.

I am grateful for the support of Martin Brusse, president of Rocky Mountain Orthodontics, for providing assistance with cephalometric tracings to illustrate this book, and for his willingness to examine and develop new ideas and concepts in treatment and diagnosis.

Twin Block Courses and Technical Support

Manuel Ponti is a dedicated publisher who first introduced me to South America by arranging for me to lecture at the International Congress in Mexico in 1982. He encouraged me for many years to write this book, and I am grateful to him for his interest and motivation.

My first exposure to large audiences in North America and Canada was organised by John Witzig, culminating in 1991 with the first ever teleconference in orthodontics, when I gave a one day course to a live audience in Chicago which was broadcast live by satellite to audiences in 25 cities throughout America and Canada. The spread of new ideas is dependent on this type of initiative.

In 1985 Don Neuenschwander organised the first Twin Block course in America outwith the universities. Since then I have come to appreciate the enormous talent and initiative shown by leaders of orthodontic laboratories throughout the world.

They have done an excellent job in providing the technical expertise that is so essential in teaching a new technique. I acknowledge their help as follows: in America, Mark Ohlendorf, Jack Skay, John Dockstader, John and Cindy Kelly, Diane Johnston, Tom McGill, Adrian Saltzer and John Jankowiak. In Canada, my thanks to Gary Robinson, Neal Russell, Emmett Griffiths and Wayne St John: in Australia to Graham Manley, and in Holland, Gerard Bosboom. In Britain I received technical support from Clive Hudson, Wayne Hallum, John Beardow and Paul Thompson.

CONTENTS

1

The Art of Orthodontics

INTRODUCTION

Orthodontics presents a philosophical challenge in that both art and science are of equal importance. A quotation of Edward Angle (1907), from the turn of the century, is still pertinent today:

> The study of orthodontia is indissolubly connected with that of art as related to the human face. The mouth is a most potent factor in making or marring the beauty and character of the face, and the form and beauty of the mouth largely depend on the occlusal relations of the teeth.
>
> Our duties as orthodontists force upon us great responsibilities, and there is nothing which the student of orthodontia should be more keenly interested than in art generally, and especially in its relation to the human face, for each of his efforts, whether he realises it or not, makes for beauty or ugliness; for harmony or inharmony; for perfection or deformity of the face. Hence it should be one of his life studies.

Although orthodontics has gained wide recognition by the general public, it can be argued that the term 'orthodontics' is self-limiting and does not describe adequately the wider aesthetic and holistic aims of a speciality that is as concerned with harmonious facial balance as with a balanced functional occlusion.

The true art of the speciality lies in its pursuit of ideals in the arrangement and function of the dentition, but never at the expense of damaging facial aesthetics. Beauty is a precious, indefinable quality that is expressed in balanced facial proportions. Facial balance and harmony are goals of orthodontic treatment, of equal importance to a balanced functional occlusion.

DENTAL CHESS

Orthodontics may be thought of as the dental equivalent of chess. The analogy is appropriate in many respects. The game is played with 32 ivory pieces that are arranged symetrically about the midline on a board in two equal and opposing armies.

The opening moves are crucial in determining the strategy of the game. From the outset, the game is won or lost depending on the strategy of development of the individual pieces. Indeed, these opening moves can determine whether the game is eventually won or lost.

It is a mistake in chess to become obsessed with the individual pieces. Rather, one must take a broader view and look at the game plan as a whole to maintain a balanced position of the pieces on the board in order to achieve mutual protection and support.

In dental chess, the board is analagous to the facial skeleton, which is of fundamental importance in supporting the individual pieces. As the orthodontic chess game progresses and the dental pieces are developed, the board may become overcrowded with pieces converging upon each other, so that even the most experienced player may at times sacrifice pieces only to realise as the game develops that the gambit was miscalculated.

Only after the passage of time, on proceeding to the end game, can the success of the strategy be evaluated. Successful treatment is judged in terms of facial balance, aesthetic harmony and functional stability in the end result. One may conclude that the objectives of treament have been achieved only when the final post-treatment balance of facial and dental harmony is observed.

ORTHODONTICS AND DENTAL ORTHOPAEDICS

An essential distinction exists between the terms 'orthodontics' and 'dental orthopaedics'. They represent a fundamental variance in approach to the correction of dentofacial abnormalities.

By definition, orthodontic treatment aims to correct the dental irregularity. The alternative term 'dental orthopaedics' was suggested by the late Sir Norman Bennett, and although this is a wider definition than 'orthodontics' it still does not convey the objective of improving facial development.

The broader description of 'dentofacial orthopaedics' conveys the concept that treatment aims to improve not only dental and orthopaedic relationships in the stomatognathic system but also facial balance. The adoption of a wider definition has the advantage of extending the horizons of the profession as well as educating the public to appreciate the benefits of dentofacial therapy in more comprehensive aesthetic terms.

A fundamental question that we must address in diagnosis is: does this patient require orthodontic treatment or orthopaedic treatment, or a combination of both, and to what degree?

An orthodontic approach aims to correct the dental irregularity and is inappropriate in the treatment of what are essentially skeletal discrepancies. By definition, orthodontics must either be combined with dentofacial orthopaedics or maxillofacial surgery in the correction of significant skeletal abnormality.

If the malocclusion is primarily related to a musculoskeletal discrepancy we should select an orthopaedic approach to treatment. It is in treatment of muscle imbalance and skeletal disproportion that functional orthopaedic appliances come into their own. Functional appliances were developed to correct the aberrant muscle environment – the jaw-to-jaw relationship – and as a result restore facial balance by improving function.

To achieve the best of both worlds it is necessary to combine the disciplines of fixed and functional appliance therapy.

THE PHILOSOPHICAL DIVIDE

In each succeeding generation the clinical approach to treatment is determined by the background of scientific research. The growth processes of the maxillofacial complex that control the response to treatment are of special significance. Since the beginning of the twentieth century, the pendulum of scientific opinion has swung back and forth in the evaluation of the 'form and function' philosophy in relation to the implementation of orthodontic and orthopaedic treatment. At the turn of the century, a division occurred in the evolution of orthodontic technique that split treatment philosophy into the separate disciplines of fixed and functional appliance therapy.

The two schools of thought had a common origin in the 'form and function' philosophy as a basis to establish treatment objectives. The general goal was to correct arch-to-arch relationships, as defined by Angle (1907), while at the same time improving the skeletal relationships through the stimulation and guidance of adaptive remodelling of bone to support those corrected dental relationships.

This philosophical divide in treatment approach can be related to geographical factors as well as to differences in socioeconomic development between the USA and Europe.

In his efforts at developing the foundations of modern US fixed appliance technique, Angle attempted to accommodate a full complement of teeth in every case, irrespective of the degree of crowding or lack of available underlying bony support. The following generation of orthodontists subsequently rejected Angle's 'form and function' philosophy as a basis for fixed appliance therapy, and discarded the functional concept of growth in favour of a concept of genetic control that dismissed the potential of environmental factors to influence growth. One dogmatic philosophy was replaced by another.

Provided skeletal development is within the range of normal, fixed appliances are ideally suited to detailing the occlusion by precise three-dimensional control of tooth movement. Fixed appliances are designed specifically to apply the optimum forces to move teeth, but they are less effective in the treatment of major muscle function imbalances or their companion jaw-to-jaw skeletal discrepancies.

THE GENETIC PARADIGM

In the development of orthodontic technique the concept of genetic control of the pattern of maxillofacial development was based on serial growth studies that came about as a by-product of the development of the cephalostat by Broadbent (1948).

These studies formed the basis for an entire philosophical approach to orthodontic treatment, where the existing skeletal framework was accepted as genetically predetermined and therefore not subject to environmental factors.

In the literature there is scant evidence of significant growth changes showing increased mandibular growth as a result of an orthodontic as opposed to an orthopaedic approach to therapy. Other studies did confirm that auxilliary orthopaedic forces restricted downward and forward maxillary growth. As a result, maxillary dental retraction became commonly accepted as a reliable method of correcting Class II malocclusion overjet problems.

However, a strict interpretation of the genetic paradigm is called into question increasingly by current research, and is no longer the only valid basis for the practice of orthodontics combined with dentofacial orthopaedics. The present findings of modern research into bone growth represent a philosophical review that once again recognises the potential of improving the existing growth pattern by altering the muscle environment and/or functional environment of the developing dentition in an orthopaedic approach to treatment.

TREATMENT CONCEPTS

A fundamental difference in approach exists between orthodontic and orthopaedic schools of thought in relation to treatment philosophy and the management of malocclusion.

In the evolution of orthodontic technique, multiband fixed appliances were developed for treatment in the permanent dentition. It was customary to delay treatment until the permanent canines and premolars had erupted, at a stage when the malocclusion was already fully developed. The concept of treatment was to retract the upper arch using the perimeter of the orthodontically corrected, albeit retruded, lower arch as a template on which to rebuild the occlusion.

However, the majority of Class II malocclusions present a laterally contracted maxilla that is often related correctly to the cranial base but is associated with an underdeveloped mandible. The fundamental skeletal problem is not correctly addressed by an approach which is designed to retract a normal maxilla to match a deficient mandible.

A skeletal mandibular deficiency is well established at an early stage of dental and facial development. The orthopaedic approach to treatment endeavours to correct the skeletal relationship before the malocclusion is fully expressed in the permanent dentition. Early diagnosis and interceptive treatment aims to restore normal function, and thereby enable the permanent teeth to erupt into correct occlusal and incisal relationships.

The concept of functional therapy is to expand and develop the upper arch to improve archform, and to use the maxilla as a template against which to reposition the retrusive mandible in a correct relationship to the normal maxilla. The functional orthopaedic approach addresses the skeletal problem of a retrusive mandible, and the malocclusion is controlled at an earlier stage of development.

Class III malocclusion is also identified by early diagnosis, and may often respond to an interceptive approach to treatment which aims to reduce the skeletal discrepancy and restore normal function in order to promote normal growth and development.

Orthodontic force

Fixed appliances are designed to apply light orthodontic forces that move individual teeth. Schwarz (1932) defined the optimum orthodontic force as 28 g per square centimetre of root surface. By applying light forces with archwires and elastic traction, fixed appliances do not specifically stimulate mandibular growth during treatment.

A bracket or 'small handle' is attached to individual teeth. Pressure is then applied to those teeth by ligating light wires to the brackets. The resulting forces applied through the teeth to the supporting alveolar bone must remain within the level of physiological tolerance of the periodontal membrane to avoid damage to the individual teeth and/or their sockets of alveolar bone.

Smith and Storey (1952), investigating optimum force levels in the edgewise appliance, found that 150 g was the optimum force for moving canines, compared to 300 g for molars. Allowance must be made, however, for frictional forces within the bracket slots themselves, in the region of 125–250 g, which must be overcome to move teeth along archwires.

Orthopaedic force

Orthopaedic force levels are not confined by the level of tolerance of the periodontal membrane but rather by the much broader tolerance of the orofacial musculature. An orthopaedic approach to treatment is not designed to move the teeth, but rather to change the jaw position and thereby correct the relationship of the mandible to the maxilla.

The forces of occlusion applied to opposing teeth in mastication are in the range of 400–500 g and these forces are transmitted through the teeth to the supporting bone. Occlusal forces form a major proprioceptive stimulus to growth whereby the internal and external structure of supporting bone is remodelled to meet the needs of occlusal function. This is effected by reorganisation of the alveolar trabecular system and by periosteal and endochondral apposition.

Considering the anteroposterior forces applied when the mandible is displaced forward in the presence of a Class II skeletal relationship, the investigations of Graf (1961, 1975) and Witt and Komposch (1971) have shown that for 1 mm of anterior displacement the forces of the stretched retractor muscles amount to approximately 100 g. A construction bite of 5–10 mm will therefore transmit considerable forces to the dentition through the functional receptors.

Orthopaedic forces would exceed the level of tolerance of the periodontal tissues if applied to individual teeth. However, these forces are spread evenly in the dental arches by appliances that are not designed to move individual teeth, but to displace the entire mandible and promote adaptation within the muscles of mastication. The muscles are the prime movers in growth, and bony remodelling is related to the functional requirements of muscle activity. The goal of functional appliances is to elicit a proprioceptive response in the stretch receptors of the orofacial muscles and ligaments, and as a secondary response to influence the pattern of bone growth correspondingly to support a new functional environment for the developing dentition.

DENTOFACIAL ORTHOPAEDICS

In contrast to the philosophical change that has accompanied the evolution of fixed appliance therapy, the form and function concept steadfastly remains the basic concept of functional therapy. The functional matrix theory of Moss (1968) supports the premise that function modifies anatomy.

By definition, the purpose of dentofacial orthopaedics is to modify the pattern of facial growth and the underlying bone structure of the face. The objective is to promote harmonious facial growth by changing the functional muscle environment around the developing dentition. The principle of functional therapy is to reposition a retrusive mandible to a forward position by constructing a removable appliance that effects a protrusive bite when the appliance is placed in the mouth. The mechanics are reversed to correct a retrusive maxilla, but the principle remains the same.

Functional appliances are designed to enhance forward mandibular growth in the treatment of distal occlusion by encouraging a functional displacement of the mandibular condyles downwards and forwards in the glenoid fossae. This is balanced by an upward and backward pull in the muscles supporting the mandible. Adaptive remodelling may occur on both articular surfaces of the temporomandibular joint to improve the position of the mandible relative to the maxilla.

In correction of mandibular retrusion, the mandible is held in a protrusive position by occlusal contact on the functional appliance. In this case a large 'handle' is attached to as many teeth as possible in both dental arches. The object of a functional appliance is not to move the individual teeth, but to displace the lower jaw downwards and forwards, and to increase the intermaxillary space in the anteroposterior and vertical dimensions. Repositioning the mandible stimulates a positive proprioceptive response in the muscles of mastication. The purpose is to encourage adaptive skeletal growth by maintaining the mandible in a corrected forward position for a sufficient period of time to allow adaptive skeletal changes to occur in response to functional stimulus.

Dentofacial orthopaedics, therefore, represents a positive approach to the treatment of craniofacial imbalance by addressing the underlying cause of the malocclusion, in an effort to maximise the natural potential for corrective growth.

REFERENCES

Angle, E.H. (1907). *Treatment of Malocclusion of the Teeth,* 7th edn. Philadelphia, S.S. White Dental Manufacturing Co.

Broadbent, B.H. (1948). *Practical Orthodontics,* ed. G.H. Anderson, 7th edn. St Louis, C.V. Mosby, p. 208.

Graf, H. (1961). In *Tecknik und Handhabung der Functionsregler,* Berlin, R. Frankel.

Graf, H. (1975). Occlusal forces during function. In *Proceedings of Symposium,* ed. N.H. Rowe. Ann Arbor, University of Michigan.

Moss, M.L. (1968). The primacy of functional matrices in profacial growth, *Dent. Practitioner,* **19**: 65–73.

Schwarz, A.M. (1932). Tissue changes incidental to orthodontics. *Austral. J. Orthod.,* **18**: 331–52.

Smith, R. & Storey, E. (1952). The importance of forces in orthodontics. *Austral. J. Dent.,* **56**: 291–304.

Witt, E. & Komposch, G. (1971). Intermaxillare Kraftwirkung bimaxillarer gerate. *Gerate. Fortschr. Kieferorhop.,* **32**: 345–52.

FURTHER READING

Moyers, R.E. (1988). Force systems and tissue responses in orthodontics and facial orthopedics. In *Handbook of Orthodontics.* Chicago, Year Book.

Sinclair, P.M. (1991). The clinical application of orthopaedic forces: Current capabilities and limitations. In *Bone Biodynamics in Orthodontic and Orthopaedic Treatment,* ed. Carlson and Goldstein, Craniofacial Growth Series, University of Michigan, Vol. 27, pp. 351–88.

Witt, E. (1966). Investigations into orthodontic forces of different appliances. *Trans. Eur. Orthod. Soc.,* 391–408.

Witt, E. (1973). Muscular physiological investigations into the effect of bi-maxillary appliances. *Trans. Eur. Orthod. Soc.,* 448–50.

2

Introduction to Twin Blocks

THE OCCLUSAL INCLINED PLANE

The occlusal inclined plane is the fundamental functional mechanism of the natural dentition. Cuspal inclined planes play an important part in determining the relationship of the teeth as they erupt into occlusion.

If the mandible occludes in a distal relationship to the maxilla, the occlusal forces acting on the mandibular teeth in normal function have a distal component of force that is unfavourable to normal forward mandibular development. The inclined planes formed by the cusps of the upper and lower teeth represent a servo-mechanism that locks the mandible in a distally occluding functional position.

Twin Block appliances are simple bite blocks that are designed for full-time wear. They achieve rapid functional correction of malocclusion by the transmission of favourable occlusal forces to occlusal inclined planes that cover the posterior teeth. The forces of occlusion are used as the functional mechanism to correct the malocclusion (**2.1 A, B**)

PROPRIOCEPTIVE STIMULUS TO GROWTH

The inclined plane mechanism plays an important part in determining the cuspal relationship of the teeth as they erupt into occlusion. A functional equilibrium is established under neurological control in response to repetitive tactile stimulus. Occlusal forces transmitted through the dentition provide a constant proprioceptive stimulus to influence the rate of growth and the trabecular structure of the supporting bone.

Malocclusion is frequently associated with discrepancies in arch relationships due to underlying skeletal and soft-tissue factors, resulting in unfavourable cuspal guidance and poor occlusal function. The proprioceptive sensory feedback mechanism controls muscular activity and provides a functional stimulus or deterrent to the full expression of mandibular bone growth. The unfavourable cuspal contacts of distal occlusion represent an obstruction to normal forward mandibular translation in function, and as such do not encourage the mandible to achieve its optimum genetic growth potential.

Functional appliance therapy aims to improve the functional relationship of the dentofacial structures by eliminating unfavourable

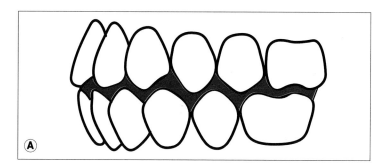

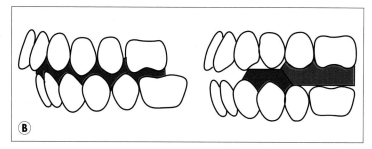

2.1 A, B The occlusal inclined plane is the functional mechanism of the natural dentition. Twin Blocks modify the occlusal inclined plane and use the forces of occlusion to correct the malocclusion. The mandible is guided forwards by the occlusal inclined plane.

developmental factors and improving the muscle environment that envelops the developing occlusion. By altering the position of the teeth and supporting tissues, a new functional behaviour pattern is established that can support a new position of equilibrium.

TWIN BLOCKS

The goal in developing the Twin Block approach to treatment was to produce a technique that could maximise the growth response to functional mandibular protrusion by using an appliance system that is simple, comfortable and aesthetically acceptable to the patient

Twin Blocks are constructed to a protrusive bite that effectively modifies the occlusal inclined plane by means of acrylic inclined planes on occlusal bite blocks. The purpose is to promote protrusive mandibular function for correction of the skeletal Class II malocclusion (**2.2 A–E**).

The occlusal inclined plane acts as a guiding mechanism causing the mandible to be displaced downwardand forward.

With the appliances in the mouth, the patient cannot occlude comfortably in the former distal position and the mandible is encouraged to adopt a protrusive bite with the inclined planes engaged in occlusion. The unfavourable cuspal contacts of a distal occlusion are replaced by favourable proprioceptive contacts on the inclined planes of the Twin Blocks to correct the malocclusion and to free the mandible from its locked distal functional position.

Twin Blocks are designed to be worn 24 hours per day to take full advantage of all functional forces applied to the dentition, including the forces of mastication. Upper and lower bite blocks interlock at a

70° angle when engaged in full closure. This causes a forward mandibular posture to an edge-to-edge position with the upper anteriors, provided the patient can comfortably maintain full occlusion on the appliances in that position. In treatment of Class II malocclusion, the inclined planes are positioned mesial to the upper and lower first molars with the upper block covering the upper molars and second premolars or deciduous molars, and the lower blocks extending mesially from the second premolar or deciduous molar region.

In the early stages of their evolution, Twin Blocks were conceived as simple removable appliances with interlocking occlusal bite blocks designed to posture the mandible forward to achieve functional correction of a Class II division 1 malocclusion. This basic principle still applies but over the years many variations in appliance design have extended the scope of the technique to treat a wide range of all classes of malocclusion. Appliance design has been improved and simplified to make Twin Blocks more acceptable to the patient without

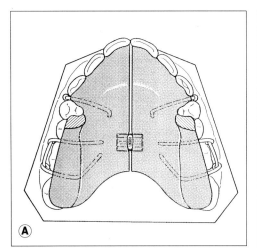
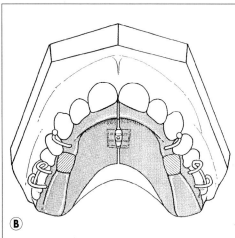
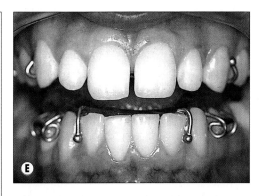
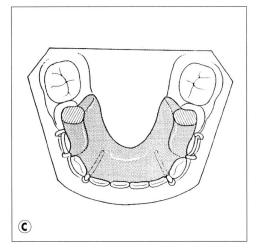
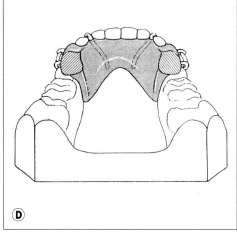
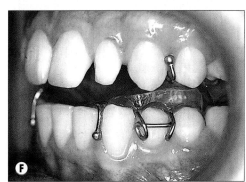

2.2 E, F Twin Blocks.

2.2 A, B Upper Twin Block – occlusal and frontal. **C, D** Lower Twin Block – occlusal and rear views. Courtesy of W. Bruden and J.A.McNamarra Jr., University of Michigan.

reducing their efficiency.

In the treatment of Class II division 2 malocclusion, appliance design is modified by the addition of sagittal screws to advance the upper anterior teeth. Control of the vertical dimension is achieved by sequentially adjusting the thickness of the posterior occlusal inclined planes to control eruption (**2.3**).

Treatment of Class III malocclusion is achieved by reversing the occlusal inclined planes to apply a forward component of force to the upper arch and a downward and distal force to the mandible in the lower molar region. The inclined planes are set at 70° to the occlusal plane with bite blocks covering lower molars and upper deciduous molars or premolars, with sagittal screws to advance the upper incisors (**2.4**).

The first principle of appliance design is simplicity. The patient's appearance is noticeably improved when Twin Blocks are fitted. Twin Blocks are designed to be comfortable, aesthetic and efficient. By addressing these requirements, Twin Blocks satisfy both the patient and the operator as one of the most 'patient friendly' of all the functional appliances.

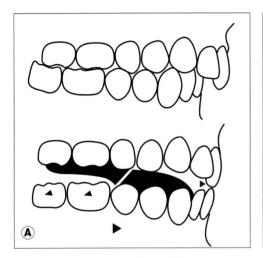
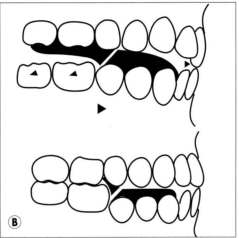
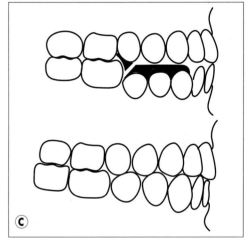

2.3 A, B, C Correction of Class II Division 2 malocclusion by advancing the mandible and proclining the upper incisors with sagittal screws.

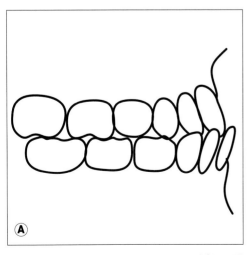
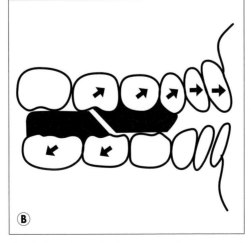
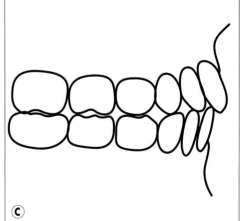

2.4 Reverse Twin Blocks for correction of Class III malocclusion with sagittal screws to advance upper incisors.

DEVELOPMENT OF TWIN BLOCKS

A clinical problem: C.G. aged 7 years 10 months

It is true that 'necessity is the mother of invention'. The Twin Block appliance evolved in response to a clinical problem that presented when a young patient, the son of a dental colleague, fell and completely luxated an upper central incisor. Fortunately, he kept the tooth, and presented for treatment within a few hours of the accident. The incisor was reimplanted and a temporary splint was constructed to hold the tooth in position (**2.5**).

Before the accident the centre line was displaced to the right and the luxated incisor had a pronounced distal angulation with a central diastema of 3 mm. When the tooth was reimplanted the socket was enlarged to reposition the incisor as near as possible to the midline. Complete correction of the midline was not possible, recognising that enlarging the socket too much might reduce the prognosis for reattachment of the tooth.

After 6 months with a stabilising splint, the tooth had partially reattached, but there was evidence of severe root resorption and the long-term prognosis for the reimplanted incisor was poor.

The occlusal relationship was Class II division 1 with an overjet of 9 mm and the lower lip was trapped lingual to the upper incisors. Adverse lip action on the reimplanted incisor was causing mobility and root resorption. To prevent the lip from trapping in the overjet it was necessary to design an appliance that could be worn full time to posture the mandible forward. At that time no such appliance was available and simple bite blocks were therefore designed to achieve this objective. The appliance mechanism was designed to harness the forces of occlusion to correct the distal occlusion and also to reduce the overjet without applying direct pressure to the upper incisors.

The upper and lower bite blocks engaged mesial to the first permanent molars at 90° to the occlusal plane when the mandible postured forward. This positioned the incisors edge-to-edge with 2 mm vertical separation to hold the incisors out of occlusion. The patient had to make a positive effort to posture his mandible forward to occlude the bite blocks in a protrusive bite. Fortunately, the young patient was successful in doing this consistently to activate the appliance for functional correction. Had he not made this effort the technique may have been stillborn.

The first Twin Block appliances were fitted on 7 September 1977, when the patient was aged 8 years 4 months. The bite blocks proved comfortable to wear and treatment progressed well as the distal occlusion corrected and the overjet reduced from 9 mm to 4 mm in 9 months.

During the course of treatment radiographs confirmed that the reimplanted incisor had severe root resorpion and an endodontic pin was placed to stabilise this tooth after 4 months treatment. This was successful in stabilising the incisor.

At a later stage, in the permanent dentition, a simple upper fixed appliance was used to complete treatment. It was not possible to correct the centre line fully in replacing the luxated tooth, and the central incisor ankylosed during the process of reattachment. Consequently, a slight displacement of the centre line had to be accepted. The reimplanted incisor was crowned successfully, and the result is stable at age 25 years.

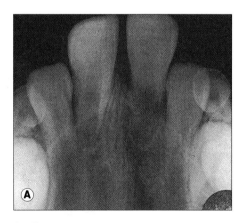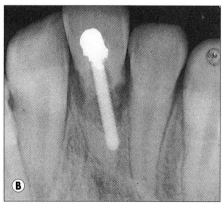

2.5 Treatment:

A, B Before treatment: 1l was completely luxated and was reimplanted. An endodontic pin was fitted to stabilise the incisor. This was successful in achieving bony reattachment.

C, D, E Profile and dental views before treatment at age 7 years 10 months.

F, G The first Twin Blocks were simple bite blocks occluding in forward posture. The blocks were angled at 90° to the occlusal plane.

H After 9 months of treatment, the overjet has reduced, and the distal occlusion is corrected.

J Profile after 9 months of treatment.

K A simple fixed appliance is used to improve alignment in permanent dentition. The damaged upper incisor is now ankylosed.

L The profile at age 24 years.

M, N, O The occlusion remains stable 5 years out of retention.

CG

MODIFICATION FOR TREATMENT OF CLASS II DIVISION 2 MALOCCLUSION

Case report: A.K. aged 11 years

Two years later, having developed a protocol for Twin Block treatment of Class II division 1 malocclusion, attention was turned to Class II division 2 malocclusion. The first patient of this type presented a severe malocclusion with an excessive overbite and an interincisal angle approaching 180° (**2.6**). As an indication of the depth of the overbite the intergingival height from the gingival margin of the upper incisors to the gingival margin of the lower incisors was 7 mm, suggesting that the upper incisors were impinging on the lower gingivae. The lower archform was good but the mandible was trapped in distal occlusion by the retroclined upper incisors.

The original Twin Block prototype appliances were modified from the standard design for correction of Class II division 1 malocclusion by the addition of springs lingual to the upper incisors to advance retroclined upper incisors. At the same time the mandible was translated forwards to correct the distal occlusion and the appliance was trimmed to encourage eruption of the posterior teeth to reduce the overbite.

The Class II division 2 Twin Blocks were worn for 6 months, at which stage brackets were fitted on the upper anterior teeth and activated with a sectional archwire to correct individual tooth alignment. This combination fixed/functional appliance treatment continued for 6 months. Completion of treatment was then effected with a simple upper fixed appliance.

AK

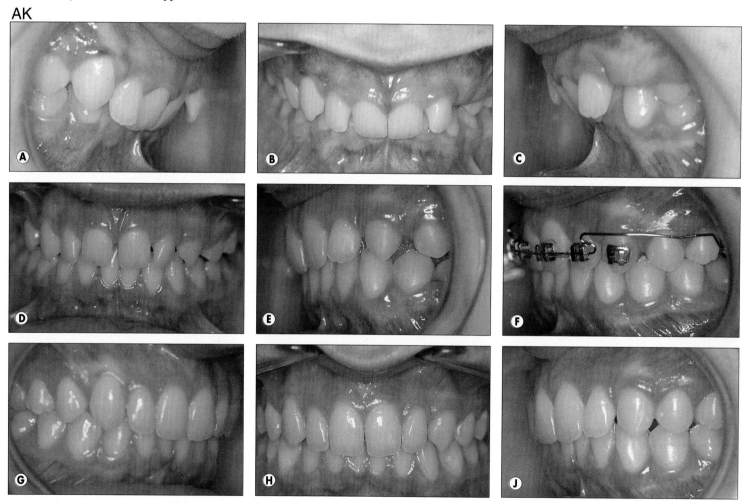

2.6 The first patient (A.K.) with a Class II division 2 malocclusion treated with Twin Blocks:
A, B, C Excessive overbite and severely retroclined incisors.
D, E After 8 months the distal occlusion is corrected and the overbite is reduced.
F A simple upper fixed appliance to correct alignment.
G, H, J The occlusion is stable 3 years later.
A diagrammatic interpretation of the treatment is given on page 19.

AK

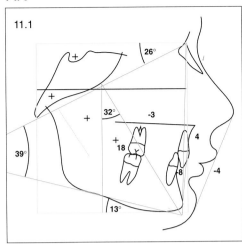

11.1

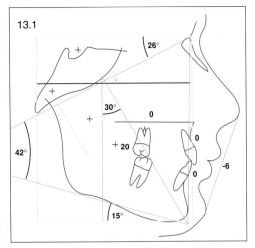

13.1

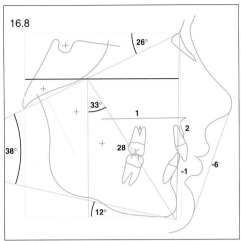

16.8

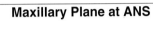

Maxillary Plane at ANS

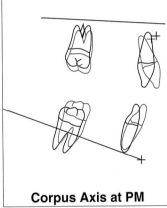

Corpus Axis at PM

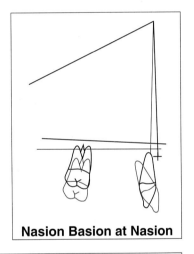

Nasion Basion at Nasion

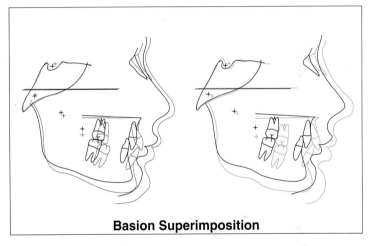

Basion Superimposition

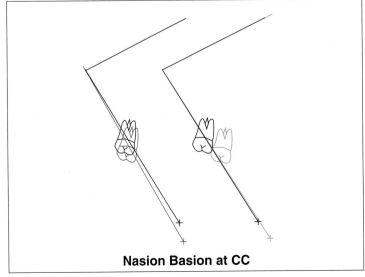

Nasion Basion at CC

A.K. -	Age	11.1	13.1	16.8	(Yr.Mon)
Cranial Base Angle		26	26	26	
Facial Axis Angle		32	30	33	
F/M Plane Angle		13	15	12	
Craniomandibular Angle		39	42	38	
Maxillary Plane		–3	0	1	
Convexity		4	0	2	
U/Incisor to Vertical		–5	22	17	
L/Incisor to Vertical		16	29	26	
Interincisal Angle		169	129	137	
6 to Pterygoid Vertical		18	20	28	
L/Incisor to A/Po		–8	0	–1	
L/Lip to Aesthetic Plane		–4	–6	–6	

Angulation of the inclined planes

During the evolution of the technique, the angulation of the inclined plane varied from 90° to 45° to the occlusal plane, before arriving at an angle of 70° to the occlusal plane as the final compromise angle that proved most suitable in the majority of cases.

As previously stated, the earliest Twin Block appliances were constructed with bite blocks that articulated at a 90° angle, so that the patient had to make a conscious effort to occlude in a forwards position. However, some patients had difficulty maintaining a forwards posture and, therefore, would revert to retruding the mandible back to its old distal occlusion position, occluding the bite blocks together on top of each other on their flat occlusal surfaces. This was detectable at an early stage of treatment when it could be observed that the patient was not posturing forwards consistently. A significant posterior open bite was caused by biting on the blocks in this fashion. This complication was experienced in approximately 30% of the earliest Twin Block cases. It was resolved by altering the angulation of the bite blocks to 45° to the occlusal plane in order to guide the mandible forwards. This was immediately successful in eliminating the problem.

An angle of 45° to the occlusal plane applies an equal downward and forward component of force to the lower dentition. The direction of occlusal force on the inclined planes encourages a corresponding downward and forward stimulus to growth. After using a 45° angle on the blocks for eight years, the angulation was finally changed to the steeper angle of 70° to the occlusal plane to apply a more horizontal component of force. It was reasoned that this may encourage more forward mandibular growth. If the patient has any difficulty in posturing forward, this is a sign that the activation should be reduced by trimming the inclined planes to reduce the amount of mandibular protrusion. It then becomes much easier for the patient to maintain a forward posture.

Bite registration

The Exactobite or Projet Bite Gauge (the name differs in the USA and Britain) is designed to record a protrusive interocclusal record or 'bite registration' in wax for construction of Twin Blocks (**2.7**). Typically, in a growing child, an overjet of up to 10 mm can be corrected on the initial activation by registering an incisal edge-to-edge bite with 2 mm interincisal clearance (**2.8 A,B**). This is provided that the patient can comfortably tolerate the mandible being protruded so the upper and lower incisors align vertically edge-to-edge. Larger overjets invariably require partial correction, followed by reactivation after the initial partial correction is accomplished.

Appliance design – standard Twin Blocks

In the correction of an uncrowded Class II division 1 malocclusion it is usually necessary to widen the upper arch to accommodate the lower arch in the corrective protrusive position. The standard design of Twin Blocks, therefore, has provision for midline expansion.

The upper appliance has delta clasps on upper first molars and additional ball ended clasps may be placed interdentally distal to the canines or between the premolars or deciduous molars.

The lower appliance is a simple bite block with delta clasps on the first premolars and ball clasps mesial to the canines (**2.9**).

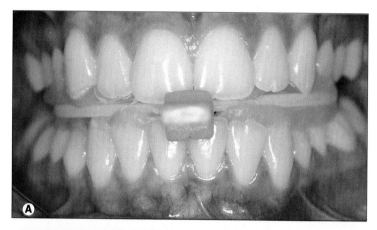

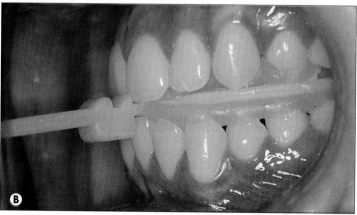

2.8 A, B The blue bite gauge registers 2 mm vertical clearance between the incisal edges of the upper and lower incisors. This generally proves to be an appropriate interincisal clearance in bite registration for most Class II division 1 malocclusions with increased overbite.

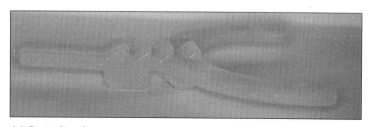

2.7 Projet Bite Gauge.

THE TWIN BLOCK TECHNIQUE – STAGES OF TREATMENT

Twin Block treatment is described in two stages. Twin Blocks are used in the active phase to correct the anteroposterior relationship and establish the correct vertical dimension. Once this phase is accomplished, the Twin Blocks are replaced with an upper Hawley type of appliance with an anterior inclined plane, which is then used to support the corrected position as the posterior teeth settle fully into occlusion.

Stage 1: active phase

Twin Blocks achieve rapid functional correction of mandibular position from a skeletally retruded Class II to Class I occlusion using occlusal inclined planes over the posterior teeth to guide the mandible into correct relationship with the maxilla. In all functional therapy, sagittal correction is achieved before vertical development of the posterior teeth is complete. The vertical dimension is controlled first by

adjustment of the occlusal bite blocks, followed by use of the previously mentioned upper inclined plane appliance.

In treatment of deep overbite, the bite blocks are trimmed selectively to encourage eruption of lower posterior teeth to increase the vertical dimension and level the occlusal plane (**2.10**).

The upper block is trimmed occlusodistally to leave the lower molars 1–2 mm clear of the occlusion to encourage lower molar eruption and reduce the overbite. By maintaining a minimal clearance between the upper bite block and the lower molars the tongue is prevented from spreading laterally between the teeth. This allows the molars to erupt more quickly. At each subsequent visit the upper bite block is reduced progressively to clear the occlusion with the lower molars to allow these teeth to erupt, until finally all the acrylic has been removed over the occlusal surface of the upper molars allowing the lower molars to erupt fully into occlusion.

Throughout this trimming sequence it is important not to reduce

2.9 Standard Twin Blocks.

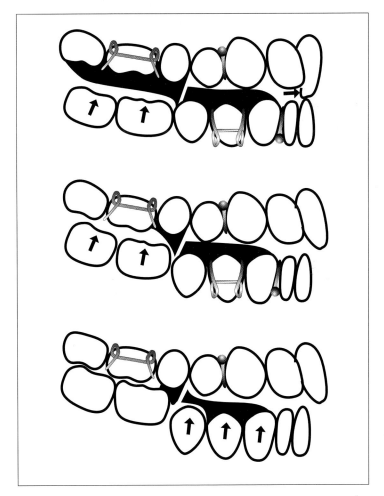

2.10 Sequence of trimming blocks.

the leading edge of the inclined plane, so that adequate functional occlusal support is given until a three point occlusal contact is achieved with the molars in occlusion.

Conversely, in treatment of anterior open bite and vertical growth patterns, the posterior bite blocks remain unreduced and intact throughout treatment. This results in an intrusive effect on the posterior teeth, while the anterior teeth remain free to erupt, which helps to increase the overbite and bring the anterior teeth into occlusion.

At the end of the active stage of Twin Block treatment the aim is to achieve correction to Class I occlusion and control of the vertical dimension by a three point occlusal contact with the incisors and molars in occlusion. At this stage the overjet, overbite and distal occlusion should be fully corrected.

Stage 2: support phase

The aim of the support phase is to maintain the corrected incisor relationship until the buccal segment occlusion is fully interdigitated. To achieve this objective an upper removable appliance is fitted with an anterior inclined plane to engage the lower incisors and canines (2.11).

The lower Twin Block appliance is left out at this stage and the removal of posterior bite blocks allows the posterior teeth to erupt. Full-time appliance wear is necessary to allow time for internal bony remodelling to support the corrected occlusion as the buccal segments settle fully into occlusion.

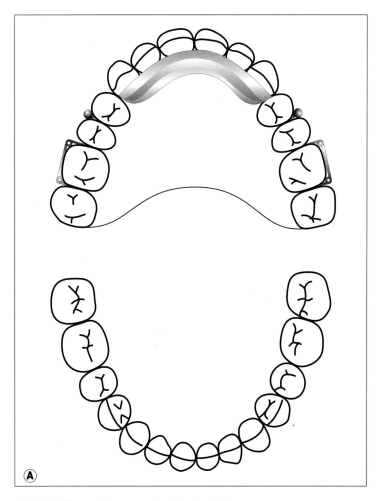

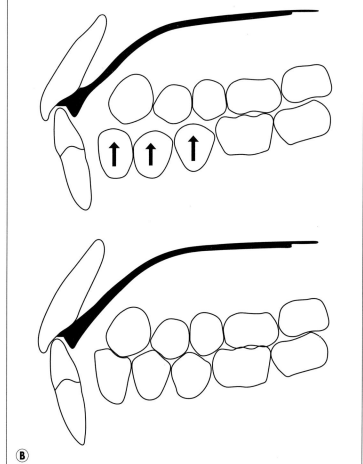

2.11 A, B Support phase – anterior inclined plane.

RETENTION

Treatment is followed by retention with the upper anterior inclined plane appliance. Appliance wear is reduced to night time only when the occlusion is fully established. A good buccal segment occlusion is the cornerstone of stability after correction of arch-to-arch relationships. The appliance-effected advanced mandibular position will not be stable until the functional support of a full buccal segment occlusion is well established.

Timetable of treatment
Average treatment time

- *Active phase*: average time 6–9 months to achieve full reduction of overjet to a normal incisor relationship and to correct the distal occlusion.
- *Support phase*: 3–6 months for molars to erupt into occlusion and for premolars to erupt after trimming the blocks. The objective is to support the corrected mandibular position after active mandibular translation while the buccal teeth settle fully into occlusion.
- *Retention*: 9 months, reducing appliance wear when the position is stabilised.

An average estimate of treatment time is 18 months, including retention.

CASE SELECTION FOR SIMPLE TREATMENT

In starting to use any new technique it is important to select suitable cases from which to learn the fundamentals of treatment without complications. This is especially important when the practitioner is not experienced in functional therapy. Case selection for initial clinical use of Twin Blocks should, therefore, display the following criteria:

- Angle's Class II division 1 malocclusion with good arch form. It is easier to learn the management of the technique first by treating uncrowded cases before progressing to crowded dentitions.
- A lower arch that is uncrowded or decrowded and aligned.
- An upper arch that is aligned or can be easily aligned.
- An overjet of 10–12 mm and a deep overbite.
- A full unit distal occlusion in the buccal segments.
- On examination of the models in occlusion with the lower model advanced to correct the increased overjet, the distal occlusion is also corrected and it can be seen that a potentially good occlusion of the buccal teeth will result. A good buccal segment occlusion is the cornerstone of stability after correction of Class II arch relationships.

- On clinical examination the profile should be noticeably improved when the patient advances the mandible voluntarily to correct the overjet. This factor is fundamental in case selection for functional appliance therapy, and is a clinical indication that the Class II arch relationship is skeletal in origin.
- To achieve a favourable skeletal change during treatment, the patient should be growing actively. A more rapid growth response may be observed when treatment coincides with the pubertal growth spurt. Conversely, the response to treatment is slower if the patient is growing more slowly. Although the rate of growth will influence progress, it is not necessary to plan treatment to coincide with the pubertal growth spurt, as the Twin Block system is effective in mixed dentition, transitional dentition and permanent dentition.

In experienced hands, Twin Blocks are very effective in the treatment of complex malocclusions that are due to a combination of dental and skeletal factors. Twin Blocks integrate more easily with fixed appliances than any other functional appliance in a combined approach to orthopaedic and orthodontic treatment.

RESPONSE TO TREATMENT

Rapid improvements in facial appearance are seen consistently even during the first few months of Twin Block treatment. These changes are characterised by the development of a lip seal and a noticeable improvement in facial balance and harmony. In growing children, the facial muscles adapt very quickly to an altered pattern of occlusal function. The changes in appearance are so significant that the patients themselves frequently comment on the improvement in the early stages of treatment.

The facial changes are soon accompanied by equivalent dental changes and it is routine to observe correction of a full unit distal occlusion within the first 6 months of treatment. The response to treatment is noticeably faster compared to alternative functional appliances that must be removed for eating.

Case report: C.H. aged 14 years 1 month

An example of treatment for a boy with an uncrowded Class II division 1 malocclusion with good archform and a full unit distal occlusion (**2.12**).

Diagnosis, skeletal classification:
- Moderate Class II.
- Facial type: moderate brachyfacial (horizontal growth).
- Maxilla: mild protrusion.
- Mandible: mild retrusion.
- Convexity = 7 mm.

Diagnosis, dental classification:
- Severe Class II division 1.
- Upper incisors: severe protrusion.
- Lower incisors: normal.
- Overjet = 12 mm.
- Overbite = 5 mm (deep).
- No crowding.

Treatment plan. Functional correction to Class I occlusion by means of a combination of maxillary retraction and mandibular advancement, with reduction of overjet and overbite.

Bite registration. The inital bite registration with the blue Exactobite aims to correct the overjet to edge-to-edge with a 2 mm interincisal clearance.

CH

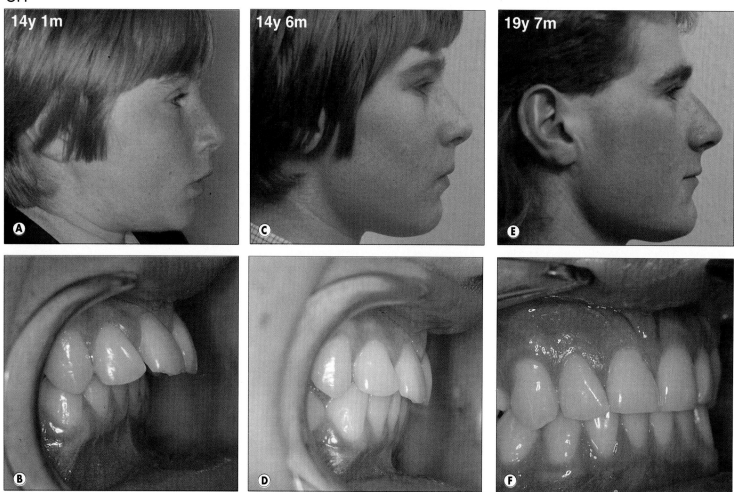

2.12 Treatment:

A, B Profile and occlusion before treatment at age 14 years 1 month.
C, D Profile and occlusal change after 5 months of treatment.

E, F Profile and occlusion at age 19 years 7 months.
A diagrammatic interpretation of the treatment is given on page 25.

CH

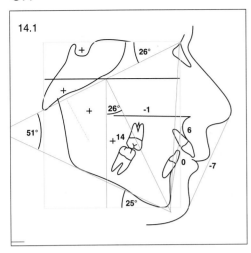

14.1

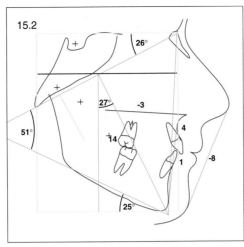

15.2

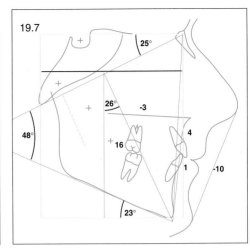

19.7

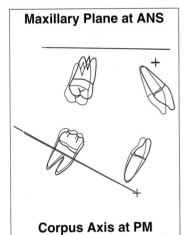

Maxillary Plane at ANS

Corpus Axis at PM

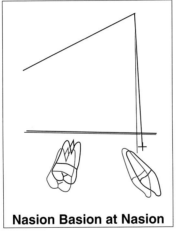

Nasion Basion at Nasion

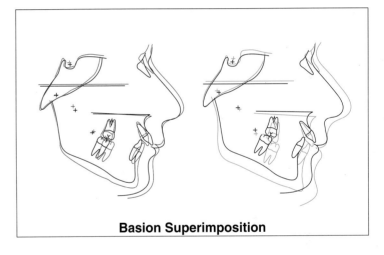

Basion Superimposition

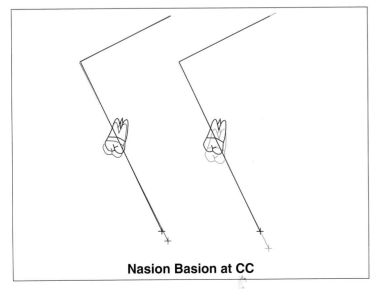

Nasion Basion at CC

C.H. -	Age	14.1	15.2	19.7	(Yr.Mon)
Cranial Base Angle		26	26	25	
Facial Axis Angle		26	27	26	
F/M Plane Angle		25	25	23	
Craniomandibular Angle		51	51	48	
Maxillary Plane		–1	–3	–3	
Convexity		6	4	4	
U/Incisor to Vertical		38	26	27	
L/Incisor to Vertical		31	30	30	
Interincisal Angle		111	124	123	
6 to Pterygoid Vertical		14	14	16	
L/Incisor to A/Po		0	1	1	
L/Lip to Aesthetic Plane		–7	–8	–10	

Appliances
- Standard Twin Blocks.

Clinical management. At the first adjustment visit 2 weeks after the appliance is fitted, it is noted that the patient is not always posturing forward, and is sometimes simply biting together on the flat occlusal surfaces of the blocks. This would tend to produce a posterior open bite, and it is important to avoid this complication by detecting this at an early stage in treatment. The problem is resolved simply by trimming the acrylic slightly from the anterior incline of the upper block until the patient bites comfortably and consistently on the inclined planes of the blocks. This reduces the initial forward activation to 7 mm with 2 mm interincisal clearance.

In spite of the slight upper block reduction, this activation reduces the overjet from 11 mm to 4 mm in 5 months. Nevertheless, as a general principle, if the overjet is greater than 10 mm it is usually necessary to correct the occlusion in a two-stage forward activation of the Twin Blocks.

After the initial partial correction, the Twin Blocks are reactivated to produce an upper to lower incisal edge-to-edge occlusion with 2 mm vertical clearance by adding cold cure acrylic to the anterior aspect of the upper inclined plane. This second activation by means of the longer upper block completes the mandibular correction to Class I occlusion. The blocks are trimmed occlusally as before to reduce the overbite and encourage vertical development.

Duration of treatment:
- Active phase: 8 months with Twin Blocks.
- Support phase and retention: 6 months.

Lower third molars were potentially impacted and on completion of treatment all four second molars were extracted to accommodate third molars, which subsequently erupted in good position.

Case report: J.McL. aged 12 years

A girl with a Class II division 1 malocclusion and mild crowding in the upper labial segment due to narrowing of the upper arch (**2.13**).

Diagnosis, skeletal classification:
- Moderate Class II.
- Facial type: mesognathic.
- Maxilla: slight protrusion, contracted laterally.
- Mandible: normal.
- Convexity = 6 mm.

Diagnosis, dental classification:
- Severe Class II division 1.
- Upper incisors: mild protrusion.
- Lower incisors: normal.
- Overjet = 9 mm.
- Overbite incomplete due to tongue thrust.

Treatment plan. Slight functional protrusion of the mandible to reduce skeletal and dental Class II relationships.

Appliances
- Standard Twin Blocks with labial bow to align the upper incisors.
- Anterior guide plane to support the corrected occlusion and retain

Bite registration. The construction bite is registered with a blue Exactobite edge-to-edge with 2 mm vertical interincisal clearance.

Clinical management. Progress in this case proved to be slow because the patient did not always posture forward. After 7 months the thickness of the blocks was increased slightly to discourage the patient from dropping out of contact with the inclined planes. This appliance adjustment was effective in completing the remaining skeletal correction and the overjet was fully reduced after 4 more months.

Duration of treatment
- Active phase: 11 months with Twin Blocks.
- Support phase and retention: 5 months.

JMcL

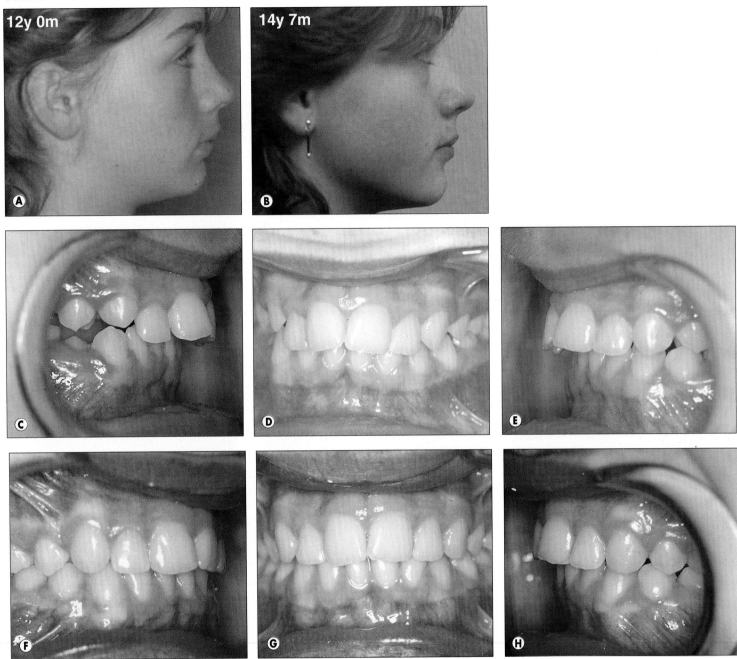

2.13 Treatment:
A Profile before treatment at age 12 years.
B Profile 1 year out of retention at age 14 years 7 months.

C, D, E Occlusion before treatment.
F, G, H Occlusion 1 year out of retention
A diagrammatic interpretation of the treatment is given on page 28.

JMcL

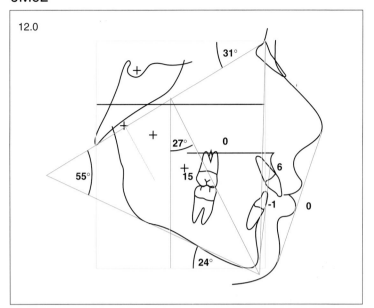

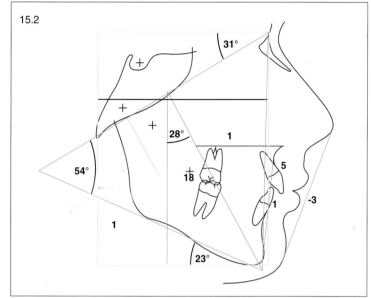

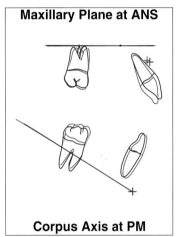

Maxillary Plane at ANS

Corpus Axis at PM

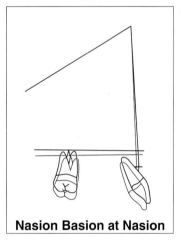

Nasion Basion at Nasion

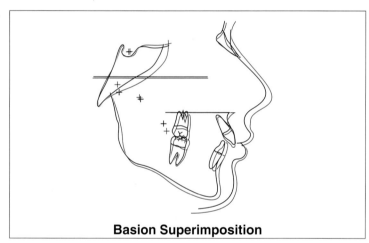

Basion Superimposition

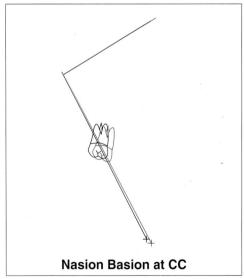

Nasion Basion at CC

J.McL-	Age 12.0	15.2 (Yr.Mon)
Cranial Base Angle	31	31
Facial Axis Angle	27	28
F/M Plane Angle	24	23
Craniomandibular Angle	55	54
Maxillary Plane	0	1
Convexity	6	5
U/Incisor to Vertical	33	28
L/Incisor to Vertical	27	25
Interincisal Angle	120	127
6 to Pterygoid Vertical	15	18
L/Incisor to A/Po	−1	1
L/Lip to Aesthetic Plane	0	−3

CHAPTER

3

Form and Function

DEVELOPMENT OF FUNCTIONAL TECHNIQUE

In the early part of the twentieth century, the 'form and function' philosophy was the fundamental basis for treatment in both fixed and functional schools of therapy. The objective of treatment was to achieve ideal correction of dental arch relationships as defined by Angle (1907) and, at the same time, improve the skeletal relationship by skeletal adaptation in response to correction of the dental relationship. However, from this common origin, fixed and functional techniques followed a divergent course of development.

Modern fixed appliance technique derives largely from the work of Angle, whose philosophy was based on the concept that compensatory growth would result from expanding the dental arches with multi-banded fixed appliances and archwires and placing the orthodontically corrected arches in perfect relationship to one another.

At the same time, a parallel development was occurring in Europe, where Pierre Robin (1902 *a,b*) first described the monobloc as the forerunner of the modern functional appliance. This was closely followed by a parallel development from Viggo Andresen (1908), who developed the activator.

A philosophical division originated when Angle attempted to accommodate a full complement of teeth to the available jaw space in every case, regardless of tooth-to-bone size discrepancy, degree of crowding or the pattern of facial growth. Nonextraction techniques were used with fixed appliances to move teeth, without significantly influencing the underlying skeletal pattern. This was followed by relapse in a high proportion of crowded dentitions treated by fixed mechanics. Consequently, nonextraction therapy fell into disrepute.

The emergence of extraction therapy

By the middle of the twentieth century, the orthodontic philosophical pendulum had swung to the other extreme as Tweed (1941) and Begg (1954) gained acceptance for the use of extractions for the relief of crowding as an integral part of orthodontic treatment planning. Hence, a mechanical approach to treatment was adopted that accepted the extraction of first premolars as standard procedure in the majority of crowded cases. The lower labial segment was thought to be in a position of natural muscle balance before treatment, and the basal perimeter of the lower arch was therefore used as a template to position the upper dentition. However, this approach made no allowance for the potential to change abnormal muscle behaviour by functional therapy.

Therapeutic limitations of the genetic paradigm

The therapeutic limitations of a genetic paradigm are significant in the treatment of Class II malocclusion due to mandibular skeletal deficiency. A philosophy that does not accept the possibility of improving mandibular growth leaves only three options in treatment of mandibular retrusion, all of which represent a biological compromise.

- *Maxillary retraction*. Reduction of forward maxillary growth by orthopaedic extraoral force has been well documented in the literature (Wieslander, 1963, 1974, 1975; Wieslander & Buck, 1974; Graber, 1969). A distal extraoral force applied to the maxillary molars by a Kloehn face bow is accompanied in some cases by a downward and backward rotation of the maxillary plane, and a secondary downward and backward rotation of the mandible. There is some evidence that maxillary expansion to free the occlusion combined with extraoral traction may help to promote mandibular growth in cases where the growth pattern is favourable. However, a distalising extraoral force is designed to retract the maxilla to match the position of a retrusive mandible and does not encourage a retrusive mandible to achieve its full genetic potential of growth.

- *Surgical correction of mandibular position*. The alternative is to correct arch alignment in a presurgical phase of treatment, followed by surgical correction to advance the mandible into correct relationship with the maxilla. Finally, a postsurgical phase of orthodontic treatment is then needed to detail the occlusion. This approach has the disadvantages of being lengthy, traumatic, complex and expensive. The long-term effects on the temporomandibular joints are unpredictable. It is not a widely viable solution.

- *Dentoalveolar compensation*. An orthodontic approach to treatment offers a simpler compromise that aims for dentoalveolar compensation, while accepting that the result will not be ideal because the skeletal discrepancy is beyond the limits of orthodontic therapy.

An orthodontic approach to treatment is most efficient in correcting Class I malocclusions or mild skeletal discrepancies.

It is in correction of malocclusion due to skeletal discrepancies that functional appliances come into their own. The timing of treatment by functional appliances lends itself to the interception of malocclusion at an earlier stage of development, attempting to resolve skeletal and occlusal imbalance by improving the functional environment of the developing dentition before the malocclusion can become fully established in the permanent dentition.

As previously stated, in contrast to the philosophical change that has accompanied the evolution of fixed appliance therapy, the form and function philosophy remains the basic concept of functional appliance treatment. The 'functional matrix' concept of Melvin Moss (1968) is a contemporary evaluation supporting the premise that function modifies anatomy.

It is commonly postulated that patients will not necessarily achieve their full growth potential if environmental factors are unfavourable during development. Malocclusion is frequently associated with unfavourable occlusal contacts and aberrant muscle behaviour, which result in a negative proprioceptive stimulus to normal growth and development.

BONE REMODELLING IN RESPONSE TO FUNCTIONAL STIMULI

The internal and external structure of bone is continuously modified throughout life by the process of bony remodelling. The sensory feedback mechanism helps the bony remodelling process to address the changing requirements of function in dentofacial development. Occlusal forces transmitted by the muscles of mastication through the teeth to the underlying bone provide a proprioceptive stimulus to influence the external form and internal trabecular structure of the supporting bone.

Unlike other connective tissue, bone responds to mild degrees of pressure and tension by changes of this nature. These changes are achieved by means of resorption of existing bone and deposition of new bone. This may take place on the surface of the bone, under the periosteum or, in the case of cancellous bone, on the surfaces of the trabeculae.

In this respect, bone is more plastic and adaptive than any other connective tissue. The internal and external structure of bone is modified by functional requirements to enable it to withstand the physical demands made upon it with the greatest degree of economy of structure. This principle is exemplified in Wolff's 'Law of transformation of bone'. The architecture of a bone is such that it can best resist the forces that are brought to bear upon it with the use of as little tissue as possible.

During mastication forces are transmitted through the teeth to the alveolar bone and to the underlying basal bone. Most of these forces are vertical, but some are transverse and anteroposterior. The external surface of the maxilla and mandible is modified precisely by function to absorb the forces of occlusion. Well-defined ridges of bone are specifically designed to absorb and transmit these force vectors.

Mastication is a function that involves the whole face, and even part of the cranium. Considerable forces are applied through the muscles of mastication to the teeth and the underlying bony structures to influence both the internal and external structure of the basal bone. It is this natural mechanism of bony remodelling by occlusal force vectors that forms the basis of functional correction by the Twin Block technique. The forces of occlusion that are applied during mastication are harnessed as an additional stimulus to growth.

Development of the temporomandibular joint

The relationship between form and function is exemplified exquisitely in the normal development of the craniofacial skeleton. As the patient matures, progressive adaptation of the intricate skeletal structures clearly exhibits the intimate relationship between skeletal form and function.

This relationship may be further demonstrated by examination of skulls to trace the stages of development of the temporomandibular joint from infancy to adulthood. Ide *et al.* (1991), in their *Anatomical Atlas of the Temporomandibular Joint,* describe the changes with age as follows:

> The size of the fossa increases by 1.2 to 1.3 times after eruption of the deciduous teeth compared to before and it increases again at the beginning of eruption of the permanent teeth. The degree of anterior inclination of the eminence changes drastically when the deciduous teeth erupt. Eventually it becomes steeper by three times in the permanent dentition than it was before the eruption of the deciduous teeth.

In the newborn child the mandible moves freely anteroposteriorly to develop suction in the primary function of breast feeding. At this stage of development the condyle is level with the gum pads, and the articular surface of the temporomandibular joint is relatively flat to allow complete freedom of movement during suckling. The form and function of the joint in the infant is similar to that of a herbivore, with flat articular surfaces that place no restriction on mandibular movement.

When a positive overbite develops as the deciduous central incisors erupt, it is then necessary for the mandible to take avoiding action by moving slightly downwards when performing a protrusive movement. This change in function is immediatly reflected in the shape of the articular surface of the temporomandibular joint. A small ridge appears that represents the first sign of an articular eminence when the deciduous incisors erupt into contact.

As yet there is no restriction on lateral movement in the joint and, at this stage, the child is still suckling. A change in function from suckling to eating solid food is related to further changes in the form and function of the temporomandibular joint to accommodate the corresponding change in masticatory function. When first deciduous molars erupt into occlusion, the form of the articular surface of the joint is modified by occlusion of the deciduous molars that now influence lateral guidance of the mandible.

As deciduous canines and molars erupt, the proprioceptive sensory feedback mechanism is responsible for continuing subtle changes in the form of the temporomandibular joint. Progressive modification of the shape of the joint articular surfaces relates to control of mandibular movement as the occlusion develops, and the joint adapts to altered function.

Still further modification of the shape of the temporomandibular articulation accompanies the transition from mixed to permanent dentition as the joint continues its adaptive development in response to the proprioceptive stimulus of a progressively more robust occlusion.

In the mature adult, the contours of the joint are fully developed and reflect the adaptive influences of the joint to the demands placed on it by the occlusion during the growth years. Occlusal guidance is directly related to condyle movement, and the shape of the joint articular surfaces in turn reflects the freedom of movement of the dentition in function. Malocclusion that presents occlusal interferences is related to restricted occlusal guidance with corresponding modification of the shape and function of the temporomandibular joint.

This correlation of form and function is also observed in the slope of the articular eminence as it relates to the occlusion. Restricted anterior movement is experienced in the Class II division 2 malocclusion, where the deep overbite necessitates a steep vertical movement of the mandible to allow the incisors to avoid occlusal interference in opening. There is an equivalent steep angulation of the articular eminence in this type of malocclusion that is related intimately to severely restricted mandibular movement in protrusive function.

Considering the aetiology of internal derangement of the temporomandibular joint, Hawthorn & Flatau (1990) observe:

> ... displacement of the meniscus anteriorly with subsequent reciprocal click in many cases is the result of confinement of mandibular movement caused by deep anterior overbite. Further degeneration or confinement of mandibular movement is brought about by developmental changes that may occur in the occlusion during the mixed dentition stage, resulting in a restrictive functional tooth angle ... it is necessary to release the mandible from a restrictive closing pathway. For long term success ... it is also necessary to provide stable, bilateral occlusal support.

Most preactivated fixed appliances in present use are designed for treatment in the permanent dentition. Late treatment of malocclusion allows adverse occlusal guidance to influence the form of the developing temporomandibular joint. The relationship between malocclusion and the development of the temporomandibular joint supports the case for early interception of malocclusion.

Functional therapy, by interceptive treatment at an earlier stage of development, attempts to achieve freedom of movement in occlusal function and thereby encourage the development of healthy joints.

The form and function philosophy is a natural progression of normal development, where functional stimuli operate through the sensory feedback mechanism to influence bone growth. In the normal sequence of growth and development, occlusal function is related directly to the functional development of the temporomandibular joint.

Evolution of functional appliance technique

It was mainly due to socioeconomic reasons that the development of functional appliances occurred almost exclusively in Europe during the major part of the twentieth century.

In the early 1900s, parallel development began in the USA and Europe in fixed and functional techniques, respectively. The Atlantic Ocean formed a geographical barrier that restricted the sharing of knowledge and experience in the fixed and functional philosophies. Integration of the two disciplines was further restricted during the First and Second World Wars, after which both cultures were committed to treatment systems that reflected their economic state.

Construction and fitting of fixed appliances by hand was time consuming and expensive. The bands were formed on the teeth and welded before attaching brackets. This procedure was beyond the economic and social circumstances of most Europeans at this stage.

The functional concept employs carefully designed removable appliances in an effort to achieve harmonious development of the dentofacial structures by eliminating unfavourable myofunctional and occlusal factors and improving the functional environment of the developing dentition. By altering the position of the teeth and supporting tissues, a new functional behaviour pattern is established to support a new position of equilibrium. This concept flourished in Europe and formed the basis of functional therapy for over a century, resulting in the development of a wide range of appliances.

The many variations in design of functional appliances that have been described since the beginning of this century bear witness to their effectiveness in correcting malocclusion and improving facial balance and harmony in the developing dentition.

OBJECTIVES OF FUNCTIONAL TREATMENT

In the natural dentition a functional equilibrium is established under neurological control in response to repetitive tactile stimuli as the teeth come into occlusion. A favourable equilibrium of muscle forces between the tongue, lips and cheeks is essential for normal development of the dental arches in correct relationship.

Any persistent deviation from normal function is associated with malocclusion. Discrepancies in arch relationships due to underlying skeletal and soft-tissue factors result in unfavourable cuspal guidance and poor occlusal function.

The purpose of functional therapy is to change the functional environment of the dentition to promote normal function. Functional appliances are designed to control the forces applied to the dentition by the surrounding soft tissues and by the muscles that control the position and movement of the mandible. A new functional behaviour pattern is established to support a new position of equilibrium by eliminating unfavourable environmental factors in a developing malocclusion.

The natural occlusal forces acting on a mandible in distal occlusion do not favour mandibular development to the patient's full potential of growth. The mandible is locked in a distal position by an unfavourable or distal driving occlusion.

Conversely, in a Class III malocclusion the maxilla is locked in a distal relationship by unfavourable occlusal forces. Altered occlusal function in this type of malocclusion has the effect of restricting maxillary development and advancing the mandible.

Functional therapy aims to unlock the malocclusion and stimulate growth by applying favourable forces that enhance skeletal development. Growth studies on experimental animals support the view that altered occlusal function produces significant changes in craniofacial growth.

Limitations of functional appliance design

All the functional appliances that have evolved from the monobloc share the limitation that the upper and lower components are joined together. As a result, the patient cannot eat, speak or function normally with the appliance in the mouth. It is also impossible to wear a one-piece functional appliance full time if it is attached to the teeth in both jaws, and the interruption to appliance wear can be a major disadvantage.

The early functional appliances were designed for night-time wear, which limited the response to treatment. It was also important to select patients who had a favourable growth pattern in order to improve the prognosis for correction, and to eliminate the uncertainty associated with night time functional appliances. There is better potential for rapid mandibular growth when the patient has a favourable horizontal growth pattern than when the facial growth vector is more vertical.

The muscles are the prime movers that modify bone growth to meet the demands of function via the proprioceptive feedback mechanism. When the appliance is removed for eating the patient reverts to functioning with the mandible in a retrusive position. The strongest functional forces are applied to the dentition during mastication, and the proprioceptive functional stimulus to growth is lost if the appliance is removed for eating.

Comfort and aesthetics are crucial in appliance design. It is essential that the patient can speak clearly with the appliance in place to avoid embarrassment. A monoblock type of appliance that is designed to fit the teeth in both jaws simultaneously interferes with speech and limits normal function. These are important factors that influence patient motivation and compliance, and are closely related to success in treatment.

The Schwarz Double Plate

The Double Plate of Martin Schwarz (1956) attempted to combine the advantages of the activator and the active plate by constructing separate upper and lower acrylic plates that were designed to occlude with the mandible in a protrusive position.

The maxillary appliance for correction of Class division 1 malocclusion carried lingual flanges that extended into the lower dental arch

to articulate with the lower appliance on an inclined plane, causing a functional mandibular displacement on closure. There were two variations in appliance design that incorporated anterior or lateral lingual flanges, respectively. The anterior lingual flange was used more commonly, and represented an extension of the principle of the anterior inclined plane, originally developed by Kingsley (1877). The Double Plate resembled a monobloc or activator constructed in two pieces.

A widely recommended variation in design was described by Muller (1962). The lateral wings were replaced by heavy gauge wires of 2 mm diameter, that extended downwards from the upper appliance at an angle of 70° to engage a groove in the lower appliance.

BITE REGISTRATION IN FUNCTIONAL THERAPY

Bite registration is a crucial factor in the design and construction of a functional appliance. The construction bite determines the degree of activation built into the appliance, aiming to reposition the mandible to improve the jaw relationship. The degree of activation should stretch the muscles of mastication sufficiently to provide a positive proprioceptive response. At the same time, activation must be within the physiological range of activity of the muscles of mastication and the ligamentous attachments of the temporomandibular joint. Bite registration should achieve a balance between these factors by providing the degree of mandibular protrusion required to achieve the optimum functional stimulus to growth.

According to Woodside (1977, p. 293) in construction of the activator as described by Andresen (1910):

> A bite registration used commonly throughout the world registers the mandible in a position protruded approximately 3.0 mm distal to the most protrusive position that the patient can achieve, while vertically the bite is registered within the limits of the patient's freeway space.

In North America, a similar protrusive bite registration is made, except that the vertical activation is 4 mm beyond the rest position.

Roccabado (pers. comm.) quantifies normal physiological temporomandibular joint movement as 70% of total joint displacement. Beyond this point, the medial capsular ligament begins to displace the disc by pulling the disc medially and distally off the condyle. This guideline allows us to measure the total mandibular displacement and relate the amount of activation to the freedom of movement of the joint for each individual patient.

Bite registration in Twin Block technique

Bite registration for Twin Blocks originally aimed for a single activation to an edge-to-edge incisor relationship with 2 mm intercisal clearance for an overjet of up to 10 mm. Allowance was made for individual variation if the patient had difficulty in maintaining an edge-to-edge position on registering the occlusion. This proved to be successful in correcting the overjet and reducing the distal occlusion in the majority of cases.

Where the overjet was greater than 10 mm, an initial advancement of 7 or 8 mm was followed by reactivation of the appliance after occlusion had corrected to the initial bite registration. Normally, a single further activation was sufficient to fully correct the overjet and distal occlusion.

In the early stages of using Twin Blocks it was noted that some patients had difficulty in maintaining the forward posture and occluding correctly on the inclined planes. These patients usually had a vertical growth pattern with weak musculature and were unable to maintain the forward mandibular posture consistently. They could be identified early in treatment as they tended to posture the mandible back and meet the blocks together behind the inclined planes. To overcome this problem the activation of the appliance was reduced slightly by trimming the inclined planes until the patient occluded comfortably and consistently in the forward position.

This difficulty can be avoided by relating bite registration to the patient's freedom of movement and by registering the protrusive path of the mandible. The George Bite Gauge has a millimetre gauge to measure the protrusive path of the mandible and to determine accurately the amount of activation registered in the construction bite.

The total protrusive movement is calculated by first measuring the overjet in centric occlusion and then in the position of maximum protrusion. The protrusive path of the mandible is the difference between the two measurements. Functional activation within normal physiological limits should not exceed 70% of the protrusive path (George, pers. comm.)(**3.1**).

By checking the protrusive path the adjustment may be related to the patient's physiological movements. The young patient usually has more freedom of movement while there is generally more restriction in the adult. In Class II division 1 malocclusion, young patients commonly have a protrusive path of 13 mm and will tolerate activation up to 10 mm. Beyond this range the muscles and ligaments cannot adapt to altered function and the patient will tend to posture out of the appliance. If the overjet is larger than 10 mm the initial activation should only partially reduce the overjet. The appliance is then reactivated during the course of treatment.

Vertical activation

The amount of vertical activation is crucial to the success of Twin Block treatment. The most common fault in Twin Block construction is to make the blocks too thin, so that the patient can posture out of the appliance, reducing the effectiveness of the treatment.

An important principle is that the blocks should be thick enough to open the bite slightly beynd the free-way space. This is necessary to ensure that the patient does not posture out of the appliance when the mandible is in the rest position.

On average the blocks are not less than 5-mm thick in the first premolar or first deciduous molar region. This thickness is normally achieved in Class II division 1 deep bite cases by registering a 2-mm vertical interincisal clearance.

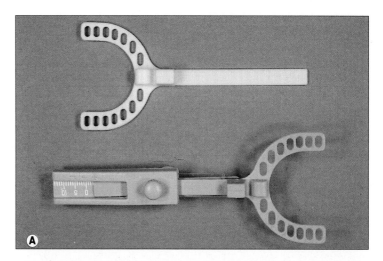

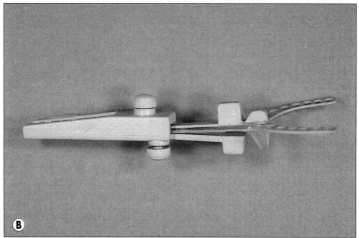

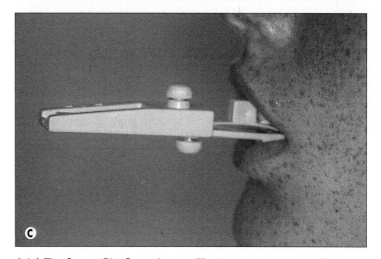

3.1 A The George Bite Gauge has a millimetre gauge to measure the protrusive path of the mandible and to determine accurately the amount of activation registered in the construction bite.

3.1 B, C Lateral views to show method of bite registration.

In Class II division 2 malocclusion with excessive overbite it is sufficient to register an edge-to-edge incisal bite registration without the additional 2-mm interincisal clearance. This is normally sufficient in this type of malocclusion to accommodate blocks of the correct thickness.

In treatment of anterior open bite it is necessary to register bite with a greater interincisal clearance to make allowance for the anterior open bite. The projet or George bite gauge has thicker versions to accommodate an interincisal clearance of 4 or 5 mm. At bite registration a judgement should be made according to the amount of vertical space between the cusptips of the first premolars or deciduous molars to achieve the correct degree of bite opening to accommodate blocks of at least 5-mm thickness.

Petrovic *et al.* (1981) found in animal experiments that a step-wise activation appeared to be the best procedure to promote orthopaedic lengthening of the mandible. Taking this into account, Falke & Frankel (1989) reduced initial activation for mandibular advancement to 3 mm, having previously registered an edge-to-edge bite unless the overjet was excessive. The concept of progressive activation for functional correction to achieve the optimum growth response has been investigated (Falke & Frankel, 1989; De Vincenzo & Winn, 1989) with differing results, and requires further investigation.

CONTROL OF THE VERTICAL DIMENSION

The mechanism of control of the vertical dimension differs in fixed and functional therapy. In fixed mechanics, the teeth remain in occlusion during the course of treatment, and the effect is limited to intrusion or extrusion of individual teeth to increase or decrease overbite and level the occlusal plane. The occlusal level is determined by occlusal contact with teeth in the opposing arch. Functional appliances have the advantage of influencing facial height to control the vertical dimension by covering the teeth with blocks or an occlusal table.

Functional appliances are designed to influence development in the anteroposterior and vertical dimensions simultaneously. Control of the vertical dimension is achieved by covering the teeth in the opposing arches and controlling the intermaxillary space. The management of the appliance differs according to whether the bite is to be opened or closed during treatment.

Opening the bite

Where a deep overbite is present it is necessary first to check that the profile is improved when the patient postures the mandible downwards and forwards. This confirms that the bite should be opened by encouraging eruption of the posterior teeth to increase the vertical dimension of occlusion.

This is achieved by placing an occlusal table between the teeth to encourage increased development of posterior facial height by growth of the vertical ramus. At the same time, the occlusion is freed between the posterior teeth to encourage selective eruption of posterior teeth to increase the vertical dimension of occlusion in the posterior quadrants.

In functional therapy anteroposterior correction is invariably achieved before vertical development in the buccal segments is complete. The overjet is reduced and the distal occlusion corrected before the buccal teeth have completely erupted into occlusion. It is common in functional therapy for a posterior open bite to develop as the overjet reduces. The upper and lower incisors come into occlusion before the posterior teeth erupt.

If a functional appliance is removed for eating, the tongue often spreads laterally between the teeth and delays eruption. Full-time appliance wear with Twin Blocks prevents the tongue from spreading between the teeth and accelerates correction of deep overbite.

Closing the bite

Reduced overbite or anterior open bite is often related to a vertical facial growth pattern. The lower facial height is already increased, and the vertical dimension must not be encouraged to increase during treatment. It is necessary to close the anterior vertical dimension, and treatment should endeavour to reduce lower facial height by applying intrusive forces to the opposing posterior teeth.

An acrylic occlusal table is designed into the appliance to maintain contact on the posterior teeth throughout treatment. This occlusal contact results in a relative intrusion of the posterior teeth while the anterior teeth are free to erupt, thereby reducing the anterior open bite.

In the Twin Block technique the intrusive forces which close the bite are increased by wearing the appliances for eating. In treatment of reduced overbite it is very important that the opposing acrylic occlusal bite block surfaces are not trimmed. All posterior teeth must remain in contact with the blocks throughout treatment to prevent eruption of posterior teeth (**3.2**)

Manipulation of the occlusal table is an important aspect of functional appliance therapy. By separating the posterior teeth it is possible to adjust the dimensions of the intermaxillary space anteroposteriorly and vertically to correct skeletal discrepancies. The concept of using occlusal inclined planes as a functional mechanism to correct distal

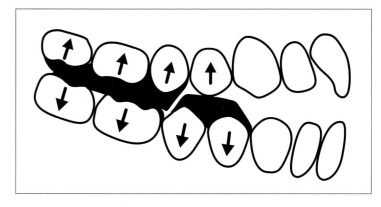

3.2 Occlusal blocks contact posterior teeth to prevent eruption.

malocclusion is the next logical step in the evolution of functional appliance technique. The mechanics can be reversed, applying the same principles for correction of Class III malocclusion.

REFERENCES

Angle, E.H. (1907). *Treatment of Malocclusion of the Teeth,* 7th edn. Philadelphia, S.S. White Dental Manufacturing Co.

Andresen, V. (1910). Beitrag zur Retention. *Z. Zahnaerztl. Orthop.,* **3**: 121–5.

Begg, P.R. (1954). Stone Age man's dentition. *Am. J. Orthod.,* **40**: 298–312; 373–83; 462–75; 517–31.

De Vicenzo, J.P. & Winn, M.W. (1989). Orthopaedic and orthodontic effects resulting from the use of a functional appliance with different amounts of protrusive activation.

Falke, F. & Frankel (1989). Clinical relevance of step by step mandibular advancement in the treatment of mandibular retrusion using the Frankel appliance. *Am. J. Orthod. Dentofac. Orthop.,* **96**: 333–41.

George, P.T. (1992). A new instrument for functional appliance bite registration. *J. Clin. Orthod.,* **26**: 721–3.

Graber (Ed.) (1969). Dento-facial orthopaedics. *Current Orthodontic Concepts and Techniques,* Vol. 2. Philadelphia, W.B. Saunders.

Hawthorn, R. & Flatau, A. (1990). Temporomandibular joint anatomy. In *A Colour Atlas of Temporomandibular Joint Surgery*, ed. J.E.DeB Norman & P.E. Bramley. London, Wolfe Publishing.

Ide, Y., Nakazawa, K., Hongo, J. & Tateishi, J. (1991). *Anatomical Atlas of the Temporomandibular Joint.* Tokyo, Quintessence Publishing Co.

Kingsley, N.W. (1877). An experiment with artificial palates. *Dental Cosmos,* **19**: 231.

Moss, M.L. (1968). The primacy of functional matrices in profacial growth, *Dent. Practitioner,* **19**: 65–73.

Muller, G.H. (1962). Die Doppelplatte mit Oberkeifer-spornfuhrung. *Fortschr. Kieferorthop.*

Petrovic, A.G., Stutzmann, J.J. & Gasson, N. (1981). The final length of the mandible: Is it genetically determined? *Craniofacial Biology,* ed. D.S. Carlson, Monograph No. 10, Center for Human Growth & Development, University of Michigan, pp. 105–26.

Robin, P. (1902*a*). Observation sur un nouvel appareil de redressement. *Rev. Stomatol.,* **9.**

Robin, P. (1902*b*). Demonstration practique sur le construction et la mise en bouche d'un nouvel appareil de redressement. *Rev. Stomatol.,* **9.**

Schwarz, A.M. (1956). *Lehrgang der Gebissregelung,* 2nd edn. Vienna, Urban & Schwarzenberg.

Tweed, C.H. (1944). Indications for the extraction of teeth in orthodontic procedure. *Am. J. Orthod. & Oral Surgery,* August.

Weislander, L. (1963). The effect of orthodontic treatment on concurrent development of the craniofacial complex. *Am. J. Orthod.,* **49**: 15–27.

Weislander, L. (1974). The effect of force on cranio-facial development. *Am. J. Orthod.,* **65**: 531–8.

Weislander, L (1975). Early or late cervical traction therapy in Class II malocclusion in the mixed dentition. *Am. J. Orthod.,* **67**: 432–9.

Weislander, L. & Buck, D.L. (1974). Physiological recovery after cervical traction therapy. *Am. J. Orthod.,* **66**: 294–301.

Woodside, D.G. (1977). The activator. In *Removable Orthodontic Appliances,* ed. T.M. Graber & B. Neumann. Philadelphia, W.B. Saunders.

FURTHER READING

Wolff, J. (1892). *Das Gesets der transformation der Knochen.* Berlin, Hirschwald.

Broadbent, J.M. (1987). Crossroads: acceptance or rejection of Functional Jaw Orthopedics. *Am. J. Orthod.,* **92**(1): 75–8.

4

Growth Studies in Experimental Animals

Animal experiments to investigate the biological response to orthodontic and orthopaedic techniques provide a basis for comparison with clinical experience, when we apply similar techniques in the treatment of patients. The findings of current research into the mechanisms that control bone growth are now examined.

The results of recent growth studies on experimental animals suggest consistently that skeletal form is adaptable to functional stimulus: Charlier *et al* (1969); Moyers *et al.* (1970); Stockli & Willert (1971); Petrovic *et al.* (1971); McNamara (1972); and Elgoyhen *et al.* (1972).

Experiments have shown that condylar cartilage is highly responsive to mechanical stimuli (Stockli & Willert, 1971) and to hormonal and chemical agents (Petrovic & Stutzmann, 1977).

Hinton (1981) reviews temporomandibular joint function to clarify past misconceptions. Clinical, experimental and biochemical data strongly suggest that the temporomandibular joint is an articulation to which forces are transmitted during normal dental function, and one that undergoes adaptive remodelling in response to these forces.

Harvold (1973) commented on research started in the University of California in 1965 to examine the changes that occur in the internal structure of bone in response to functional stimulus:

> The pilot studies demonstrated that an alteration in pressure distribution on the maxilla caused rapid resorption of the existing trabecular system within two months. Another few months were necessary before the stabilised pressure distribution was manifested in a new, functionally orientated trabecular system. These pilot experiments indicated that only stimuli that were relatively uniform for a period of several months could contribute to the development of a trabecular system.

THE OCCLUSAL INCLINED PLANE IN ANIMAL EXPERIMENTS

Moss (1980), investigating the effects of the inclined plane in six adult ferrets, concluded:

> The results of this simple experiment illustrate the profound effect that a biting force on an inclined plane can have on the whole of the dental arch, including the condylar head, the muscle attachments and teeth remote from the tooth being moved. Even in the adult animal, the whole of the stomatognathic system, including the soft tissues, adapts to re-establish an efficient masticatory system.

FUNCTIONAL REGULATION OF CONDYLAR CARTILAGE GROWTH RATE

The theory of functional regulation of condylar cartilage growth rate is supported by recent evidence from animal experiments (Stutzmann & Petrovic, 1979; McNamara 1980).

Fixed occlusal inclined planes have been used to alter the distribution of occlusal forces in animal experiments investigating the effects of functional mandibular displacement on mandibular growth and on adaptive changes in the temporomandibular joint (McNamara, 1980; Stutzmann & Petrovic, 1979). Results have demonstrated improved mandibular growth in experimental animals compared to control animals (**4.1A–D**).

A fundamental study of the relationship between form and function was carried out in animal experiments at the University of Michigan, and the results were summarised by McNamara (1980). The studies evaluated changes in muscle function and related changes in bone growth in the rhesus monkey by a comparison of experimental and control animals as monitored by electromyographic (EMG), cephalometric and histological studies. McNamara concluded:

> These studies demonstrated the close relationship between the functional and structural components of the craniofacial region.

The findings were based on the use of fixed occlusal inclined planes that were designed to cause a forward postural displacement of the mandible in all active and passive muscle activity. The pattern of muscle behaviour during the experimental period showed a cyclical change in response to functional mandibular propulsion. Each animal was used as its own control to register muscle activity by a series of control records prior to appliance placement. This established the level of muscle activity before treatment.

Initial placement of the appliance produced an increase in the overall activity of the muscles of mastication as the animal sought to find a new occlusal position. A distinct change in muscle activity occurred within 1–7 days. This was characterised by a decrease in the activity of the posterior head of temporalis, an increase in activity of the masseter muscle, and most significantly an increase in function of the superior head of the lateral pterygoid muscle.

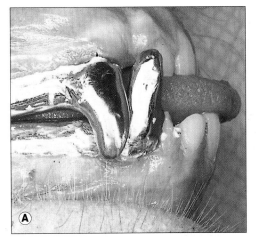
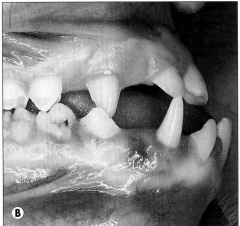
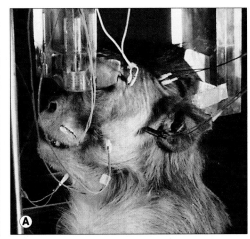

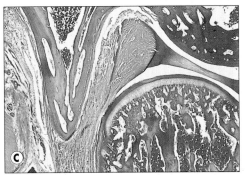
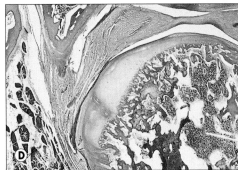
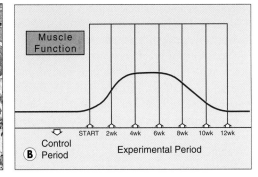

4.1 A, B Fixed inclined planes produced a Class III dental relationship in monkeys.
C, D Proliferation of condylar cartilage in experimental animals demonstrated compared to controls.
Courtesy of J.A. McNamara Jr.

4.2 A, B Electromyographic study shows the cycle of change in muscle behaviour.
Courtesy of J.A. McNamara Jr.

After 3 weeks a new plateau of muscle activity was reached at a higher level of activity than the pretreatment record. This level of activity persisted for 4 weeks before a further decline in muscle activity over a period of 4 weeks to the level recorded before treatment. The cycle of changes was completed in a 3-month period (**4.2**).

These changes are consistent with an equilibrium of muscle activity before treatment which is disturbed by placement of the appliance. The level of muscle activity increases accordingly until, after a period of adjustment, a new equilibrium is reached at a higher level of activity. Further adaptation within the muscles over a period of time results in a reduction of muscle activity when a new equilibrium is again established at the same level that existed before treatment.

A similar experimental study at the University of Toronto came to different conclusions on the effect of placement of a functional appliance on muscle activity (Sessle *et al.*, 1990). This study used chronically implanted EMG electrodes to identify a statistically significant decrease in postural EMG activity of the superior and inferior heads of the lateral pterygoid, and the superficial masseter muscles, which persisted for 6 weeks and returned to pretreatment levels during a subsequent 6-week period. Progressive mandibular advancement of 1.5–2 mm every 10–15 days did not prevent the decrease in postural EMG activity.

The clinical implication of these differing results is that the question of activation of a functional appliance by a single large mandibular displacement or a progressive series of smaller activations is still to be resolved.

It is not established whether active muscle contraction or passive muscle tension is the primary stimulus to growth in functional therapy.

CENTRAL CONTROL OF ADAPTIVE RESPONSE

Neuromuscular and skeletal adaptations

In principle, the muscles are the prime movers in promoting skeletal adaptation in response to proprioceptive sensory stimulus. Adaptive skeletal changes in the structure and form of bone is a secondary response to alterations in sensory and muscle function. Essentially, skeletal changes occur to support the alteration in load and functional requirements, assuming that the alterations in occlusal function are within the biological limits of tolerance of the organism.

McNamara (1980) summarises the adaptive responses observed in functional protrusion experiments as follows:

> The placement of the appliance results in an immediate change in the stimuli to the receptors in the orofacial region, particularly those in the tongue, gingiva, palate, dentition and temporo-mandibular joint region. This alteration in stimuli is transmitted to the central nervous system that ... mediates changes in muscle activity. This alteration in muscle function leads to a forward positioning of the jaw. These muscular changes are very rapid and can be measured in terms of minutes, hours and days.
>
> Structural adaptations are more gradual in nature. Structural adaptations occur throughout the craniofacial region ... As structural balance is restored during the weeks and months following appliance placement, the need for altered muscle activity is lessened, and there is a gradual return to more typical muscle patterns. This experimental model provides a clear illustration of the relationship between form and function in the growing individual.

McNamara concluded that a rapid neuromuscular response is followed by a more gradual skeletal adaptation. Structural harmony can be restored by a combination of mechanisms including dentoalveolar movement or condylar growth. The exact nature of the skeletal adaptations depends upon the age of the animal.

In growing monkeys, increased growth of the mandibular condyle is shown following functional protrusion. As a result of mandibular hyperpropulsion, the dental relationship changed in the experimental animals from normal to Class III occlusion.

The following factors may all contribute to the development of a Class III molar relationship:

- Restriction of maxillary skeletal growth.
- Inhibition of downward and forward migration of maxillary dentition.
- Mesial migration of mandibular dentition.
- Increased mandibular skeletal growth.
- Adaptations in other regions.

The study concluded that the Class III dental relationship could not be explained by adaptations in any single craniofacial structure or region, but was a result of both pronounced and subtle adaptations throughout the structures of the craniofacial complex.

ADAPTATION IN BONE GROWTH IN RESPONSE TO FUNCTIONAL STIMULUS

Research on bone growth at the University of Toronto has examined adaptive changes in bone in response to functional stimulus. Woodside *et al.* (1983) hypothesised that the movement of bone into new positions within a muscle system results in rearrangement of the stress distribution and reorganisation of shape and internal structure. To test the hypothesis, clinical and animal experiments involving the use of posterior occlusal bite blocks, Herbst appliances and temporal and masseter muscle stimulation were undertaken.

This study concluded:

> Chronic or continuous alteration in mandibular position within the neuromuscular environment with the posterior occlusal bite block and the Herbst appliance in a sample of monkeys produced extensive condylar remodeling and change in mandibular size.

These experiments demonstrate the principle that:

> consistent changes in bone shape and internal structure are obtained when the alteration in neuromuscular activity is continuous

and that:

> changing the muscle activity will affect the bone morphology.

In further experiments Woodside *et al.* (1987) examined: 'The influence of functional appliance therapy on glenoid fossa remodeling', following a period of progressively activated and continuously maintained advancement using the Herbst appliance. They concluded: 'In adult, adolescent and juvenile primates, continuous and progressive mandibular protrusion produces extensive anterior remodeling of the glenoid fossa.'

In all experimental animals, including, most importantly, the mature adult, a large volume of new bone had formed in the glenoid fossa, especially along the anterior border of the postglenoid spine. With this bone formation, and the resorption along the posterior border of the postglenoid spine, the glenoid fossa appeared to be remodelling anteriorly. Expert histopathologists agreed that the newly forming bone had a normal appearance.

The new bone formation appeared to be localised in the primary attachment area of the posterior fibrous tissue of the articular disc. The deposition of the finger-like woven bone seemed to correspond to the direction of tension exerted by the stretched fibres of the posterior part of the disc.

This study further concluded that the proliferation of condylar tissue may be age- or sex-related, and was seen only in the juvenile primate. Proliferation of the posterior part of the fibrous articular disc was also described, splinting the condyle eccentrically in the glenoid fossa. The skeletal jaw relationship may be altered by both glenoid fossa remodelling and condylar extension in young primates, and thereafter by glenoid fossa relocation. This result may be related to age, sex and the amount of mandibular protrusion.

A REVIEW OF THE PARADIGM OF GENETIC CONTROL

It is never too late to give up your prejudices.

Henry David Thoreau

The paradigm of strict genetic control of growth mechanisms is reviewed in a paper by Petrovic *et al.* (1981), entitled: 'The final length of the mandible: is it genetically predetermined?':

Our concept of orthopaedically modulable growth in the mammalian condylar cartilage was confirmed by Stockli & Willert (1971); McNamara *et al.* (1975); Graber (1975) and Komposh & Hocenjos (1977). Only experiments by Gaumond (1973, 1975) in the rat fail to support the possibility that the mandible can be lengthened by orthopaedic forces.'

The orthodontic community began to accept the idea that it is possible to change not only growth direction, but also growth rate (Graber, 1972; Linge, 1977). The idea that the final length of the mandible is "genetically preprogrammed" has been the prevalent concept for the past 40 years, even if not specifically substantiated (Brodie, 1941; Bjork, 1955; Ricketts, 1952; Hiniker & Ramfjord, 1964; Joho, 1968; Harvold, 1968). Indeed, this concept is widely accepted as part of the doctrine underlying fixed appliance ideology.

Petrovic et al. (1981) conclude:

First:

Appropriate orthopaedic appliances placing the rat mandible in a forward position increase the condylar cartilage growth rate, and growth amount, i.e. the mandible becomes longer than that of control animals. ... No genetically predetermined length of the mandible could be detected in these experiments.

Secondly, Petrovitch recommends a step-wise functional activation to produce the most effective lengthening of the mandible:

Periodic increases in the thickness of the postural hyperpropulsar results in new increases in lateral pterygoid muscle activity as recorded electromyographically, and, consequently, brings about a new increase in the rate and amount of condylar cartilage growth.

Thirdly:

When the appliance was removed after the growth of the animal was completed, no relapse was observed. When the appliance was removed before growth was completed no significant relapse was detected if a good intercuspation had been achieved during the experimental phase; if a good intercuspation had not been achieved, the "comparator" of the servosystem imposed an increased or decreased condylar growth rate until a state of intercuspal stability was established.

Fourthly:

How can a clinician use concepts and theories formulated from animal experiments? It is out of the question to extrapolate automatically from one mammalian species to another one. A concept or theory, that has been established using rats as the experimental model and corroborated using monkeys must be tested in humans. ... Appliances used in the child and aimed to produce effects similar to those produced in the rat should be appropriate.

A comparison of Twin Block response with animal experiments

The clinical response observed after fitting Twin Blocks is closely analogous to the changes observed and reported in animal experiments using fixed inclined planes. Harvold (1983) confirms from histological study in animal experiments that rapid adaptive changes occur in the tissues surrounding the condyle when a full-time functional appliance is fitted:

The placement of appliances results in an immediate change in the neuromuscular proprioceptive response ... the resulting muscular changes are very rapid, and can be measured in terms of minutes, hours and days. Structural alterations are more gradual and are measured in months, whereby the dentoskeletal structures adapt to restore a functional equilibrium to support the altered position of muscle balance.

Harvold has demonstrated in animal experiments the tissue changes that occur as a result of altered occlusal function. When the mandible postures downwards and forwards a vacuum is not created distal to the condyle. Above and behind the condyle is an area of intense cellular activity described as a 'tension zone' that is quickly invaded by proliferating connective tissue and capillary blood vessels, when the mandible functions in a protrusive position. These changes occur within hours and days, rather than weeks and months of the appliance being fitted.

These tissue changes are reflected in the clinical signs after fitting Twin Blocks. The patient experiences adaptation of muscle function immediately on insertion of the appliances, in response to altered occlusal function. When an occlusal inclined plane is fitted, a rapid initial conscious adaptation occurs to avoid traumatic occlusal contacts.

Within a few days the patient experiences pain behind the condyle when the appliance is removed. From the studies of histological changes in animal experiments, it may be deduced that retraction of the condyle results in compression of connective tissue and blood vessels and that ischaemia is the principal cause of pain.

A new pattern of muscle behaviour is quickly established whereby the patient finds it difficult and later impossible to retract the mandible into its former retruded position. After a few days, it is more comfortable to wear the appliance than to leave it out. This change in muscle activity has been described by McNamara as the 'pterygoid response' which results from altered activity of the medial head of the lateral pterygoid muscle in response to mandibular protrusion. It is extremely rare for such a response to be observed with functional appliances that are not worn full time.

The initial response to functional mandibular protrusion is, therefore, a change in the muscles of mastication to establish a new equilibrium in muscle behaviour. Volumetric changes behind the condyle result in cellular proliferation at this stage. When the altered muscle function is established the proprioceptive sensory mechanism initiates compensatory bone remodelling to adapt to the altered function.

The muscles are the prime movers in growth, followed by bone remodelling as a secondary response to altered muscle function. Muscle function must be altered over a sufficient period of time to allow adaptive bone remodelling changes to occur to reposition the condyle in the glenoid fossa.

SUMMARY

Over the past 30 years many animal experiments investigating the orthopaedic effects of functional mandibular protrusion have come to consistent conclusions. Electromyographic, cephalometric and histological studies in animal experiments provide a better understanding of the biological changes that result from orthopaedic technique. Controlled experiments confirm that the mandibles of monkeys and rats are responsive to functional stimuli, and that bone remodelling occurs in the glenoid fossa, and in muscles and ligaments and their attachments at sites which are remote from the dentoalveolar areas normally associated with a response to orthodontic treatment.

That the conclusions drawn from these experiments differ from traditional views relating to orthodontic treatment only serves to underline that different mechanical systems do not produce an identical biological response.

Animal growth studies are of direct relevance to clinical practice. As one evaluates the biological and histological changes produced by appliance mechanisms in experimental animals, a better understanding is gained of the changes observed clinically in patients. The growth response in animals has been measured through full-time appliances using inclined planes as the functional mechanism. It is now possible to conduct equivalent growth studies for patients with an identical appliance mechanism using the occlusal inclined plane. Growth studies of consecutively treated patients against untreated control values form a basis for comparison with the results of animal growth studies.

REFERENCES

Brodie, A.G. (1941). On the growth pattern of the human head from the third month to the eighth year of life. *Am. J. Anatomy,* **68**: 209–62.

Bjork, A. (1955). Facial growth in man studied with the aid of metallic implants. *Acta Odont. Scand.,* **13**: 9–34.

Charlier, J.P., Petrovic, A. & Stutzmann, J. (1969). Effects of mandibular hyperpropulsion on the prechondroblastic zone of the young rat condyle, *Am. J. Orthod.,* **55**: 71–4.

Elgoyen, J.C., Moyers, R.E., McNamara, Jr, J.A. & Riolo, M.L. (1972). Craniofacial adaptation to protrusive function in juvenile Rhesus monkeys. *Am. J. Orthod.,* **62**: 469–80.

Gaumond, G. (1973). Les effets d'une force extraorale de traction sur la croissance mandibulaire de jeune rats. *L'Orthodontie Française,* **44**: 213–27.

Gaumond, G. (1975). Effets d'un sopareil d'hyperpropulsion fonctionelle sur la croissance mandibulaire de jeune rats. *L'Orthodontie Française,* **46**: 107–28.

Graber, L.W. (1975). The alterability of mandibular growth. In *Determinants of Mandibular Form and Growth,* ed. J.A. McNamara Jr, Monograph No. 4, Craniofacial Growth series, University of Michigan, pp. 229–41.

Graber, T.M. (1972). *Orthodontics: Principles and Practice,* 3rd edn. Philadelphia, W.B. Saunders.

Harvold, E.P. (1968). The role of function in the etiology and treatment of malocclusion. *Am. J. Orthod.,* **54**: 883.

Harvold, E.P. (1983). Altering craniofacial growth: force application and neuromuscular–bone interaction. In *Clinical Alteration of the Growing Face,* Monograph 14, Craniofacial Growth Series, University of Michigan.

Hiniker, J.J. & Ramfjord, S.P. (1964). Anterior displacement of the mandible in adult rhesus monkey.*J. Dent. Res.,* **43**: suppl., 811.

Hinton, R.H. (1981). Form and function in the temporomandibular joint. *Craniofacial Biology,* ed. D.S. Carlson, Monograph 10, Craniofacial Growth Series, University of Michigan.

Joho, J.P. (1968). Changes in the form of the mandible in the orthopaedically treated Macaca virus (an experimental study). *Eur. Orthod. Soc.,* **44**: 161–173.

Komposh, G. & Hocenjos, Cl. (1977). Die Reaktionsfahigkeit des temporomandibularen Knorpels. *Fortschr. Kieferorthopadie,* **38**: 121–32.

Linge, L. (1977). Klinishe Relevanz tierexprimenteller Untersuchungen (Korreferat Zum Vortrag Petrovic). *Fortschr. Kieferorthopadie,* **38**: 253–60.

McNamara, Jr, J.A. (1972). *Neuromuscular and skeletal adaptations to Altered Function in the Orofacial Region.* Monograph No. 1, Craniofacial Growth Series, University of Michigan.

McNamara, Jr, J.A. (1980). Functional determinants of craniofacial size and shape. *Eur. J. Orthod.,* **1**: 131–59.

McNamara, Jr, J.A., Connelly & T.G., McBride, M.C. (1975). Histological studies of temporomandibular joint adaptations. In *Control mechanisms in Craniofacial Growth,* ed. J.A. McNamara Jr, University of Michigan, pp. 209–27.

Moss, J.P. (1980). The soft tissue environment of teeth and jaws. *Brit. J. Orthod.,* **7**: 127–37, 205–16.

Moyers, R.E., Elgoyhen, J.C. & Riolo, M.L. (1970). Experimental production of class III malocclusion in Rhesus monkeys. *Trans. Eur. Orthod. Soc.,* **46**: 61.

Petrovic, A. & Stutzmann, J. (1977). Further investigations into the functioning of the 'comparator' of the servosystem (respective positions of the upper and lower dental arches) in the control of the condylar cartilage growth rate and of the lengthening of the jaw. In *The Biology of Occlusal Development,* ed. J.A. McNamara Jr, Monograph No. 6, Craniofacial Growth series, Center for Human Growth & Development, University of Michigan, pp. 225–91.

Petrovic, A. & Stutzmann, J. & Lavergne (1971). Mechanisms of craniofacial growth and modus operandi of functional appliances: A cell-level and cybernetic approach to orthodontic decision making.

Petrovic, A.G., Stutzmann, J.J. & Gasson, N. (1981). The final length of the mandible: Is it genetically determined? *Craniofacial Biology,* ed. D.S. Carlson, Monograph No. 10, Center for Human Growth & Development, University of Michigan, pp. 105–26.

Ricketts, R.M. (1952). A study of the changes in temporomandibular relations associated with the treatment of Class II malocclusion (Angle). *Am. J. Orthod.,* **38**: 918.

Sessle, B.J. *et al.* (1990). Effect of functional appliances on jaw muscle activity. *Am. J. Orthod. Dentofac. Orthop.,* **98**: 222–30.

Stockli, P.W. & Willert, H.G. (1971). Tissue reactions in the temporomandibular joint resulting from the anterior displacement of the mandible in the monkey. *Am. J. Orthod.,* **60**: 142–55.

Stutzmann, J. & Petrovic, A. (1979). Intrinsic regulation of condylar cartilage growth rate. *Eur. J. Orthod.,* **1**: 41–54.

Woodside, D.G., Altuna, G., Harvold,E. & Metaxas, A. (1983). Primate experiments in malocclusion and bone induction. *Am. J. Orthod.,* **83**: 460–8.

Woodside, D.G., Metaxas, A. & Altuna, G. (1987). The influence of functional appliance therapy on glenoid fossa remodelling. *Am. J. Orthod. Dentofac. Orthop.,* **92**: 181–98.

CHAPTER

5

Diagnosis and Treatment Planning

CLINICAL EXAMINATION

Orthodontic records

Successful orthodontic treatment is dependent on a disciplined approach to record taking and diagnosis, as well as careful monitoring of progress in treatment. Inadequate records may be reflective of a poor standard of treatment.

The essentials for orthodontic records are a diagnostic report supported by study models, x-rays and photographs to establish the condition of the case before treatment and to record progress during treatment.

Radiographic examination is necessary to identify and locate all unerupted teeth. This is accomplished routinely by a panoral x-ray with intraoral films if required for individual teeth. Temporo-mandibular joint x-rays are also extremely important, especially in today's litigious society, to establish the condition of the joint before treatment. Cephalometric analysis of a lateral skull x-ray gives detailed information to support clinical diagnosis. Important clinical guidelines in treatment planning for Class II division 1 malocclusion are now considered.

Clinical guidelines

Clinical examination provides the fundamental guideline in case selection for functional therapy. If the facial profile improves when the mandible is advanced with the lips lightly closed, then functional mandibular advancement is the treatment of choice. The change in facial appearance is a preview of the anticipated result of functional treatment. This clinical impression is even more important than lines and angles drawn on a cephalometric x-ray. This does not negate or diminish the value of cephalometric analysis, but adds a three-dimensional view to support and confirm the diagnosis (**5.1**).

Photographic records

Facial and dental photographs are an invaluable diagnostic aid to establish the objectives of treatment and to monitor progress.

Photographs are used to predict the change in facial appearance that will result from treatment. Profile and full-face photographs with

SW

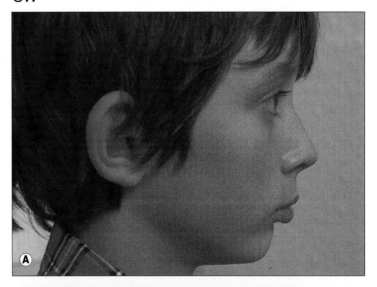

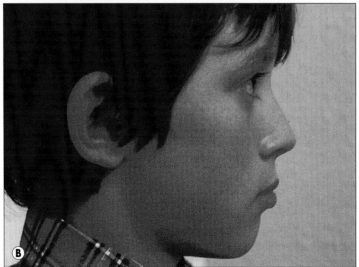

5.1 S.W. aged 14 years 2 months:
A, B The immediate profile change on the day the appliance is fitted is a preview of the result of treatment.

SW

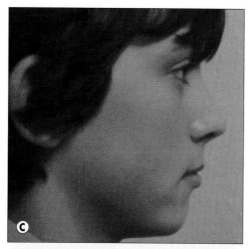

5.1 C Profile after 11 months of treatment.
D Overjet before treatment.
E Inclined planes guide the mandible forwards.
F Occlusion is corrected after 11 months.

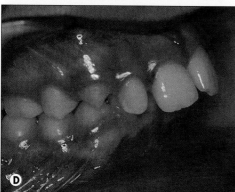

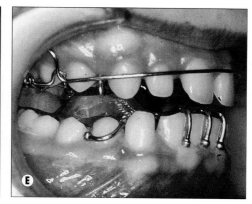

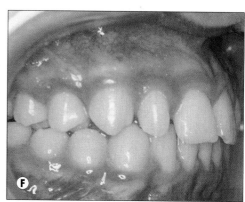

the mandible in the retrusive position show the appearance before treatment, and are repeated with the mandible advanced to give the projected optimum improvement in facial appearance.

An additional set of photographs for the patient, from a simple polaroid camera, improves motivation by allowing the patient to observe the rapid improvement in appearance during the first few months of treatment.

EXAMINATION OF MODELS

An equally simple guideline helps to predict occlusal changes by checking the occlusion resulting when the mandible postures downwards and forwards to reduce the overjet. This can be observed directly in the mouth, but is best confirmed on study models by sliding the lower model forwards and observing the articulation of the mandibular dental arch with that of the upper model.

In an uncrowded Class II division 1 malocclusion with an overjet of 10 mm or more, it can be seen that a good buccal segment occlu-

sion will result from advancing the mandible and, at the same time, laterally expanding the maxilla to match the width of the mandibular dental arch in the projected advanced position.

If the arches are crowded with irregular teeth, the upper and lower models will often not fit when the lower model is advanced. Depending on the degree of irregularity, a first phase of arch development may be necessary to correct archform before the mandible can be advanced to correct the occlusion. Alternatively, appliance design may be modified to improve archform during the Twin Block phase, if the irregularity is less severe.

If the upper incisors prevent the lower model from advancing into a Class I buccal segment occlusion, provision must be made to advance the upper incisors with springs or screws to accommodate the mandible in correct occlusion (**5.2**). This often applies in a Class II malocclusion when an overjet of less than 9 mm is present with a full unit distal occlusion. It is necessary to procline the upper incisors to release the mandible forwards. The same restriction applies in Class II division 2 malocclusion, and appliance design must be modified accordingly.

GD

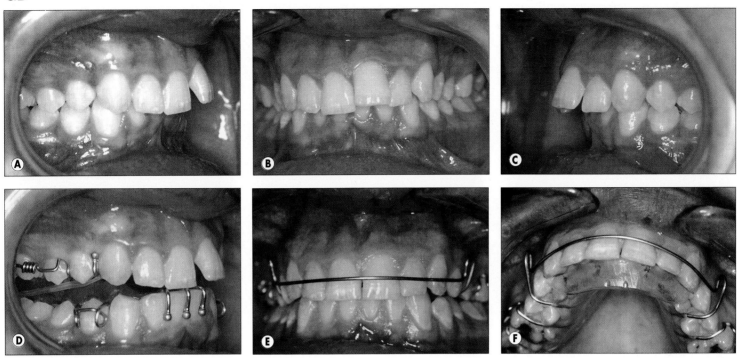

5.2 G.D. aged 14:
A, B, C Retroclined incisors must be proclined with springs or screws on the upper Twin Block to release the mandible forwards.
D Aesthetic design. Light Class II elastics are optional.
E, F Anterior inclined plane to support the corrected incisor relationshiop and to allow the lower premolars and canines to erupt into occlusion.
G, H A flat occlusal stop on the incline plane engages the incisors to maintain the vertical dimension as premolars and canines erupt.

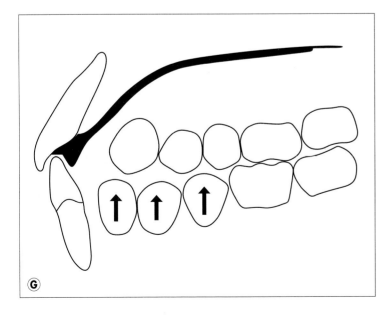

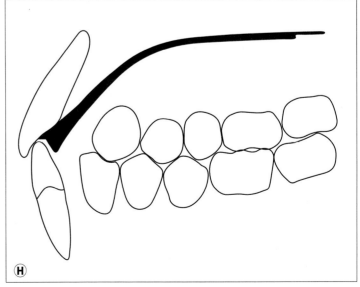

GD

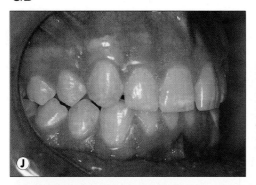

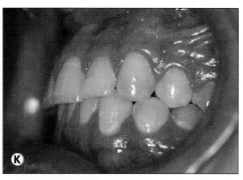

5.2 J, K After 12 months the occlusion has settled and the same appliance serves as a retainer.

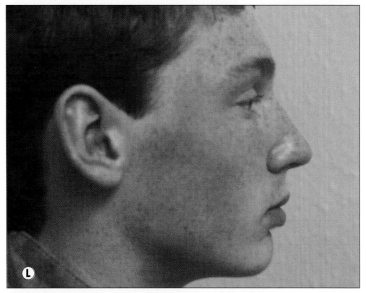

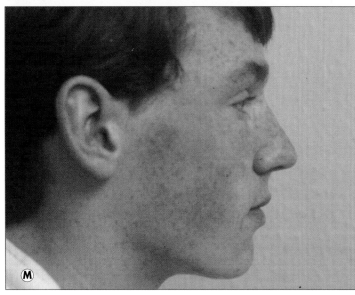

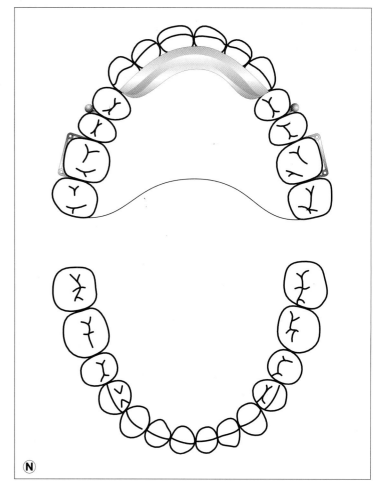

5.2 L, M Profile change after 1 year.
N The anterior inclined plane extends to the canine region to engage all six lower anterior teeth.

GD

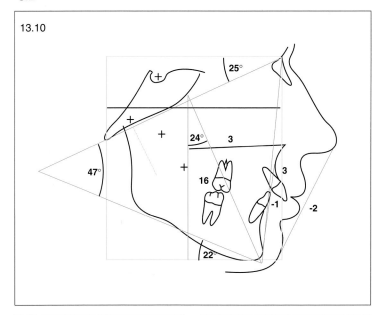

13.10

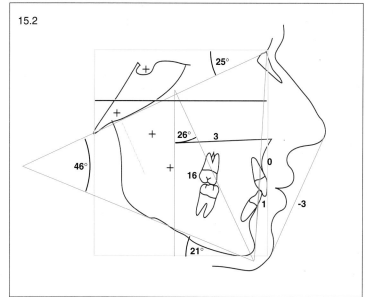

15.2

Maxillary Plane at ANS

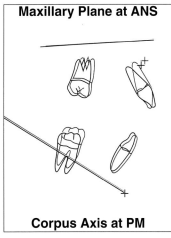

Corpus Axis at PM

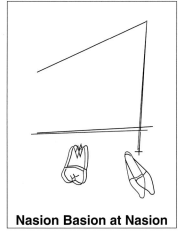

Nasion Basion at Nasion

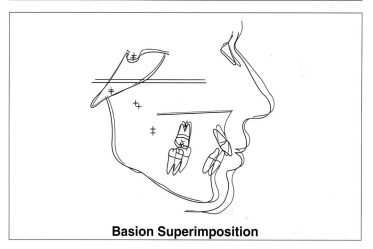

Basion Superimposition

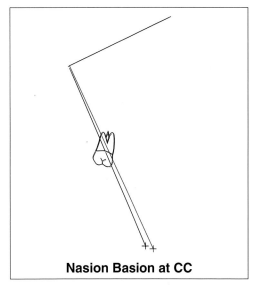

Nasion Basion at CC

G.D. -	Age	13.10	15.2	(Yr.Mon)
Cranial Base Angle		25	25	
Facial Axis Angle		24	26	
F/M Plane Angle		22	21	
Craniomandibular Angle		47	46	
Maxillary Plane		3	3	
Convexity		3	0	
U/Incisor to Vertical		36	20	
L/Incisor to Vertical		32	33	
Interincisal Angle		112	127	
6 to Pterygoid Vertical		16	16	
L/Incisor to A/Po		−1	1	
L/Lip to Aesthetic Plane		−2	−3	

CHAPTER
6

The Clark Cephalometric Analysis

You who wish to describe by words the form of man and all aspects of the ways his parts are put together, drop that idea. For the more minutely you describe, the more you will confuse the mind of the reader and the more you will prevent him from the knowledge of that which you describe. So it is necessary to ***draw and describe****.*

Leonardo Da Vinci, *Notebooks*
Translation by Robert E. Moyers

THE JIGSAW PUZZLE

The jaw bone's connected to the head bone

Popular song

Consider the jigsaw puzzle: the aim is to assemble all the pieces into a recognisable pattern, but the method of achieving this objective is rather haphazard. We examine the shape and form of each piece of the puzzle as a separate entity. By concentrating our attention on the detail of the individual pieces we may fail to recognise the underlying pattern. Only when all the pieces are assembled in a unified framework can we clearly understand the puzzle. Current methods of cephalometric analysis resemble a jigsaw puzzle.

Cephalometric analysis attempts to define the pattern of craniofacial growth by examining the angular and linear relationships of clearly defined skeletal landmarks on cephalograms. Having defined a series of reference points and planes, the most common analytical method is to compare a series of unrelated measurements with means and standard deviations to evaluate the diagnostic significance of areas of deficient or excessive craniofacial growth in the aetiology of malocclusion. The lack of correlation of measurements makes it more difficult to arrive at a clear perception of the diagnostic significance of each factor in order to resolve the puzzle.

No existing method of analysis correlates all the linear and angular measurements in a common framework. There is no specific orientation of reference points in space. Current methods of analysis essentially examine each piece of the jigsaw puzzle as a separate entity without attempting to assemble the component parts into a unified

pattern to define the relationship of the pieces. It is impossible to isolate the component parts of the craniofacial skeleton, and the principle of analysis by fragmentation is of limited value as a means of illustrating the pattern of craniofacial growth.

An alternative approach is to examine reciprocal relationships in the pattern of craniofacial development by a correlative method of cephalometric analysis. The logical basis for this approach is that the component parts of the craniofacial complex are mutually interdependent so that variation of one component has a reciprocal effect on the others. If a reliable registration framework is established using horizontal and vertical axes it is then possible to observe reciprocal variations in the pattern of craniofacial growth of the individual, with less dependence on unrelated corporate or average values.

A new approach to cephalometric analysis is derived from principles expressed in three previous analytical methods. These are the Ricketts (1960), McNamara (1984) and Bimler (1977) analyses. Having used and studied these analyses the author has adapted features of these methods to arrive at a system which aims to simplify and clarify the analytical method for diagnostic purposes.

Since the early cephalometric studies of Broadbent (1948) and Brodie (1940, 1941, 1946), the teaching of cephalometric analysis has been based largely on the concept that the face grows downwards and forwards from the base of the skull along the Y-axis or facial axis. Structures in the anterior cranial base were selected for superimposition of serial cephalometric tracings to demonstrate growth changes.

Assessment of facial growth by superimposition in the anterior cranial base is equivalent to judging the growth of a tree by sitting in its branches. This would give the impression that the earth grows downwards. Only when we stand away from the tree do we realise from a new perspective that the tree grows upwards. This analogy applies with equal logic to our concepts of facial growth.

Coben (1955) has spent 40 years of research on cephalometric analysis, with particular reference to growth of the cranial base. Coben observes that superimposition of tracings in the anterior cranial base has the major disadvantage of ignoring growth at the primary growth site in the base of the skull, the spheno-occipital synchondrosis, which has a fundamental influence on facial growth. The growth and angulation of the cranial base inevitably affects the structure of the face. Growth of the head is observed more accurately by superimposition at basion as recommended by Coben.

The head is suspended on the vertebral column and grows in a radial direction from its fulcrum of attachment. Basion is the closest point to this fulcrum that can be used in cephalometric analysis as a base point to establish growth of the face Superimposition at basion gives a new perspective on growth of the face, and this represents an improved interpretation of our present concepts of facial growth.

Coben (1961) retraced the tracings used in the Bolton growth study (Broadbent, 1937) to show growth changes from childhood to adulthood. Comparison with Bolton tracings reveals a more regular pattern of facial growth, illustrated by superimposing the tracings at the basion with the Frankfort plane horizontal. This is a more accurate method of evaluating growth vectors in facial development.

Coben's concept of facial growth is, that the wedge of the face opens by growth upwards and forwards along the cranial base, and downwards and forwards along the mandibular plane. The opening of the facial wedge increases facial height to accommodate growth in height of the nasal sinuses and to accommodate the successional teeth from deciduous to permanent dentition. Frankel & Frankel (1989) subsequently used Coben's concept in his book to analyse the results of treatment with the function regulator. Superimpositions are made at the basion with the Frankfort plane horizontal.

The Clark analysis lends itself well to the expression of Coben's interpretation of facial growth by horizontal orientation of the head and evaluation of growth changes from basion. The same method of superimposition has been selected to demonstrate facial growth changes with Twin Block treatment in this book, using basion as a fulcrum point for analysis of growth changes in the facial rectangle, with Frankfort plane horizontal.

VISION, BALANCE AND POSTURE

Our perception of the world is based on horizons that are dependent on a highly developed mechanism of vision, balance and posture. To demonstrate this clearly, we need only tilt our head to one side, or forwards or back, to realise that we cannot function comfortably for long in this posture. While freedom of movement is necessary in function, in more prolonged postural activity it is necessary that the face is directed approximately to the front in a vertical plane to maintain anatomical and physiological balance. A limited range of visual acuity ensures that body posture is adapted accurately to our area of attention.

It is no accident that the facial plane lies approximately in the vertical plane. This is a necessary physiological feature in humans as an accommodation to an upright stature. A similar principle applies in the midsagittal plane of the head, which approximates to the vertical plane, and also to the midtransverse plane which passes through the head and down through the shoulders. These characteristics ensure that in normal posture the eyes lie in a horizontal plane, and are directed forwards,

in the same direction as the feet, to assist in balance and locomotion. The weight of the head is evenly balanced on the vertebral column with the minimum of muscular effort. Vertical and horizontal axes therefore represent an important adaptation in anatomical and physiological function to allow humans to adopt an erect posture.

Facial architecture

In cephalometric analysis, the significance of horizontal and vertical reference planes in relation to facial balance, and the resulting implications in treatment planning, has not yet been fully realised. Visual appreciation of aesthetic balance is clearly evident in good architectural design. The architect, who is involved in planning the construction of inanimate objects, makes constant reference to horizontal and vertical planes in order to achieve structural balance. The same principle applies in the analysis of facial form and the planning of reconstructive treatment of the face.

In many respects, the orthodontist is a facial architect who can alter the structure and balance of the face. Orthodontic and dentofacial orthopaedic techniques have the potential to produce dramatic changes in facial appearance that may be beneficial or detrimental according to the quality of treatment planning. Successful treatment depends on accurate analysis of the facial growth pattern before treatment, and prediction of the future growth trend to select the appropriate technique to produce the best long-term functional and aesthetic result within the growth potential of the individual patient.

PARALLELISM IN DENTOFACIAL DEVELOPMENT

A major advantage of a correlative approach using horizontal and vertical axes is the resulting simplification in the interpretation of results. The existence of parallelism in dentofacial development transforms a complex subject. It immediately becomes easier to teach and understand.

Parallelism has been referred to before in cephalometric analysis. Bimler (1957) and others have noted the parallel relationship that often exists between the Frankfort and maxillary planes. Similarly, Ricketts (1960) referred to the parallel development of the facial axis, the condyle axis and the upper incisor. Ricketts recommended that the upper incisor should be positioned parallel to the facial axis for stability and balance after treatment. These features may be interpreted as indicating harmony in facial development, and are usually evident in aesthetically pleasing, well-balanced faces (6.1).

Ricketts expressed the view that growth and development followed the fundamental rules of physics, resulting in the recurrence of the divine proportion in facial development. This can be illustrated using a device to measure the proportions of the face and the facial features. The principle of incremental archial growth was described to account for the natural balance in facial contours. A balanced relationship of form and function in facial development is expressed in aesthetic harmony.

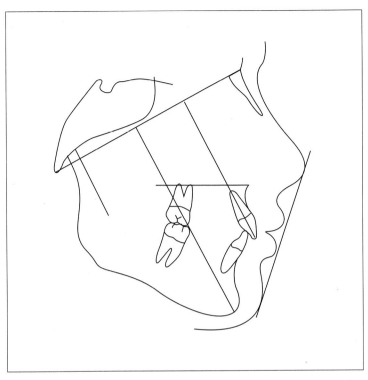

6.1 Tracing (P.G.) to show facial axis, condyle axis and upper incisor parallel, indicating balance in facial development.

A REGISTRATION FRAMEWORK FOR CEPHALOMETRIC ANALYSIS

The jigsaw concept of cephalometric analysis has the disadvantage that the component parts of the puzzle are not correlated. This complicates both the understanding and the teaching of the principles of analysis, which remain incomprehensible to a large proportion of the profession.

To return to the jigsaw puzzle, the best technique in assembling a puzzle is first to establish the outer framework, usually a rectangle, by constructing the edges to define the outer limits of the puzzle. This provides a guide as a basis for examination and definition of structures within the framework.

The fundamental principle of framing an object in order to define balance and contour is well exemplified in the world of art. The concept is of equal value in examining facial contours, and as a means of evaluating the underlying skeletal structures in aesthetic and scientific terms. Essentially, the principles of cartography are applied to cephalometric analysis to study the relationship of the craniofacial structures.

On a cephalogram the face is represented in simple terms as a wedge-shaped triangle superimposed on a rectangle. In the upright position, the facial features lie approximately in the anterior vertical plane. A rectangle provides an ideal framework to examine the position and dimensions of the craniofacial structures in cephalometric analysis.

Ricketts triangle: the facial wedge

The Ricketts triangle defines the face in profile as a wedge-shaped triangle attached to the undersurface of the cranial base (**6.2**)

- The base of the triangle extends from basion to nasion and defines the cranial base plane.
- The facial plane extends from nasion tangent to the chin at the pogonion to define the angulation of the face in the anterior plane.
- The mandibular plane is the third leg of the triangle defining the angulation of the lower border of the mandible.
- The triangle is bisected by the facial axis, extending from pterygoid to gnathion to define the direction of growth of the chin.

The facial wedge defined by the Ricketts triangle is superimposed on the facial rectangle to provide a good visual representation of the face with the component parts orientated in a common framework. A few key angular measurements define the pattern of craniofacial growth and the relationship of the cranial, maxillary and mandibular structures. It is easy to identify correlations that exist within the craniofacial complex by visual reference to the facial rectangle.

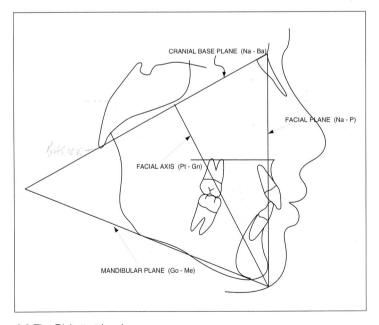

6.2 The Ricketts triangle.

THE FACIAL RECTANGLE

A facial rectangle is formed to frame the face. The formation of a facial rectangle helps to define the relative position and angulation of cranial, maxillary, mandibular and dentoalveolar structures. The rectangular framework makes it easier to identify areas where growth departs from normal in the facial pattern. Perhaps the most obvious feature of the analysis is the visual simplification of the underlying pattern that results from placing the face in a rectangle. It is easier to recognise the pattern of the jigsaw puzzle when the pieces are fitted together in a recognisable framework.

The same principle lends itself to three-dimensional analysis.

Horizontal registration plane

The facial rectangle is constructed to define the upper, lower, anterior and posterior limits of the face. No single anatomical plane consistently relates exactly to the true horizontal in every case. Either a skeletal plane or the true horizontal may be selected to construct the upper registration plane of the facial rectangle (**6.3**).

For practical purposes in most cases the Frankfort horizontal is suitable, except where porion or orbitale cannot be identified clearly, or when the Frankfort plane diverges significantly from the true horizontal. The true horizontal may be selected as an alternative when the cephalogram is taken in the natural head position. The selected plane is used as a horizontal base line to construct the facial rectangle. The following description uses the Frankfort plane as the registration plane.

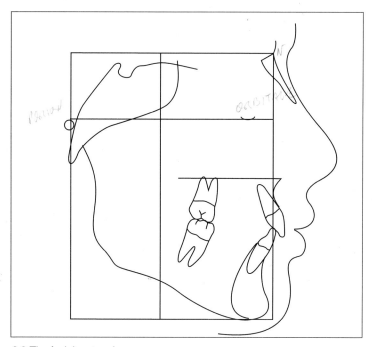

6.3 The facial rectangle

Frankfort plane: porion to orbitale

The Frankfort horizontal has the advantage that it can be located on external examination of the face, and it may be defined on a photograph. This is increasingly important as we relate analysis of the underlying bony strucures to the facial contours in computer-imaging technology. A further significant advantage of the Frankfort plane is that it has been widely taught and so it is familiar to the majority of the profession.

Nasion horizontal
A line is drawn through nasion parallel to the Frankfort plane. This defines the upper limit of the face and the anterior point of union with the cranium.

Menton horizontal
A tangent through menton on the lower border of the symphysis parallel to the Frankfort plane. This defines the lower limit of the face.

Nasion vertical
A perpendicular line is drawn to the Frankfort plane through nasion. This line defines the anteroposterior relationship of the maxilla and the mandible relative to the anterior cranial base.

Basion vertical
A perpendicular through basion defines the posterior limit of the face. Basion is an important anatomical point in the midline on the foramen magnum, marking the anterior point of union between the cervical column and the base of the skull.

Pterygoid vertical
A perpendicular line to the Frankfort plane through the pterygoid point. This midfacial perpendicular line was selected by Ricketts because it is in a stable area of growth, being close to the point of emergence of the trigeminal nerve from the base of the skull.

The facial rectangle now defines the upper, lower, anterior and posterior limits of the face, with the addition of a midfacial vertical line. This construction facilitates measurement of all factors relative to vertical and horizontal axes. The spatial relationship of the key structures in facial development can now be observed and related to common vertical and horizontal axes.

BALANCED FACIAL PROPORTIONS

If the structure of the face is superimposed on a rectangular framework with horizontal and vertical axes, certain consistent criteria must be fulfilled in order to achieve the harmonious facial balance that is characteristic of the classical straight profile. Excellent facial balance results in the face growing correctly into the facial rectangle, so that the facial features relate closely to the anterior vertical (**6.4**).

To achieve ideal facial proportions, the integral parts of the facial structure must be well related in size, shape and position. In well-balanced faces the Frankfort and maxillary planes are approximately parallel to the upper maxillary plane and optic plane, and relate closely to the true horizontal in the natural head position. This signifies parallel development of the anterior cranial base and the floor of the nose. Functional balance of the craniofacial and cervical components may be expressed in a favourable equilibrium of muscle forces acting on the underlying skeletal structures to produce a balanced growth response to the forces of gravity and posture. By comparison, divergence of the horizontal planes is an expression of functional imbalance in facial development that can be recognised in cephalometric analysis, and is significant in the aetiology and treatment of malocclusion.

The relative angulation of the upper incisor, the facial axis, the axis of the condyle, and the nasal outline are easily compared as they are all related to the vertical axis. A direct comparison of these measurements is useful in evaluating the aetiology of the malocclusion in structural and positional terms, and is helpful in diagnosis and treatment planning. In a well-balanced face with a good occlusion these structures show approximately parallel development. In treatment, one aims to align these structures to improve facial balance.

A unique feature of this method of analysis is the close correlation of the mean values of all key factors involved in the determination of facial type. The mean values express balance and harmony in facial proportions, and departure from the mean is often related to occlusal imbalance of skeletal origin in the aetiology of malocclusion. The value of a common mean for key factors is that deviation is immediately obvious, and we can identify easily the areas where the pattern departs from the norm. Disproportion in one area is reflected in reciprocal changes in other areas when we examine facial proportions in the facial rectangle. When we assemble all the pieces within a unified framework a pattern in the jigsaw puzzle begins to be emerge.

Definition of skeletal planes

A further construction is now made to define the main facial and dental characteristics by defining points (**6.5**) and planes:

1. *Cranial base plane:*
   nasion (N) to basion (Ba).
2. *Mandibular base plane:*
   menton (ME) to gonion (Go).
3. *Facial plane:*
   nasion to pogonion (P).
4. *Facial axis:*
   pterygoid point (Pt) to gnathion (Gn).
5. *Condyle axis:*
   centre of the condyle to Xi-point.
6. *Maxillary plane:*
   anterior nasal spine (ANS) to posterior nasal spine (PNS).
7. *A to Po:*
   A-point to pogonion (P).

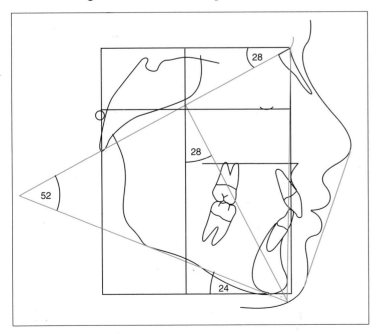

6.4 Patient P.G. showing a mesognathic pattern with good facial balance.

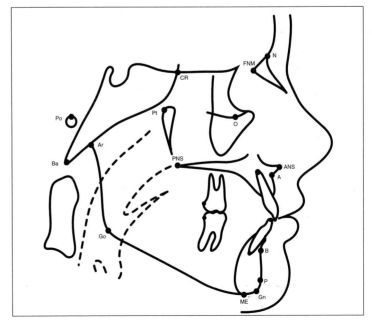

6.5 Location of points. See text above for key.

Dental planes

1. *Functional occlusal plane:*
   distal the intersection of the first molars to the intersection of the first premolars.
2. The long axis of the upper incisor.
3. The long axis of the lower incisor.

Soft-tissue planes

- *Nasal plane:* the outline of the nose from root to tip.
- *Aesthetic plane:* the tangent to the nose and chin.

A CORRELATIVE CEPHALOMETRIC ANALYSIS

Measurement relative to common vertical and horizontal axes reveals a surprising consistency in the mean angulation of key structures in cephalometric analysis. This confirms the structural interdependence between key parts of the craniofacial skeleton that leads to balanced facial development.

Key factors in craniofacial angular analysis

1. *Cranial base angle:*
   Cranial base plane to horizontal registration plane.
   Norm = 27°; clinical deviation ± 3°; ideal = 29–30°.
   The angulation of the cranial base to the horizontal is of fundamental importance in determining facial type.

2. *Mandibular plane angle:*
   Angle of mandibular plane to horizontal.
   Norm = 27°; clinical deviation ± 4°.
   A measure of vertical or horizontal growth potential.

3. *Craniomandibular angle:*
   Angle of cranial base plane to mandibular base plane.
   Norm = 54°; clinical deviation + 5°.
   A measure of facial height.
   Equals the sum of the cranial base angle and the mandibular base angle.

4. *Facial plane angle:*
   Angulation of facial plane to nasion vertical.
   Norm = –3°; clinical deviation = 3°.
   Determines the degree of mandibular prognathism or retrognathism.

5. *Facial axis angle:*
   Facial axis to pterygoid vertical.
   Norm 27°; clinical deviation ± 3°; ideal = 29–30°.
   Determines the direction of growth of the chin.
   An important indicator for prognosis related to growth direction.

6. *Condyle axis angle:*
   Condyle axis to pterygoid vertical.
   Norm = 27°; clinical deviation ± 4°.
   Relate to the facial axis angle for balance in facial development.

7. *Mandibular arc:*
   Angulation of condyle axis to body of mandible (Xi to Pm).
   Norm = 26° at age 8; clinical deviation = 4°.
   Increases by 0.5° per year.
   High angles > square mandible/deep bite/prognathic.
   Low angles > open bite/retrognathic.

8. *Craniomaxillary angle:*
   Cranial base plane to maxillary plane.
   Norm = 27°; clinical deviation = 3°.
   Relates the cranial base angle to maxillary deflection.

9. *Maxillary deflection:*
   Angulation of maxillary plane to horizontal.
   Norm = 0°; clinical deviation ± 3°.
   Determines the proportions of upper and lower facial height.

Dental analysis

The dental relationship may be defined by the following measurements:

The upper and lower incisors are related to the anterior vertical

10. *Upper incisor angle:*
    Upper incisor to anterior vertical.
    Norm = 25°; clinical deviation ± 7°.

11. *Lower incisor angle:*
    Lower incisor to anterior vertical.
    Norm = 25°; clinical deviation ± 4°.
    This is equivalent to 65° to the Frankfort horizontal in Tweed's analysis.

12. *Interincisal angle:*
    Angle between upper and lower incisal axes.
    Norm = 128°; clinical deviation = 6°.

Position of dentition

13. *Position of upper dentition:*
    Distal of upper molar to pterygoid vertical.
    Norm = patient's age ± 3 mm.
    Indicates whether or not to distalise upper molars.

14. *Position of lower dentition:*
    Lower incisor to A–Po line.
    Norm = +1 mm; clinical deviation + 2 mm.
    An important indicator of stability of the lower incisor position.
    A key guideline for extraction or nonextraction therapy.
    Review value after functional therapy.

Soft tissue analysis

15. *Nasal angle:*
    Angulation of nose to anterior vertical.
    In a harmonious face, the nasal plane is nearly parallel to the facial axis.

16. *Lower lip to E-plane:*
    Distance of lower lip from a line tangent to nose and chin.
    Norm –2 mm at age 8; decreases by 0.2° per year.
    Determines the degree of protrusion or retrusion of the lips.

These key factors normally complete the diagnostic analysis. If a more detailed analysis is required for research or diagnostic purposes, additional factors may be considered.

Assessment of functional balance

Functional guidance of upper and lower incisors is determined by the relationship of the tips of the incisors and the hinge axis of the mandible and can be measured relative to the horizontal axis. The interincisor guidance angle may indicate anterior or posterior occlusal interferences.

1. *Maxillary incisal guidance angle:*
   Maxillary incisor/hinge axis: angle to horizontal.
   Line from tip of upper incisor to hinge axis.
   Norm = 27°; clinical deviation ± 3°.
   Determines incisal guidance in protrusive function.

2. *Mandibular incisal guidance angle:*
   Mandibular incisor /hinge axis: angle to horizontal.
   Line from tip of lower incisor to hinge axis.
   Norm = 27°; clinical deviation ± 3°.
   Determines mandibular guidance in protrusive function.

3. *Interincisor guidance angle:*
   Angle between upper and lower incisal guidance axes.
   Measures freedom of mandibular movement in protrusive function.
   An increased positive angle indicates incisal interference.
   An increased negative angle indicates posterior interference.

4. *Occlusomaxillary plane angle:*
   Functional occlusal plane to maxillary plane.
   Norm = 12°; clinical deviation ± 3°.

5. *Occlusomandibular plane angle:*
   Norm =14°; clinical deviation ± 3°.
   Affects the prognosis for opening or closing the bite.
   A high angle is favourable for opening the bite.
   A low angle is favourable for closing the bite.

Craniofacial linear analysis

Cranial, maxillary and mandibular length are compared by measurement from the basion, which represents the fulcrum of craniofacial growth. Cranial length and mandibular length should relate closely to a 1/1 ratio and maxillary length should be 10 mm less for ideal proportions. An increase or decrease in these ratios indicates prognathic or retrognathic tendencies.

1. Cranial length: basion to nasion:
   Mean = 105.7 mm at age 8; S.D. = 4.5 mm; increases by 1.3 mm per year.

2. Maxillary length: basion to A-point:
   Mean = 94.5 mm at age 8; S.D. = 4.75 mm; increases by 1.25 mm per year.

3. Mandibular length: basion to pogonion:
   Mean = 103.5 mm at age 8; S.D. = 5.5 mm; increases by 2.3 mm per year.

For ideal proportions the mandibular corpus and the anterior cranial base should also be close to a 1/1 ratio. A decrease or increase of mandibular corpus length relates to a Class II or Class III skeletal tendency.

4. Anterior cranial base length: sella to nasion:
   Mean = 74 .0 mm at age 8; S.D. = 3.3 mm; increases by 0.75 mm per year.

5. Mandibular corpus length: gonion to pogonion:
   Mean = 70.8 mm at age 8; S.D. = 0.0 mm; increases by 1.65 mm per year.

6. Maxillary position: A-point to nasion vertical:
   Mean = 0 mm in mixed dentition; mean = +1 mm in adult.

7. Mandibular position: pogonion to nasion vertical:
   Mean = –10 mm at age 8; decreases by 0.75 mm per year.

8. Convexity: A-point to facial plane:
   Mean = 2.5 mm at age 8; decreases by 0.1 mm per year.
   Increased convexity is Class II skeletal; decrease is Class III skeletal.

DESCRIPTIVE TERMS IN CEPHALOMETRIC ANALYSIS

Definition of facial type

Mesognathic. A normal relationship of the maxilla and mandible to the cranial base.

Prognathic. Prominence of jaw position relative to the cranial base.

Retrognathic. Retrusion of jaw position relative to the cranial base.

Where the relationship of the maxilla and mandible to the cranial base is not the same, the terms normal, protrusive and retrusive are used to describe the individual jaw relationship.

Mesofacial. Describes a well-balanced face with harmonious musculature and a pleasant soft-tissue profile.

Brachyfacial. The face is typically short and square with a reduced mandibular plane angle and strong musculature. It describes a horizontal growth pattern (Ricketts, 1960) with a deep overbite of skeletal origin. A mild brachyfacial tendency is favourable for normal dental development. A strong brachyfacial growth pattern is accompanied by retrusion of the lips in the profile. Anchorage is good and non-extraction therapy is indicated.

Dolichofacial. The face is typically long and narrow with a high mandibular plane angle and weak musculature. It describes a vertical growth pattern (Ricketts, 1960) with an anterior open bite tendency. Patients are likely to exhibit nasorespiratory problems with incompetent or strained lip musculature. The alveolar processes are long and thin due to increased lower facial height. There is frequently dental crowding associated with narrow archform. Natural anchorage is poor and these patients present difficulties in treatment. Extraction therapy may be indicated for relief of crowding.

Note. Confusion arose in terminology when Bimler (1977) used the anthropological terms dolichoprosopic and leptoprosopic to relate facial depth to facial height, while Ricketts combined Latin and Greek roots in his terminology. A detailed expanation of the origin of this confusion is given by Witzig & Spahl, 1989 (Chapter 3, pp 118–31).

To avoid further confusion, because of the use of Ricketts' triangle in the Clark analysis, the terminology used in this book is as defined by Ricketts.

NATURAL HEAD POSITION

It is fully realised that the selection of a single horizontal skeletal plane for the purpose of head orientation in the living subject is a compromise, because the vertical location of landmarks varies among individuals. This limitation was accepted when the Frankfort horizontal was defined after much debate in Germany (1884) to approximate to a standardised head position of the living, in order to orient skulls for craniometric research. In orientating the head relative to the true vertical, therefore, there is good reason to consider alternative skeletal planes for registration, to compensate for individual variation in the position of skeletal landmarks.

Determination of natural head position in relation to the true vertical is a starting point in the aesthetic examination of the facial profile. This method has been used for the purpose of serial cephalometric radiography, as described by other authors in previous studies. The classic natural head position is a reproducible, standardised position of the head, whereby the individual looks at a point in the distance at eye level. The visual axis is horizontal.

This concept cannot always be achieved in a clinical setting, and an alternative is to place the patient standing or seated in an upright position opposite a vertically mounted mirror that is 150 cm in front of the ear rods, so that the patient can observe his eyes in the mirror (**6.6**) The patient is positioned carefully in the cephalostat with the head tilted neither forwards nor backwards, and the true vertical is

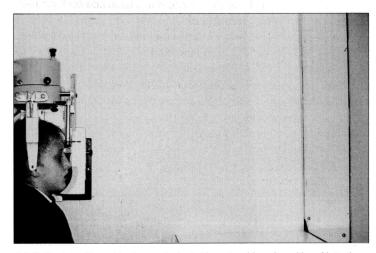

6.6 Patient positioned in the cephalostat in natural head position. Note the vertically mounted mirror.

registered as a plumb line suspended over the cassette holder in the occipital region. Investigation has established a method error of 2.3° for variability of head posture recorded by auxilliaries for head position to the true vertical. (Solow & Tallgren, 1971; Siersbaek-Neilsen & Solow, 1982).

Positioning the patient in the cephalostat

First the ear-plug must be raised or lowered to engage the ear canal at the correct height, with the head in an upright position. One ear-plug is then engaged in the ear and the patient is instructed to look directly into his or her own eyes in the mirror without tilting the head forwards or backwards. The proprioceptive balance mechanism is used to establish a visual cue in positioning the patient in a natural and relaxed position in the cephalostat. When this position is established the other ear-plug is engaged.

The patient's eye is checked to confirm that the pupil is central in the cornea when the head is positioned in the cephalostat. The angulation of the Frankfort plane is checked by extraoral examination and the patient is viewed through the colimator before positioning the x-ray tube. Some recent cephalostats incorporate a light beam that can be orientated correctly to the Frankfort horizontal as a consistent means of orientating the patient in the cephalostat. The true vertical can be registered on the x-ray by suspending a thin chain over the x-ray cassette in the occipital region, so as not to obscure important structures to be examined in analysis. Careful positioning of the patient in the cephalostat allows one to relate head and neck position to true horizontal and vertical lines.

A frequent source of error in cephalometric radiography is the use of plastic ear-rods with vertical and circular plastic supports. This design obscures anatomical porion, and plastic should be replaced with wood or another radiolucent material. Porion is an important point in our diagnosis, which should not be obscured by inadequate design of cephalometric x-ray equipment.

FACIAL CHANGE IN TWIN BLOCK TREATMENT

Treatment of uncrowded Class II division 1 malocclusion

This section illustrates examples of treatment of different facial types with Twin Blocks to compare the response to treatment.

Case report: K.H. aged 9 years 7 months (6.7)

Diagnosis, skeletal classification:
- Mild Class II.
- Facial type: severe brachyfacial – horizontal growth.
- Prognathic facial pattern.
- Maxilla: mild prognathic.
- Mandible: normal.
- Convexity = 5 mm.

Diagnosis, dental classification:
- Severe Class II division 1.
- Upper incisors: mild protrusion.
- Lower incisors: mild retrusion.
- No crowding.
- Overjet = 10 mm.
- Overbite incomplete.

Treatment plan. Cephalometric analysis indicates maxillary protrusion and a prognathic tendency. However, clinical examination confirms that the profile improves when the mandible is advanced slightly. When the patient postures downwards and forwards, the resulting change in the profile is a preview of the change which will be produced by functional therapy. Clinical guidelines therefore indicate a functional approach to treatment in spite of the prognathic facial tendency. Guiding the mandible forwards to match the protrusive position of the maxilla will improve the profile in this case.

Appliances. Standard Twin Blocks for functional correction followed by support and retention by an anterior inclined plane.

Adjustment. The screw is turned to expand the maxilla for 3 months. The upper Twin Block includes a spring to advance the lingually displaced 2|. The occlusal bite blocks are progressively trimmed in the usual way to reduce the overbite.

KH

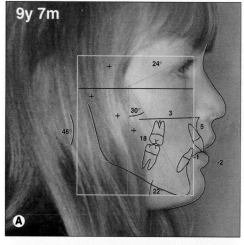

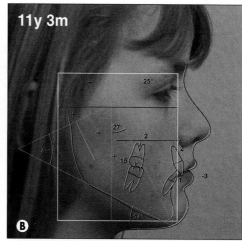

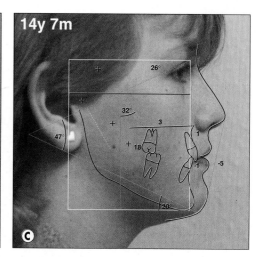

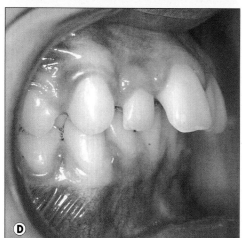

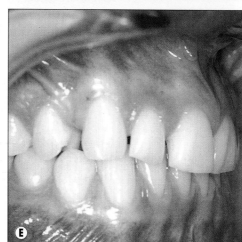

6.7 Treatment:
A Profile at 9 years 7 months.
B Profile at 11 years 3 months.
C Profile at 14 years 7 months.
D Occlusion before treatment at 9 years 7 months.
E Occlusion 3 years out of retention at age 14 years 7 months.

Treatment duration:
- Active phase: 5 months with Twin Blocks, when the overjet is overcorrected from 10 mm to an edge-to-edge occlusion.
- Support and retention: 3 months.
- Total treatment time: 8 months, including retention.

Treatment is uncomplicated thanks to good archform, and the response to treatment is rapid due to the strong horizontal skeletal growth pattern. As a general rule the profile will continue to straighten as the patient matures when there is a prognathic facial pattern with horizontal growth.

KH

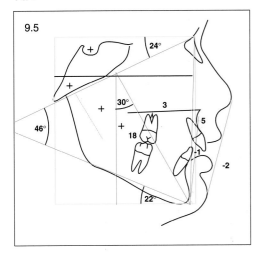

9.5

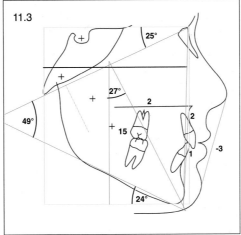

11.3

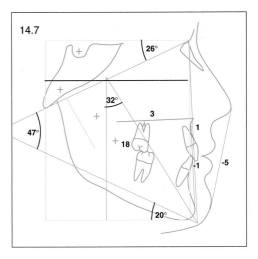

14.7

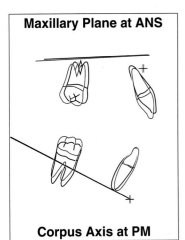

Maxillary Plane at ANS

Corpus Axis at PM

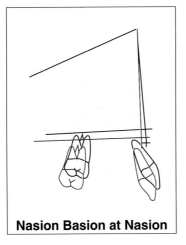

Nasion Basion at Nasion

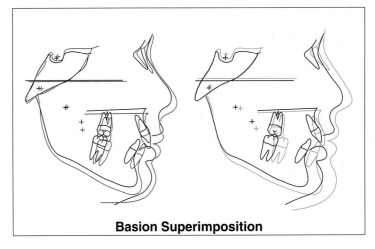

Basion Superimposition

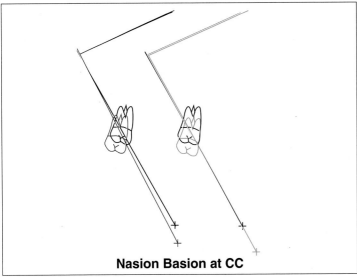

Nasion Basion at CC

K.H. -	Age	9.5	11.3	14.7	(Yr.Mon)
Cranial Base Angle		24	25	26	
Facial Axis Angle		30	27	32	
F/M Plane Angle		22	24	20	
Craniomandibular Angle		46	49	47	
Maxillary Plane		3	2	3	
Convexity		5	2	1	
U/Incisor to Vertical		29	19	22	
L/Incisor to Vertical		32	29	26	
Interincisal Angle		119	132	132	
6 to Pterygoid Vertical		18	15	18	
L/Incisor to A/Po		−1	1	−1	
L/Lip to Aesthetic Plane		−2	−3	−5	

ME

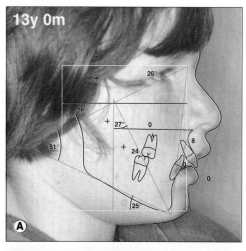

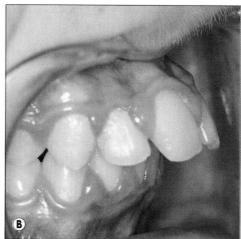

6.8 Treatment:
A, B Profile and occlusion before treatment at age 13 years.
C, D Profile and occlusion at age 17 years.

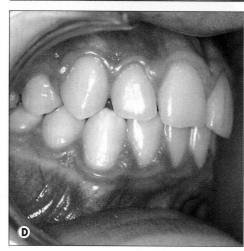

Case report: M.E. aged 13 years (6.8)

Diagnosis, skeletal classification:
* Severe Class II.
* Facial type: mild brachyfacial.
* Maxilla: normal.
* Mandible: severe retrusion.
* Facial convexity = 8 mm.

Diagnosis, dental classification:
* Severe Class II division 1.
* Upper incisors: severe protrusion.
* Lower incisors: normal.
* Overjet = 13 mm.
* Overbite = 8 mm (excessive)

Treatment plan. Functional correction to retract the maxilla and advance the mandible.

Appliances:
* Active phase: standard Twin Blocks.
* Support and retention: anterior inclined plane.

Adjustment. Screw to expand the maxilla operates for 3 months. The overjet reduces from 11 mm to 2 mm in 3 months, and the distal occlusion is corrected by the initial activation of the Twin Blocks.

Duration of treatment:
* Active phase: Twin Blocks for 6 months.
* Support phase: 4 months with anterior inclined plane.
* Retention: anterior inclined plane – 4 months at night only.
* Total treatment time: 14 months, including retention.

Final records. 2 years 10 months out of retention at age 17 years.

ME

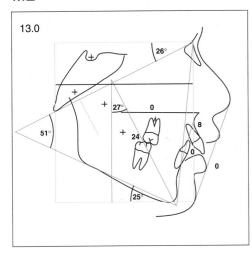

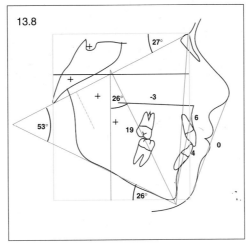

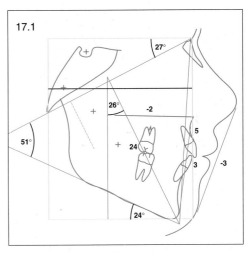

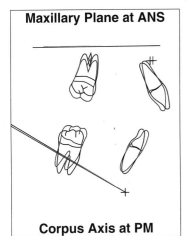

Maxillary Plane at ANS

Corpus Axis at PM

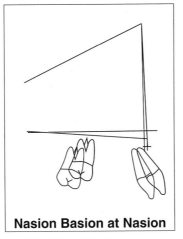

Nasion Basion at Nasion

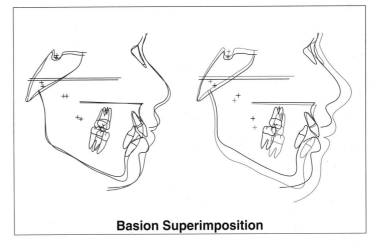

Basion Superimposition

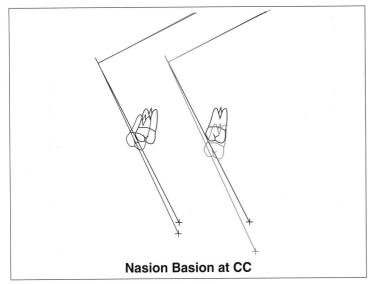

Nasion Basion at CC

M.E-	Age	13.0	13.8	17.1	(Yr.Mon)
Cranial Base Angle		26	27	27	
Facial Axis Angle		27	26	26	
F/M Plane Angle		25	26	24	
Craniomandibular Angle		51	53	51	
Maxillary Plane		0	−3	−2	
Convexity		8	6	5	
U/Incisor to Vertical		31	22	24	
L/Incisor to Vertical		26	36	26	
Interincisal Angle		123	122	122	
6 to Pterygoid Vertical		24	19	24	
L/Incisor to A/Po		0	4	3	
L/Lip to Aesthetic Plane		0	0	−3	

PMcL

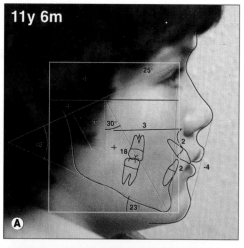

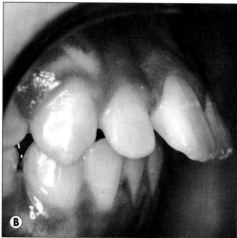

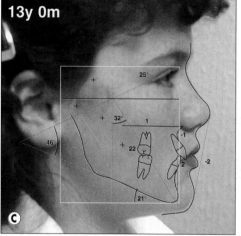

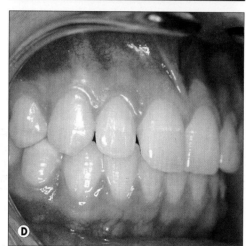

6.9 Treatment:
A, B Profile and occlusion before treatment at age 11 years 6 months.
C, D Profile and occlusion after treatment at age 13 years.

Case report: P.McL. aged 11 years 6 months

This girl has a Class II division I malocclusion on a Class I skeletal base relationship. An incomplete overbite is associated with a forward tongue thrust. (**6.9**)

Diagnosis, skeletal classification:
- Class I.
- Facial type: moderate brachyfacial.
- Maxilla: normal.
- Mandible: normal.
- Convexity =1 mm.

Diagnosis, dental classification:
- Severe Class II division 1.
- Upper incisors: severely proclined.
- Lower incisors: normal.
- Overjet = 11 mm.
- Overbite = 1 mm (incomplete).
- Anterior tongue thrust.
- Facial asymmetry.
- Lower centre line displaced to the left.

Treatment plan. Control the tongue thrust and achieve dental correction by functional therapy, with minimal anteroposterior activation to limit skeletal change.

Appliances. Twin Blocks to reduce the overjet with a tongue guard and spinner to discourage tongue thrust.

Bite registration. The construction bite registers an overjet of 3 mm with 2 mm interincisal clearance and the centre lines correct.

Clinical management. The tongue guard and spinner are effective in controlling the tongue thrust. The overjet reduces from 10 mm to 2 mm in 7 months. After the distal occlusion is corrected, the occlusal cover is gradually reduced over the posterior teeth to allow the buccal teeth to come into occlusion.

Duration of treatment:
- Active phase: 7 months with Twin Blocks.
- Support phase: 5 months with Twin Blocks to support the corrected occlusion.
- Retention: 9 months with a simple night-time retainer.
- Total treament time: 21 months, including retention.

PMcL

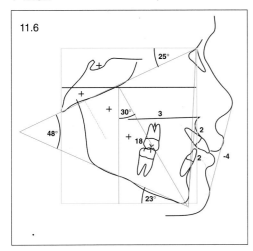
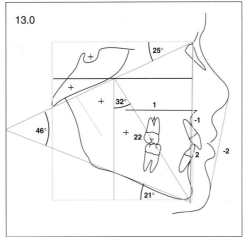
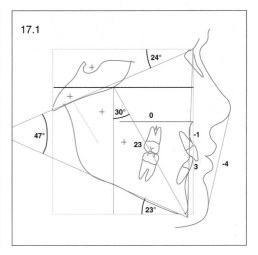

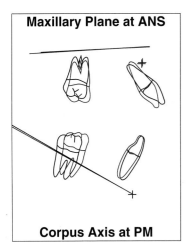

Maxillary Plane at ANS

Corpus Axis at PM

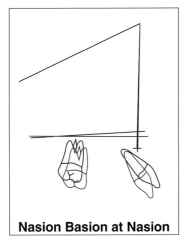

Nasion Basion at Nasion

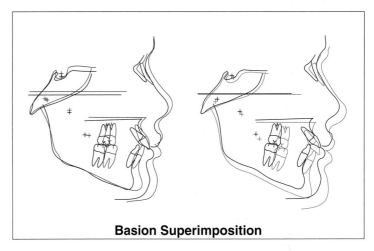

Basion Superimposition

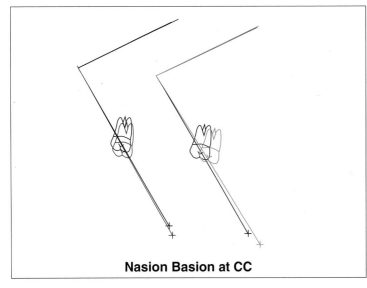

Nasion Basion at CC

P.McL.-	Age	11.6	13.0	17.1	(Yr.Mon)
Cranial Base Angle		25	25	24	
Facial Axis Angle		30	32	30	
F/M Plane Angle		23	21	23	
Craniomandibular Angle		48	46	47	
Maxillary Plane		3	1	0	
Convexity		2	−1	−1	
U/Incisor to Vertical		44	31	31	
L/Incisor to Vertical		28	28	28	
Interincisal Angle		108	121	121	
6 to Pterygoid Vertical		18	22	23	
L/Incisor to A/Po		2	2	3	
L/Lip to Aesthetic Plane		−4	−2	−4	

EF

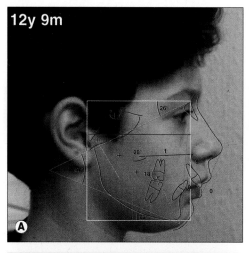

12y 9m

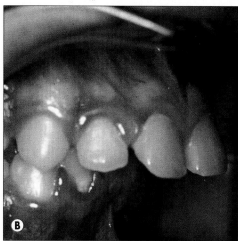

15y 0m

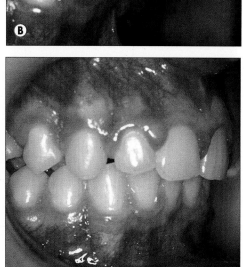

6.10 Treatment:
A, B Profile and occlusion before treatment at age 12 years 9 months.
C, D Profile and occlusion after treatment at age 15 years.

Case report: E.F. aged 12 years 9 months

A girl with good archform and mild crowding in the lower arch and with impaction of a lower second premolar (**6.10**).

Diagnosis, skeletal classification:
- Moderate Class II.
- Facial type: severe brachyfacial.
- Maxilla: normal.
- Mandible: severe retrusion.
- Convexity = 5 mm.

Diagnosis, dental classification:
- Severe Class II division I.
- Overjet = 14 mm.
- Overbite = 4 mm.
- Upper incisors: severe protrusion.
- Lower incisors: normal.
- Mild crowding lower left quadrant with impaction $\overline{5}$.
- Lower centre line displaced to the left.

Treatment plan. Advance the mandible to correct the distal occlusion and reduce convexity. Open space for impacted $\overline{5}$.

Appliances.
- Standard Twin Blocks. A lower Twin Block with a screw to open space to accommodate $\overline{5}$.
- Anterior guide plane to support the corrected occlusion and retain.

Bite registration. Because the overjet is in excess of 10 mm the construction bite is registered with a blue exactobite for a forward activation of 8 mm with 2 mm vertical interincisal clearance. It is planned to complete correction of the overjet and distal occlusion by a second activation of the Twin Blocks during the course of treatment.

Clinical management. Cooperation and appliance wear in this case was inconsistent, so this is an example of a result achieved with relatively poor cooperation. The overjet reduced from 13 mm to 5 mm in 8 months, and the Twin Blocks were reactivated into edge-to-edge with 2 mm vertical clearance by adding cold cure acrylic to the anterior incline of the upper Twin Block. The overjet was fully reduced after a further 6 months, and the position was then supported and retained for a year.

Duration of treatment:
- Active phase: 14 months with Twin Blocks.
- Support phase and retention: 12 months.
- Total treatment time: 26 months, including retention.

EF

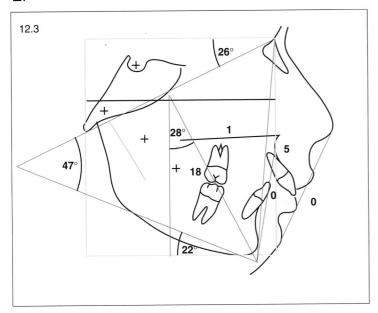

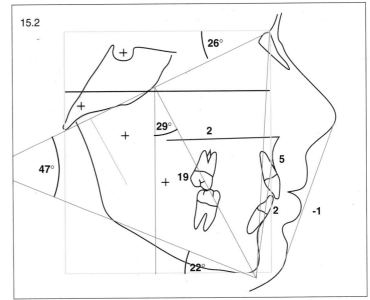

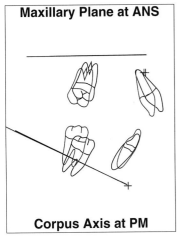

Maxillary Plane at ANS

Corpus Axis at PM

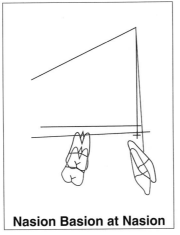

Nasion Basion at Nasion

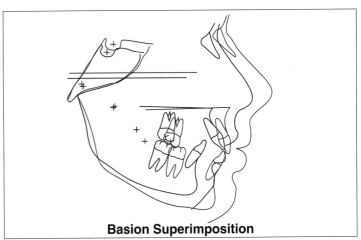

Basion Superimposition

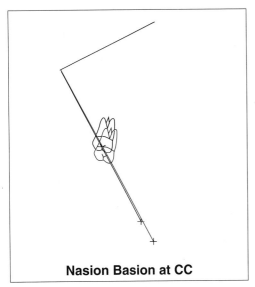

Nasion Basion at CC

E.F.-	Age 12.3	15.2 (Yr.Mon)
Cranial Base Angle	26	26
Facial Axis Angle	28	29
F/M Plane Angle	22	22
Craniomandibular Angle	47	47
Maxillary Plane	1	2
Convexity	5	5
U/Incisor to Vertical	32	19
L/Incisor to Vertical	39	34
Interincisal Angle	109	127
6 to Pterygoid Vertical	18	19
L/Incisor to A/Po	0	2
L/Lip to Aesthetic Plane	0	–1

WL

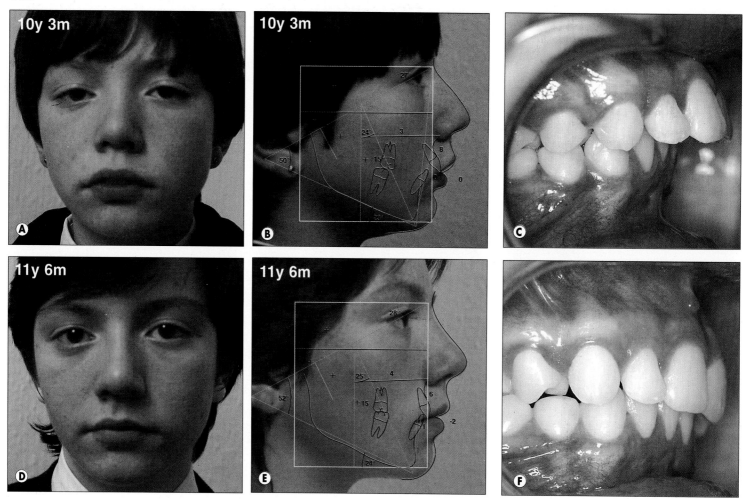

6.11 Treatment:

A, B, C Appearance and occlusion before treatment at age 10 years 3 months.

D, E, F Appearance and occlusion at age 11 years 2 months.

•   Total treatment time: 26 months, including retention.

Case report: W.L. aged 10 years 3 months (6.11)

Diagnosis, skeletal classification:
•   Severe Class II.
•   Facial type: Mild brachyfacial
•   Maxilla: normal.
•   Mandible: severe retrusion
•   Convexity = 8 mm.

Diagnosis, dental classification:
•   Severe Class II division 1.
•   Overjet = 9 mm.
•   Deep overbite.
•   Upper incisors: protrusive.

•   Lower incisors: normal.
•   Molar relationship: full unit Class II.

Treatment plan. The maxilla is normal and the mandible is retrusive. Mandibular advancement is indicated to improve the facial profile.

Appliances:
•   Active phase: standard Twin Blocks.
•   Support and retention: anterior inclined plane.

Adjustment. Screw to expand the maxilla; operates for 3 months. The overjet reduces from 9 mm to 3 mm in 4 months, and the distal occlusion is corrected by the initial activation of the Twin Blocks.

Duration of treatment:
•   Active phase: Twin Blocks for 11 months.
•   Support phase: 6 months with anterior inclined plane.

WL

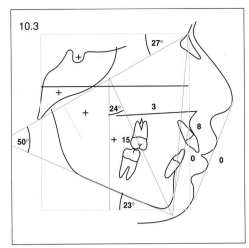

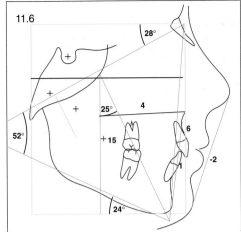

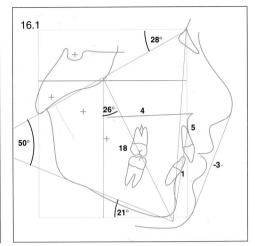

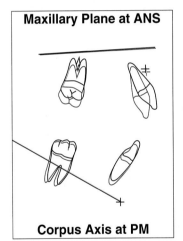

Maxillary Plane at ANS

Corpus Axis at PM

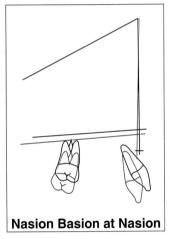

Nasion Basion at Nasion

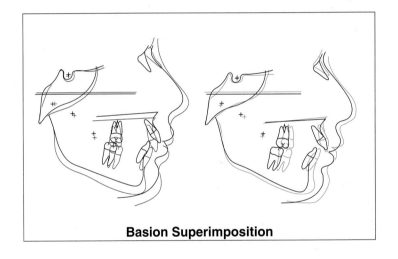

Basion Superimposition

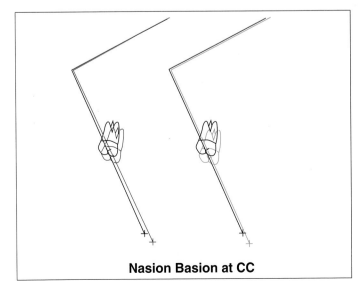

Nasion Basion at CC

W.L.-	Age	10.3	11.6	16.1	(Yr.Mon)
Cranial Base Angle		27	28	28	
Facial Axis Angle		24	25	26	
F/M Plane Angle		23	24	21	
Craniomandibular Angle		50	52	49	50
Maxillary Plane		3	4	4	
Convexity		8	6	5	
U/Incisor to Vertical		31	21	14	
L/Incisor to Vertical		34	42	36	
Interincisal Angle		115	117	140	
6 to Pterygoid Vertical		15	15	18	
L/Incisor to A/Po		0	1	1	
L/Lip to Aesthetic Plane		0	–2	–3	

AF

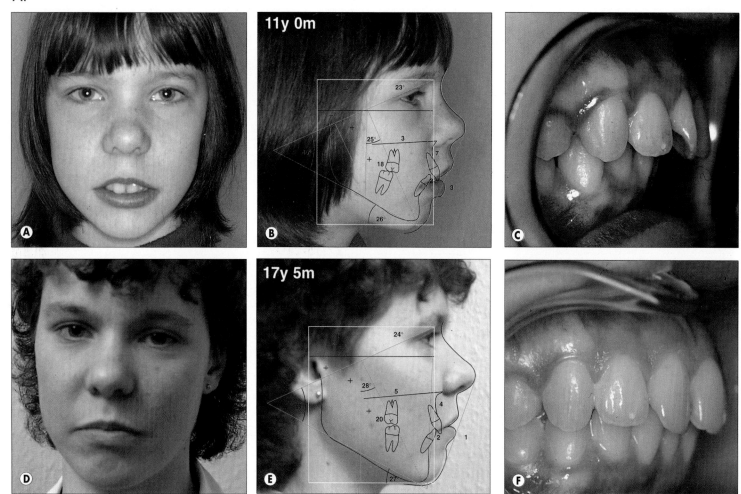

6.12 Treatment:
A, B, C Appearance and occlusion before treatment at age 11 years.
D, E, F Appearance and occlusion 4 years out of retention at age 17 years 5 months.

Case report: A.F. aged 11 years (6.12)

Diagnosis, skeletal classification:
- Severe Class II.
- Facial type: moderate dolichofacial.
- Maxilla: normal.
- Mandible: severe retrusion.
- Convexity = 7 mm.

Diagnosis, dental classification:
- Severe Class II division 1.
- Overjet = 9 mm.
- Overbite increased but incomplete due to tongue thrust.
- Upper incisors: protrusive.
- Lower incisors: protrusive.
- Mild upper and lower incisor crowding.

Duration of treatment:
- Orthopaedic phase: 6 months with Twin Blocks.
- Orthodontic phase: 3 months with a simple upper fixed appliance to complete treatment.
- Retention: 12 months.
- Total treatment time: 24 months.

Pericision was carried out on 1/1 to stabilise their position after correction of rotations. All second molars were extracted to reduce the risk of recrowding and to avert potential impaction of the third molars.

AF

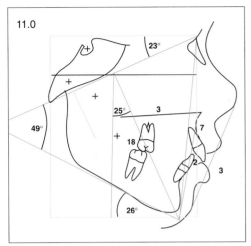

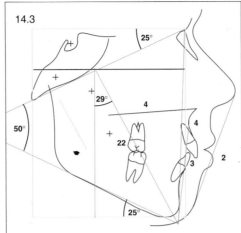

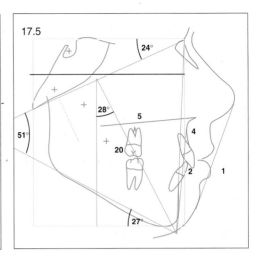

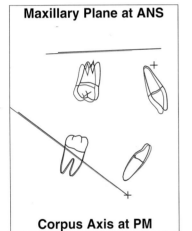

Maxillary Plane at ANS

Corpus Axis at PM

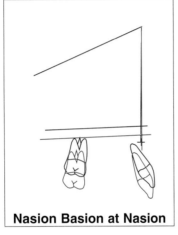

Nasion Basion at Nasion

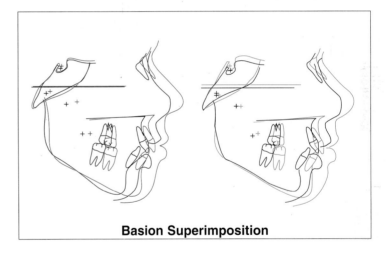

Basion Superimposition

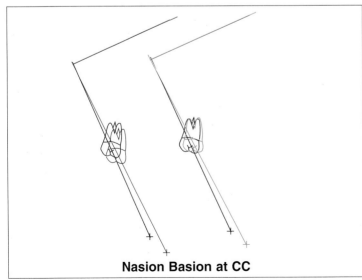

Nasion Basion at CC

A.F.-	Age	11.0	14.3	17.5	(Yr.Mon)
Cranial Base Angle		23	25	24	
Facial Axis Angle		25	29	28	
F/M Plane Angle		26	25	27	
Craniomandibular Angle		49	50	51	
Maxillary Plane		3	4	5	
Convexity		7	4	4	
U/Incisor to Vertical		27	23	23	
L/Incisor to Vertical		37	32	30	
Interincisal Angle		116	125	127	
6 to Pterygoid Vertical		18	22	20	
L/Incisor to A/Po		2	3	2	
L/Lip to Aesthetic Plane		3	2	1	

LC

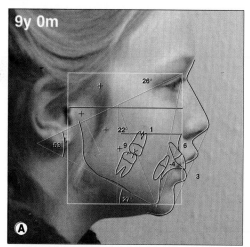

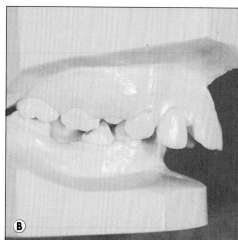

6.13 Treatment:
A, B Appearance and occlusion before treatment at age 9 years.
C, D Appearance and occlusion out of retention at age 14 years 11 months.

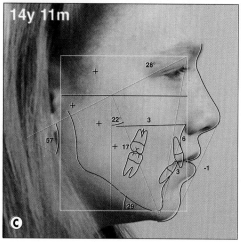

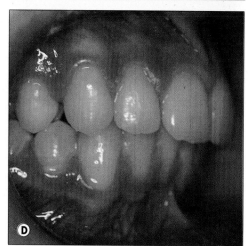

Case report: L.C. age 9 years (6.13)

Diagnosis, skeletal classification:
- Severe Class II.
- Facial type: dolichofacial – vertical growth.
- Maxilla: mild retrognathic.
- Mandible: severe retrognathic.
- Convexity = 6 mm.

Diagnosis, dental classification:
- Severe Class II division I.
- Overjet = 14 mm.
- Excessive overbite.
- Upper incisors: protrusive.
- Lower incisors: moderate retrusion.

Duration of treatment:
- Orthopaedic phase: 16 months with Twin Blocks.
- Support phase: 12 months – a lower fixed appliance completed correction in the lower arch during the support phase.
- Total treatment time: 28 months.

LC

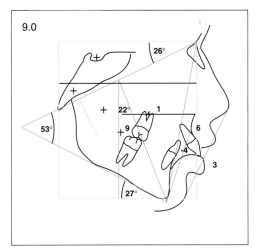

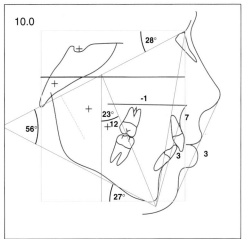

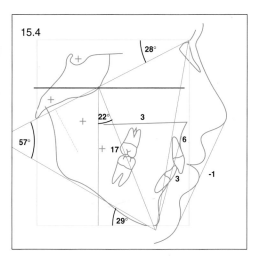

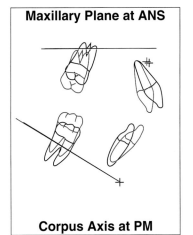

Maxillary Plane at ANS

Corpus Axis at PM

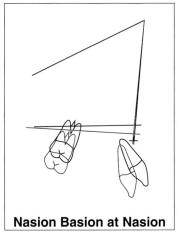

Nasion Basion at Nasion

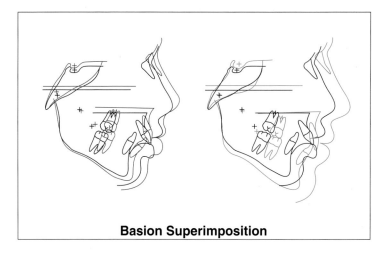

Basion Superimposition

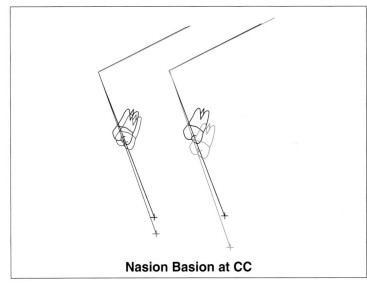

Nasion Basion at CC

L.C.-	Age	9.0	10.0	15.4	(Yr.Mon)
Cranial Base Angle		26	28	28	
Facial Axis Angle		22	23	22	
F/M Plane Angle		27	27	29	
Craniomandibular Angle		53	56	57	
Maxillary Plane		1	−1	3	
Convexity		6	7	6	
U/Incisor to Vertical		32	15	13	
L/Incisor to Vertical		30	42	40	
Interincisal Angle		118	123	127	
6 to Pterygoid Vertical		9	12	17	
L/Incisor to A/Po		−4	3	3	
L/Lip to Aesthetic Plane		3	3	−1	

FUNCTIONAL TREATMENT OBJECTIVE

The functional treatment objective uses the same principles employed in functional therapy of guiding the mandible forwards and bringing the lips together. This is the natural reaction of the patient when a functional appliance is fitted.

Preparing a treatment objective for functional therapy presents the problem of forecasting the response to functional mandibular protrusion and anticipating the facial changes that will result from functional therapy (**6.14**).

The 'functional treatment objective' may be used to predict the change in facial profile as a result of functional treatment. The method is suitable for use with visual imaging techniques using superimposition of cephalometric and photographic records.

The best clinical guideline in case selection for functional therapy is to establish that the profile is noticeably improved when the patient postures the mandible forwards with the lips closed. Photographic and cephalometric records in this position provide a functional treatment objective that shows the anticipated facial change, based on the patient's individual response to treatment.

Photographs and cephalometric films are used to record the position before treatment. An estimate of facial change resulting from mandibular protrusion is then made by registering the occlusion with the mandible closed, first in the existing retrusive, then in a protrusive position.

- A normal pre-treatment cephalogram is taken in centric occlusion.
- A tracing is completed showing the outlines of the cranial base, maxilla and mandible and the outlines of the incisors and molars.
- A template of the mandible and lower teeth is drawn on a second tracing that also registers the cranial base for reference.
- Where the upper or lower incisors are proclined or retroclined, an additional step positions the incisor at the correct angulation. The template is advanced to place the incisor teeth in correct contact with the lower incisors occluding on the base point of the upper incisor.
- The lip outline is redrawn with the lips closed and the mandible forwards. This method is not intended to illustrate growth change, but rather to use pretreatment records to predict the changes in facial appearance that should result from functional therapy.

A more sophisticated version of the functional treatment objective may use a visual imaging system to combine photographic and cephalometric records to predict the results of functional orthopaedic treatment. The method may be combined with computer programming for growth increments to predict growth changes as a result of a functional orthopaedic approach to treatment.

The patient is photographed with the mandible in retrusive and protrusive positions and cephalometric values are overlayed to predict the anticipated change in the facial profile. The predicted changes can be illustrated in colour on computer and may be printed out for record purposes.

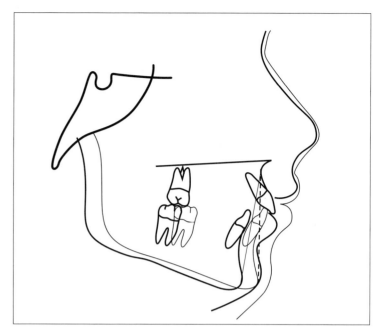

6.14 Functional Treatment Objective predicts the facial change that will result from mandibular advancement. The lower incisor translates forward relative to the A-Po line.

REFERENCES

Bimler, H.P. (1957). A roentgenoscopic method of quantifying the facial proportions. *Trans. Eur. Orthod. Soc.*, **1957**: 241–53

Bimler, H.P. (1977). *Removable Orthodontic Appliances*, ed. T.M. Graber & B. Neumann. Philadelphia, W.B. Saunders.

Broadbent, B.H. (1937). The face of the normal child. *Angle Orthod.*, **76**: 183–208.

Broadbent, B.H. (1948). *Practical Orthodontics*, ed. G.H. Anderson, 7th edn. St Louis, C.V. Mosby, p. 208.

Brodie, A.G. (1940). Some recent observations on growth of the face and their implications to the orthodontist. *Am. J. Orthod. & Oral Surgery*, **26**: 741–57.

Brodie, A.G. (1941). On the growth pattern of the human head from the third month to the eighth year of life. *Am. J. Anatomy*, **68**: 209–62.

Brodie, A.G. (1946). Facial patterns: a theme and variations. *Angle Orthod.*, **16**: 75–87.

Coben, S.E. (1955). The integration of facial skeleton variants. *Am. J. Orthod.*, **41**: 407–34.

Coben, S.E. (1961). Growth concepts. *Angle Orthod.*, **31**: 194–201.

Coben, S.E. (1979). Basion coordinate tracing film. *J. Clin. Orthod.*, 194–201.

Frankel, R. & Frankel, Ch. (1989). *Orthofacial Orthopedics with the Function Regulator*. Basle, Munich, Karger.

McNamara, Jr, J.A. (1984). A method of cephalometric evaluation. *Am. J. Orthod.* **86**: 449–69.

Ricketts, R.M. (1960). A foundation for cephalometric communication. *Am. J. Orthod.* **46**: 330–57.

Ricketts, R.M., Roth, R.H., Chaconas, S.J., Schulhof, R.J. & Engel, G.A. (1982). Orthodontic diagnosis and planning. *Rocky Mountain Orthodontics*.

Solow, B. & Tallgren, A. (1971). Natural head position in standing subjects. *Acta Odont. Scand.*, **29**: 591–607.

Siersbaeck-Neilson, S. & Solow, B. (1982). Intra and inter-examiner variability in head posture recorded by dental auxilliaries. *Am. J. Orthod.*, **82**: 50–57.

Witzig, J.W. & Spahl, T.J. (1989). *The Clinical Management of Basic Maxillofacial Orthopedic Appliances*, Vol. 2, Diagnostics. Massachusetts, PSG Publishing Co., pp. 130–1.

CHAPTER

7

Appliance Design and Construction

Comfort and aesthetics are the two most important factors in appliance design. It is important to design appliances that are 'patient friendly' to remove any obstacles to compliance and to motivate the patient to cooperate in treatment.

Twin Blocks have the advantage of versatility of design. They meet a wide range of requirements for correction of different types of malocclusion for patients throughout the age range from childhood to adulthood. Because the upper and lower appliances are separate components, the design can be adapted to resolve problems in both arches independently.

The component parts of Twin Block appliances are common to conventional removable appliances with the addition of occlusal inclined planes. Appliance design is modified by the addition of screws and springs or bows to move individual teeth. Arch development can proceed simultaneously with correction of arch relationships in the horizontal and vertical dimensions.

EVOLUTION OF APPLIANCE DESIGN

The earliest Twin Blocks were designed with the following basic components:

- A midline screw to expand the upper arch.
- Occlusal bite blocks.
- Clasps on upper molars and premolars.
- Clasps on lower premolars and incisors.
- A labial bow to retract the upper incisors.
- Springs to move individual teeth and to improve the archform as required.
- Provision for extraoral traction in some cases.

Twin Block appliances are tooth and tissue borne. The appliances are designed to link teeth together as anchor units to limit individual tooth movement, and to maximise the orthopaedic response to treatment. In the lower arch, peripheral clasping combined with occlusal cover exerts three-dimensional control on anchor teeth, and limits tipping and displacement of individual teeth. When indicated, additional clasps may be placed on lower incisors but, in practice, it is found that clasps mesial to the lower canines are equally effective in controlling the lower labial segment. An example of an early design with a labial bow, lower incisor clasps and provision for extraoral traction, which is no longer used to reinforce anchorage, is shown in **7.1 A, B**.

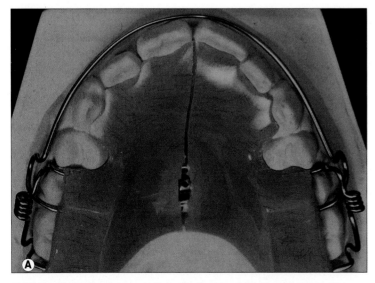

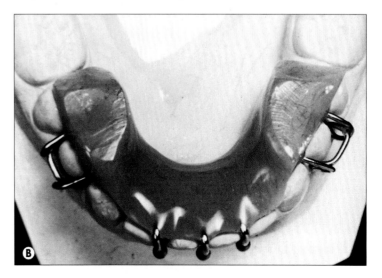

7.1 A, B Example of an early Twin Block with a labial bow, lower incisor clasps and provision for extraoral traction, which is no longer used to reinforce anchorage.

STANDARD TWIN BLOCKS

Standard Twin Blocks are essentially for treatment of an uncrowded Class II division 1 malocclusion with a good archform and an overjet large enough to allow unrestricted forward translation of the mandible to allow full correction of distal occlusion.

Labial bow

In the early stages of development, the upper Twin Block invariably incorporated a labial bow. It was observed that if the labial bow engaged the upper incisors during functional correction it tended to overcorrect incisor angulation. It was, therefore, routinely adjusted out of contact with the upper incisors. Retracting upper incisors prematurely limits the scope for functional correction by mandibular advancement. This led to the conclusion that a labial bow is not always required unless it is necessary to upright severely proclined incisors, and even then it must not be activated until full functional correction is complete and a Class I buccal segment relationship is achieved. If a labial bow is included in the appliance design, and it is activated prematurely to retract upper incisors, this will act as a brake to limit the functional correction by mandibular advancement. In many cases, the appliance is more effective for functional correction without a labial bow.

In Twin Block treatment a good lip seal is achieved naturally without additional lip exercises, as the appliance is worn for eating and drinking, making it necessary to form a good anterior seal. The lips act like a labial bow and lip pressure is effective in uprighting upper incisors, making a labial bow superfluous. In many cases, the absence of a labial bow improves aesthetics without reducing the effectiveness of the appliance (**7.2 A–D**).

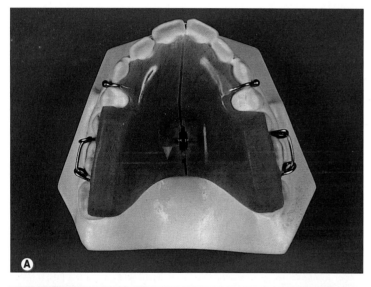
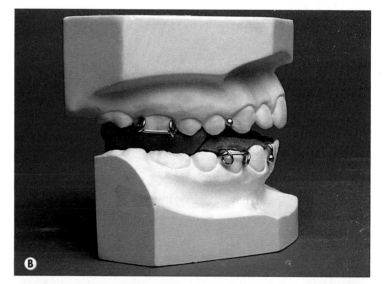
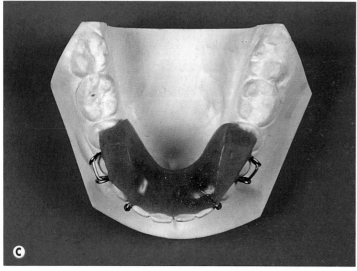
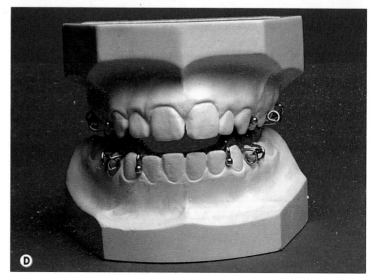

7.2 A–D Standard Twin Blocks.

TWIN BLOCK CONSTRUCTION

The laboratory requires a good set of impressions and an accurate construction bite to record the activation to be built into the appliance The construction bite should be taken in modelling wax that retains its dimensional stability after it is removed from the mouth.

Any excess wax extending over the buccal surfaces of the teeth should be removed to allow the models to seat correctly into the construction bite. The models are then mounted on an articulator. A plasterless articulator may be used, with adjustable screws to position the models.

THE DELTA CLASP

The delta clasp was designed by the author to improve the fixation of Twin Blocks. The delta clasp is similar to the Adams clasp (Adams, 1970) in principle, but incorporates new features to improve retention, reduce metal fatigue and minimise the need for adjustment. The retentive loops were originally triangular in shape (from which the name 'delta' is derived), or alternatively the loops may be circular, both types having similar retentive properties.

The delta clasp retains the basic elements of the Adams clasp, that is, interdental tags, retentive loops and a buccal bridge. The crucial difference is that the retentive loops are shaped as a closed triangle or circle as opposed to an open U-shaped arrowhead as in the Adams clasp. The advantage of the closed loop is that the clasp does not open with repeated insertion and removal and, therefore, maintains its shape better and requires less adjustment, and is less subject to breakage. A further advantage is that the clasp gives excellent retention on lower premolars, and is suitable for use on most posterior teeth (**7.3**).

According to the area of best retention there are two possible methods of construction for the delta clasp. The first is similar to the Adams clasp, with the retentive loop angled to follow the curvature of the tooth into mesial and distal undercuts. This design is appropriate if the tooth is favourably shaped, with good undercuts mesially and distally.

If the individual teeth are not favourably shaped, the loop of the clasp may be directed interdentally. The loop is then constructed at right angles to the bridge of the clasp, so that it passes into the interdental undercut to gain retention from adjacent teeth.

In the permanent dentition, delta clasps are placed routinely on upper first molars and on lower first premolars. They may also be used on deciduous molars. Additional interdental ball-ended clasps or C-shaped clasps may be placed to improve retention and provide resistance to anteroposterior tipping.

Ball-ended clasps are routinely employed mesial to lower canines and in the upper premolar or deciduous molar region to gain interdental retention from adjacent teeth. C-clasps are useful in mixed dentition where they can be used for peripheral clasping on deciduous molars and canines (**7.4**).

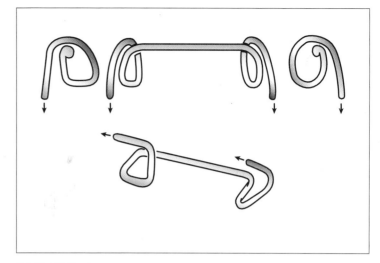

7.3 The Delta clasp .

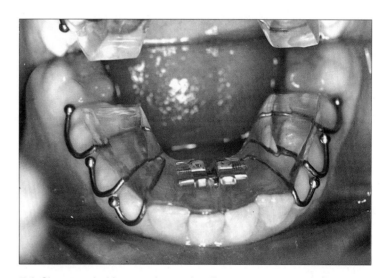

7.4 Clasps on deciduous molars and canines

ADJUSTMENT OF THE DELTA CLASP

The delta clasp may be adjusted gingivally into an interdental undercut by placing pliers on the wire as it emerges from the acrylic interdentally. Bird beak or 139 pliers have a short round beak that is placed under the wire and the square beak is placed on top. A slight adjustment extends the retentive loop of the clasp into the gingival or interdental undercut.

The other method of adjustment is to grasp the arrowhead from the buccal aspect and twist the retentive loop inwards towards the tooth to adjust into a mesial or distal undercut.

THE BASE PLATE

Appliances may either be made with heat cure or cold cure acrylic. Heat cure acrylic has the advantage of additional strength and accuracy. Making the appliances in wax first allows the blocks to be formed with greater precision.

Cold cure acrylic has the advantage of speed and convenience, but sacrifices something in strength and accuracy. It is essential to use a top-quality cold cure acrylic to avoid problems with break-age, especially in the later stages of treatment, after trimming the blocks to allow eruption in treatment of deep overbite. The inclined planes can lose their definition as a result of wear if a soft acrylic is used.

The disadvantages of cold cure acrylic can be overcome by using preformed blocks made from a good-quality heat cured acrylic. This has the important advantage of making construction easier and increasing the accuracy of the inclined planes by providing a consistent angle for occlusion of the blocks (**7.5 A–E**).

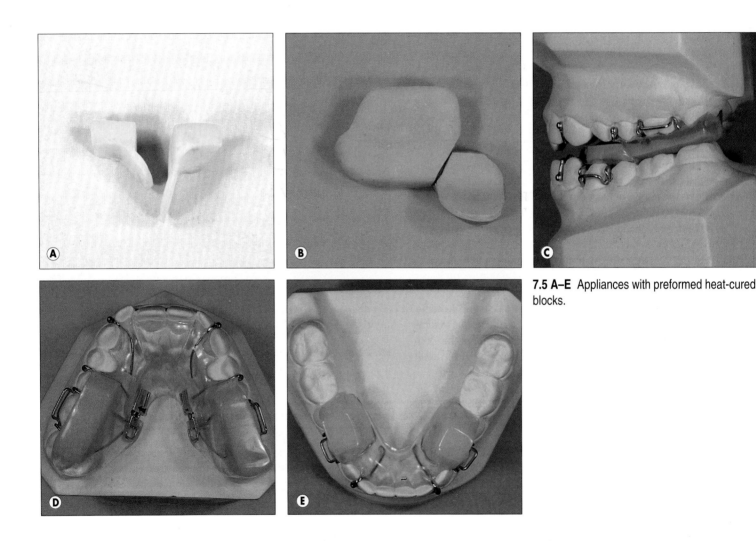

7.5 A–E Appliances with preformed heat-cured blocks.

OCCLUSAL INCLINED PLANES

The position and angulation of the occlusal inclined planes is crucial to efficiency in correcting arch relationships. In most cases, the inclined planes are angled at 70° to the occlusal plane, although the angulation may be reduced to 45° if the patient fails to posture forwards consistently and thereby to occlude the blocks correctly.

The position of the inclined plane is determined by the lower block and is critical in treatment of deep overbite. It is important that the inclined plane is clear of mesial surface contact with the lower molar, which must be free to erupt unobstructed in order to reduce the overbite. The inclined plane on the lower bite block is angled from the mesial surface of the second premolar or deciduous molar at 70° to the occlusal plane. The lower block does not extend distally to the marginal ridge on the lower second premolar or deciduous molar. This allows the leading edge of the inclined plane on the upper appliance to be positioned mesial to the lower first molar so as not to obstruct eruption. Buccolingually the lower block covers the occlusal surfaces of the lower premolars or deciduous molars to occlude with the inclined plane on the upper Twin Block (**7.6**).

The flat occlusal bite block passes forwards over the first premolar to become thinner buccolingually in the lower canine region. The full thickness of the blocks need not be maintained in the canine region. Reducing the bulk in this area is important, as speech is improved by allowing the tongue freedom of movement in the phonetic area.

As this can be the most vulnerable part of the appliance, the lingual flange of the lower appliance in the midline should be sufficiently thick to give adequate strength to avoid breakage.

The upper inclined plane is angled from the mesial surface of the upper second premolar to the mesial surface of the upper first molar. The flat occlusal portion then passes distally over the remaining upper posterior teeth in a wedge shape, reducing in thickness as it extends distally.

Because the upper arch is wider than the lower, it is only necessary to cover the lingual cusps of the upper posterior teeth, rather than the full occlusal surface. This has the advantage of making the clasps more flexible and allows access to the interdental wires of the clasps for adjustment.

In constructing the blocks a decision must be made concerning the angulation of the blocks in relation to the line of the arch. There are two alternatives, both of which are effective in practice.

First, the blocks may be aligned in each quadrant at right angles to the line of the arch in the same pattern as the teeth are aligned. Alternatively, the lower blocks may be aligned at right angles to the midline bisecting the arch. The upper blocks would be constructed to match this angulation. This second method has the advantage that the blocks maintain the same angulation relative to each other even if the midline screws are turned to widen the archform.

The author has observed many basic errors in appliance design and construction that often ignore the fundamental principles of clinical management. Mistakes in appliance construction can lead to treatment failure. It should be emphasised that problems in clinical management can be avoided by quality in appliance construction. Every effort has been made to work with laboratories to teach details of construction and appliance design. Experienced orthodontic laboratories should be used so that appliances are constructed correctly.

Appliance design has been progressively simplified over the years and additional designs have been developed to treat different types of malocclusion.

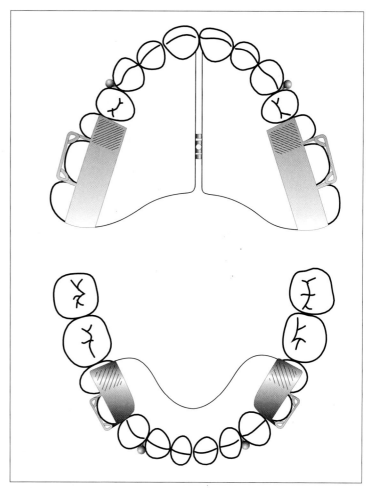

7.6 Occlusal view of standard Twin Blocks.

TWIN BLOCKS FOR ARCH DEVELOPMENT

Transverse development

Upper and lower Schwarz appliances (Schwarz & Gratzlinger, 1966) were commonly used in the past for transverse development in mixed dentition. It is now possible to combine transverse arch development simultaneously with sagittal and vertical correction of arch relationships by combining Twin Block and Schwarz appliances (**7.7**).

Screws may be incorporated in the upper and lower Twin Blocks to develop the archform in mixed dentition. This allows independent control of archwidth in both arches to improve anterior crowding or correct posterior crossbite. An upper transpalatal arch or lower Jackson design (Jackson, 1887) may be used as an alternative to screws for arch development (**7.8**)

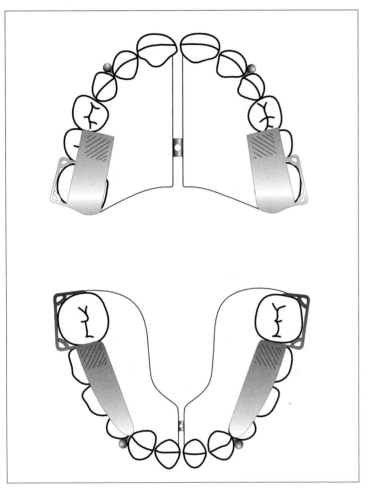

7.7 Twin Block Schwarz appliances.

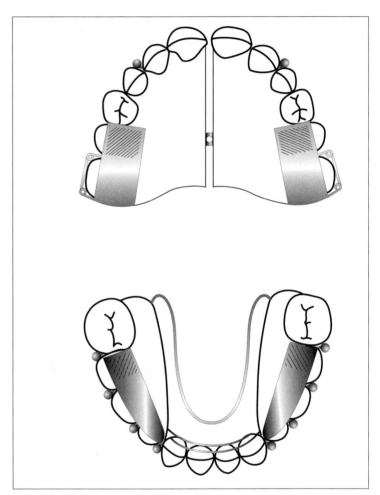

7.8 Upper, transpalatal arch/ Lower Jackson Twin Block.

The Twin Block Crozat appliance (Crozat, 1920) provides a useful alternative that is suitable for adult treatment with minimum palatal and lingual coverage. This appliance requires careful adjustment to maintain symmetry (**7.9**).

SAGITTAL DEVELOPMENT

Twin blocks to open the bite

Twin Block sagittal appliance
Sagittal arch development is required when upper or lower incisors are retroclined with deep overbite. As the name implies, the Twin Block sagittal appliance is designed primarily for anteroposterior arch development by positioning two screws which are aligned anteroposteriorly in the palate. Some oblique movement is also pos-

sible by offsetting the angulation of the screws to achieve an additional component of buccal expansion. Normally, the palatal screws are angled to drive the upper posterior segments distally along the line of the arch.

The anteroposterior positioning of the screws and the location of the cuts determines whether the appliance acts mainly to move upper anterior teeth labially or to distalise upper posterior teeth. The position of the anterior cut determines how many teeth are included in the anterior segment. If only the central incisors are retroclined, a cut distal to the central incisors will move only these teeth labially or, alternatively, the lateral incisors may also be advanced by placing the cut distal to the lateral incisors. The incisor teeth are then pitted against the posterior teeth to advance the labial segment (**7.10**).

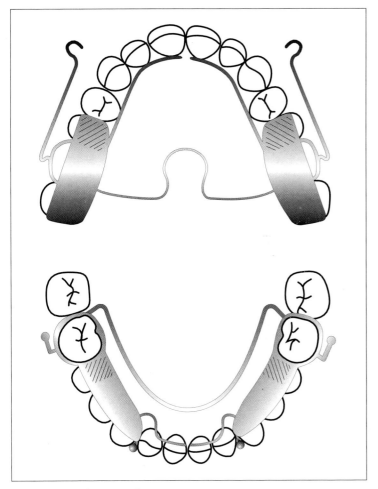

7.9 Twin Block Crozat appliances.

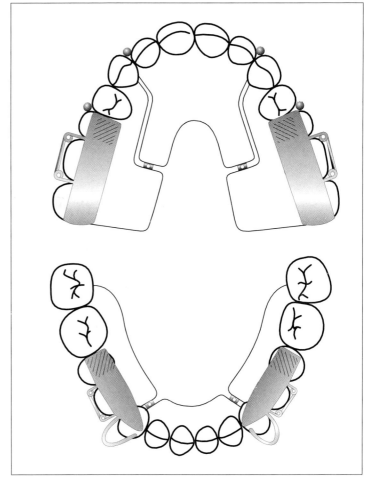

7.10 Twin Block sagittal appliance.

In cases with asymmetrical arch development, if more distal movement is required unilaterally the screw on one side may be activated more than the other. If the cut is positioned distal to the canines or premolars the distalisation of posterior teeth increases in proportion to the number of teeth included as anchorage in the anterior segment.

In placing the screws in the palate it is important that they are set in the horizontal plane, and not inclined downwards anteriorly, which would cause the appliance to ride down the anterior teeth, reducing its effectiveness.

The lower Twin Block sagittal appliance applies similar principles in the lower arch. To advance the lower labial segment, curved screws are placed in the lower canine region, or to open premolar spaces straight screws are placed in the second premolar region.

Transverse and sagittal development

Some cases require a combination of transverse and sagittal development. A three-way screw incorporates two screws in a single housing and allows independent activation for transverse and sagittal expansion, although it is fairly bulky in the anterior part of the palate and therefore interferes with speech (**7.11**).

The three-screw sagittal appliance achieves this objective with an additional midline screw which can be positioned anteriorly or posteriorly in the palate to achieve a similar objective (**7.12A** and **7.12B**).

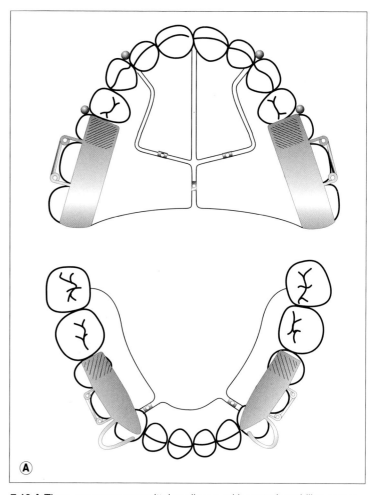

7.12 A Three-screw upper sagittal appliance, with posterior midline screw.

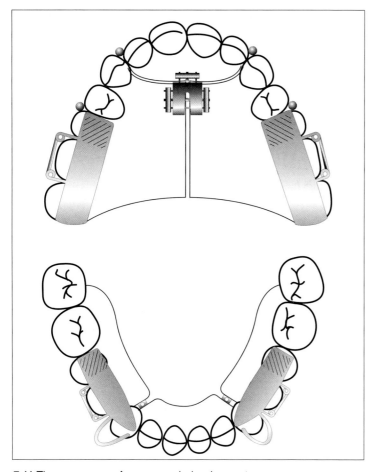

7.11 Three-way screw for upper arch development.

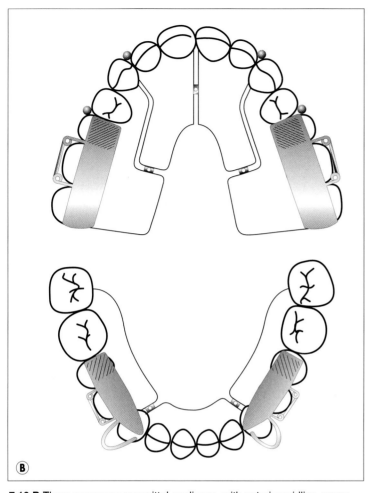

7.12 B Three-screw upper sagittal appliance, with anterior midline screw.

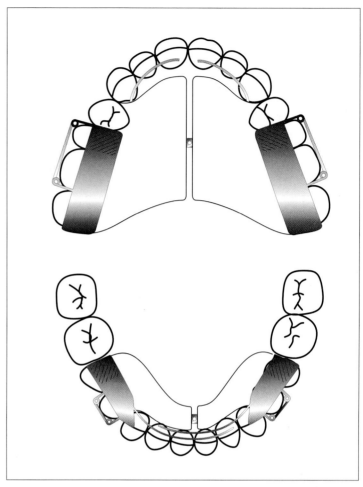

7.13 Twin Blocks to open the bite and advance anterior teeth; springs to advance upper and lower incisions.

Alternatively, a midline screw may be combined with lingual wires to advance and align upper and lower incisors. This design of appliance may be used in both arches to advance retroclined upper and lower incisors and to open the bite in treatment of bimaxillary retrusion (**7.13**)

Twin blocks to close anterior open bite

Twin Blocks are designed to close an anterior open bite by applying an intrusive force to the posterior teeth. Occlusal contact of the bite blocks on all the posterior teeth is essential to prevent eruption, which would open the bite. Similar principles apply in designing both upper and lower appliances to achieve these objectives (**7.14**).

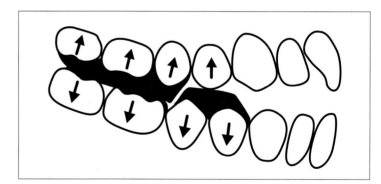

7.14 Twin Blocks to close the bite.

The upper appliance must extend distally to cover all the upper posterior teeth including second molars to prevent overeruption. Occlusal rests should extend distally to control second molars if they are about to erupt. Prevention is better than cure, as failure to control second molars will increase the open bite and cause treatment to fail.

The design of the lower appliance is modified for anterior open bite to prevent eruption of posterior teeth by placing clasps on lower molars and first premolars or deciduous molars to give good stability to the appliance. There is no need to add additional clasps in the lower labial segment.

It is not necessary to extend acrylic anteriorly to contact the lingual surfaces of the upper and lower anterior teeth, leaving them free to erupt to reduce the anterior open bite. A labial bow may be added to upright proclined upper incisors and help reduce the anterior open bite. Tongue thrust may be controlled by the addition of a spinner or tongue guard. In some cases, both may be indicated (**7.15**).

REVERSE TWIN BLOCKS

The position of the bite blocks is reversed compared with that of Twin Blocks for treatment of Class II malocclusion. The occlusal blocks on the upper appliance are positioned over the deciduous molars to occlude distally with blocks placed over the lower first permanent molars.

The addition of two sagittal screws in the palate provides a means of activation to advance the upper incisors, and the reciprocal force on the inclined planes uses anchorage in the lower arch to drive the upper arch labially. Apart from the reverse position of the blocks and inclined planes, the design of the upper appliance is similar in principle to the sagittal design used in treatment of Class II division 2 malocclusion and the same principles apply in relation to positioning the screws.

A contracted maxilla frequently requires three-way expansion. This is achieved by a three-screw sagittal design or the three-way screw to combine transverse and sagittal arch development (**7.16 A, B**)

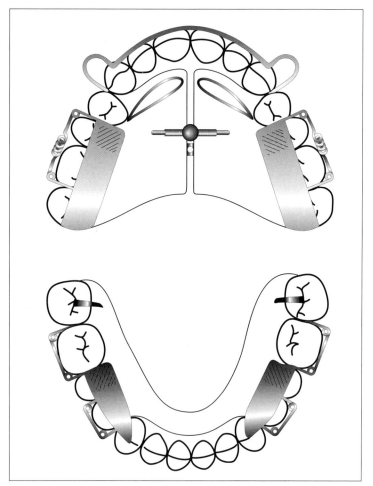

7.15 Spinner to control tongue thrust – Clasps on lower first molars; occlusal rests to prevent eruption of second molars – E.O.T. tubes.

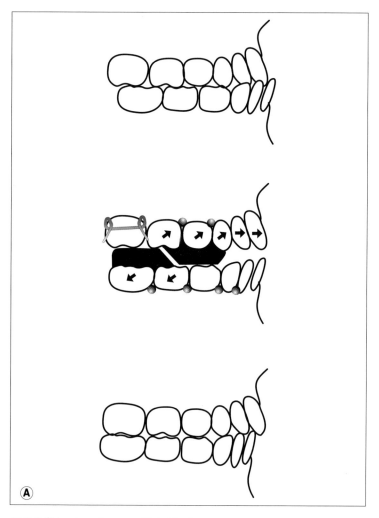

7.16 A Side view of reverse Twin Blocks.

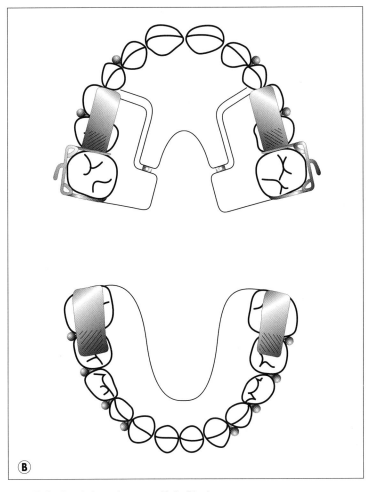

7.16 B Occlusal view of reverse Twin Blocks.

REFERENCES

Adams, C.P. (1970). *The Design and Construction of Removable Orthodontic Appliances*, 4th edn. Bristol, John Wright & Sons Ltd.

Crozat, G.B. (1920). Possibilities and use of removable labio-lingual spring appliances. *Int. J. Oral Surg.*, **6**: 1–7.

Jackson, V.H. (1887). Some methods of regulating. *Dent. Cosmos*, **29**: 373–87.

Schwarz, A.M. & Gratzinger, M. (1966). *Removable Orthodontic Appliances*. Philadelphia, W.B. Saunders.

CHAPTER
8

Treatment of Class II Division 1 Malocclusion Deep Overbite

CLINICAL MANAGEMENT OF TWIN BLOCKS

After a century of development of functional techniques it is surprising that the forces of occlusion have not been used to any significant extent as a functional mechanism to correct malocclusion. Twin Blocks adapt the functional mechanism of the natural dentition, the occlusal inclined plane, to harness the forces of occlusion to correct the malocclusion.

The Twin Block is a natural progression in the evolution of functional appliance therapy. It represents a fundamental transition from a one-piece appliance that restricts normal function to twin appliances that promote normal function.

Twin Blocks are designed on aesthetic principles to free the patient of the restrictions imposed by a one-piece appliance made to fit the teeth in both jaws. With Twin Blocks the patient can function quite normally. Eating and speaking can be accomplished without overly restricting normal movements of the tongue, lips and mandible. This means that the patient eats with the appliances in the mouth and the forces of mastication are harnessed to maximise the functional response to treatment.

Bite registration

The procedure of bite registration for construction of Twin Blocks for a Class II division 1 malocclusion with deep overbite is described in greater detail.

The Exactobite or Projet Bite Gauge is designed to record a protrusive bite for construction of Twin Blocks. The blue bite gauge registers 2 mm vertical clearance between the incisal edges of the upper and lower incisors, which is an appropriate interincisal clearance for bite registration in most Class II division 1 malocclusions with increased overbite.

The incisal portion of the bite gauge has three incisal grooves on one side that are designed to be positioned on the incisal edge of the upper incisor and a single groove on the opposing side that engages the incisal edge of the lower incisor. The appropriate groove in the bite gauge for bite registration is selected depending on the ease with which the patient can posture the mandible forwards.

In Class II division 1 malocclusion a protrusive bite is registered to reduce the overjet and the distal occlusion on average by 5–10 mm on initial activation, depending on the freedom of movement in protrusive function. The length of the patient's protrusive path is determined by recording the overjet in centric occlusion and fully protrusive occlusion. The activation should not exceed 70% of the protrusive path.

In the growing child with an overjet of up to 10 mm, provided the patient can posture forwards comfortably, the bite may be activated edge-to-edge on the incisors with a 2 mm interincisal clearance. This allows an overjet of up to 10 mm to be corrected on the first activation, without further activation of the Twin Blocks. Larger overjets invariably require partial correction, followed by reactivation after the initial correction is complete.

It is best first to rehearse the procedure of bite registration, with the patient using a mirror. The patient is instructed to close correctly into the bite gauge before applying the wax. When the patient understands what is required, softened wax is applied to the bite gauge from a hot water bath. The clinician then places the bite gauge in the patient's mouth to register the bite. After removing the registration bite from the mouth, the wax is chilled in cold water and should now be firm and dimensionally stable.

In registering the bite the wax is kept clear of the incisors, so that the operator has an unobstructed view of the anterior teeth. This helps the laboratory to position the models correctly in the squash bite (**8.1 A–C**). Silicone putty may be used as an alternative to wax to register the bite, but the elasticity of the material can make it more difficult to locate the models correctly in the construction bite.

Centre lines should be coincident provided no dental asymmetry is present. To reduce the overjet when the lower incisors close into the incisal guidance groove on the underside of the bite gauge, the bite gauge is positioned with the upper incisors occluding in the appropriate groove. It is essential that the patient bites 'fully home' into the bite gauge to register the correct vertical opening for the occlusion.

In the vertical dimension a 2-mm interincisal clearance is equivalent to an approximately 5 or 6 mm clearance in the first premolar region. This usually leaves 3 mm clearance distally in the molar

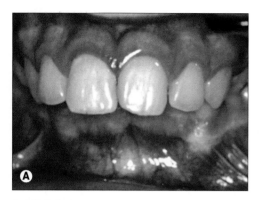
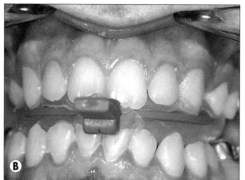
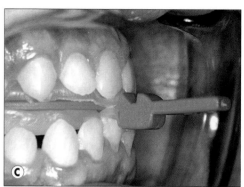

8.1 A–C Construction bite for deep overbite with the projet.

region, and ensures that space is available for vertical development of posterior teeth to reduce the overbite.

It is very important to open the bite slightly beyond the clearance of the free-way space to encourage the patient to close into the appliance rather than allow the mandible to drop out of contact into rest position, which is one of the disadvantages of making the blocks too thin.

APPLIANCE DESIGN: TWIN BLOCKS TO OPEN THE BITE

In designing Twin Blocks to open the bite the inclined planes must be positioned carefully to achieve vertical control by selective eruption of posterior teeth. The inclined planes must be clear of the lower molars so that they can erupt without obstruction (**8.2**).

Fitting Twin Blocks: Instructions to the patient

Patient motivation is an important aspect of all removable appliance therapy. The process of patient education and motivation continues when the patient attends to have Twin Blocks fitted. It is often helpful to the patient if the clinician demonstrates Twin Blocks on models to confirm that it is a simple appliance system and is easy to wear, with no visible anterior wires.

Simply biting the blocks together guides the lower jaw forwards to correct the bite. The appliance system is easily understood even by young patients, who can see that biting the blocks together corrects the jaw position. It is important to emphasise positive factors and to motivate the patient before treatment.

The patient is shown how to insert the Twin Blocks with the help of a mirror, pointing out the immediate improvement in facial appearance when the Twin Block is fitted and explaining that the appliances will produce this change in a few months, provided they are worn full time.

A removable appliance only corrects the teeth when it is in the mouth, not in the pocket. Both appliances must be worn full time,

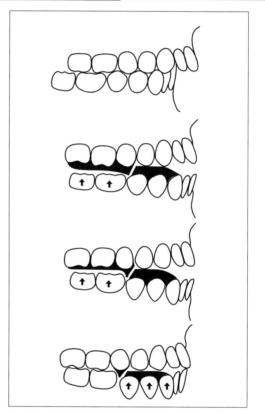

8.2 Twin Blocks to open the bite – side view.

especially during eating, and removed only for cleaning. Exceptions may be made for swimming and contact sports.

At first the appliance will feel large in the mouth, but within a few days it will be very comfortable and easy to wear. Twin Blocks cause much less interference to speech than a one-piece functional appliance. For the first few days speech will be affected, but will steadily improve and should return to normal within a week.

When the patient has learned to insert and remove the appliance, instruction is given on operating the expansion screw, one quarter turn per week, explaining the necessity to widen the upper arch as the lower arch is advanced to correct the bite. The screw should be turned for the first time after a few days, when the appliances have settled in comfortably.

As with any new appliance it is normal to expect a little initial discomfort. But it is important to encourage the patient to persevere and keep the appliance in the mouth at all times except for hygiene purposes. The patient should also be instructed not to hesitate to contact the office if it is not comfortable within a few days.

The patient may be advised to remove the appliance for eating for the first few days. Then it is important to learn to eat with the appliance in the mouth. The force of biting on the appliance corrects the jaw position, and learning to eat with the appliances in is important to accelerate treatment. In a few days, patients should be eating with the Twin Blocks and, within a week, should be more comfortable with the appliance in the mouth than they are without it.

It is necessary to check the initial activation and confirm that the patient closes consistently on the inclined planes with the mandible protruded in its new position. The overjet is measured with the mandible fully retruded and this measurement should be recorded in the patient's notes and checked at every visit to monitor progress.

FULL-TIME APPLIANCE WEAR

Temporary fixation of Twin Blocks

The most crucial time to establish good cooperation with the patient is in the first few days after fitting the Twin Blocks, when he or she is learning to adjust to the new appliance. Twin Blocks have the unique advantage compared to other functional appliances in that they can be fixed to the teeth. Such temporary fixation guarantees full-time wear, 24 hours per day, and excellent cooperation is established at the start of treatment.

The technique for fixing the appliances in place is simple. The teeth should first be fissure sealed and treated with topical fluoride as a preventive measure prior to fixation. There are two alternative methods of fixation of Twin Blocks:

- The appliances may be fixed to the teeth by spreading cement on the tooth-bearing areas of the appliance but not on the gingival areas. The appliance is then inserted and secured in place with cement adhering to the teeth. Zinc phosphate or zinc oxide cement is suitable for temporary fixation. Alternatively, a small quantity of glass ionomer cement may be used, taking care to ensure that the appliance can be freed easily from the teeth (**8.3**).
- Twin Blocks may also be bonded directly to the teeth by applying composite around the clasps. This is a useful approach in mixed dentition when ball clasps may be bonded directly to deciduous molars to improve fixation.

After a few days, when the patient has adapted to the Twin Block and is wearing it comfortably, the appliance can be removed by freeing the clasps with a sickle scaler. Sharp edges of composite can be smoothed over, leaving some composite attached to the teeth. The altered contour of the deciduous teeth will improve the retention of the appliance.

If cooperation is doubtful at any stage of treatment, the operator should not hesitate to fix the appliance in for 10 days to regain control and restore full-time wear. After 10 days full-time wear the patient is more comfortable with the appliance in the mouth than without it.

MANAGEMENT OF DEEP OVERBITE

Overbite reduction is achieved by trimming the occlusal blocks on the upper appliance, so as to encourage eruption of the lower molars. A progressive sequence of trimming aims to encourage selective eruption of posterior teeth to increase the vertical dimension. The objective is to increase lower facial height and improve facial balance by controlling the vertical dimension (**8.4**). Provided the correct sequence of trimming is carried out to control eruption, closure of a posterior open bite is accelerated in Twin Block treatment compared with a one-piece functional appliance, which is removed for eating, and allows the tongue to spread between the teeth and prevent eruption of the posterior teeth. Posterior support is established as the molars erupt into occlusion before relieving the appliance over the premolars until they also are free to erupt into occlusion.

The management of deep overbite begins even before the appliance is fitted – by placing elastic separators in the molar region. When the appliance is fitted, the separators are removed and the appliance is adjusted to encourage the molars to erupt.

In the treatment of deep overbite, it is important to encourage vertical development of the lower molars from the start of treatment, by trimming the upper bite block occlusodistally to allow the lower molars to erupt.

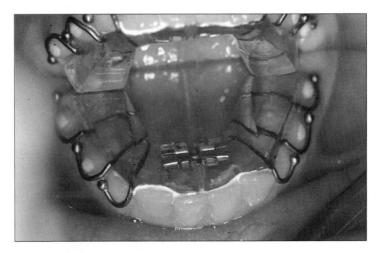

8.3 Twin Blocks cemented in position.

The upper bite block is progressively trimmed at each visit over several months, leaving only a small vertical clearance of 1 or 2 mm over the lower molars to allow them to erupt into occlusion. The clearance between the upper appliance and the lower molars is checked by inserting a probe (or explorer) between the posterior teeth to establish that the lower molars are free to erupt. At each subsequent visit for appliance adjustment the occlusion is cleared by sequentially trimming the upper block occlusodistally to allow further eruption of the lower molars, again checking that the clearance is correct.

This sequence of adjustment does not allow the tongue to spread laterally between the teeth to prevent eruption of lower molars, and results in a more rapid development of the vertical dimension. The molars will erupt into occlusion normally within 6–9 months.

It is important that the mandible continues to be supported in a protruded position throughout the sequence of trimming the blocks. The leading edge of the inclined plane on the upper bite block remains intact, leaving a triangular wedge in contact with the lower bite block.

When the molars have erupted into occlusion, a lateral open bite is present in the premolar region because the lower bite block is still intact. The final adjustment at the end of the Twin Block stage aims to reduce the lateral open bite by trimming the upper occlusal surface of the lower bite block over the premolars by 2 mm. To maintain adequate inclined planes to support the corrected arch relationships, the lower bite block is shaped into a triangular wedge distally in contact with the upper block.

Relieved of occlusal contact, the lower premolars erupt, carrying the lower appliance up into occlusion. The occlusal height of the upper premolars is maintained by interdental clasps that effectively prevent their eruption. The lateral open bite in the premolar region now reduces and the occlusal plane begins to level.

ESTABLISHING THE CORRECT VERTICAL DIMENSION

The intergingival height
A simple guideline is used to establish the correct vertical dimension during the Twin Block phase of treatment. The intergingival height is measured from the gingival margin of the upper incisor to the gingival margin of the lower incisor when the teeth are in occlusion (**8.5**).

This measurement has proved to be beneficial for temporomandibular joint practitioners who use the intergingival height to establish the vertical dimension in a restorative approach to rebuild the occlusion in treatment of patients with temporomandibular joint dysfunction.

The 'comfort zone' for intergingival height for adult patients is generally found to be 17–19 mm. This is equivalent to the combined heights of the upper and lower incisors minus an overbite within the range of normal. Patients whose intergingival height varies significantly from the 'comfort zone' are at greater risk of developing temporomandibular joint dysfunction. This applies both to patients with a deep overbite, whose intergingival height is significantly reduced,

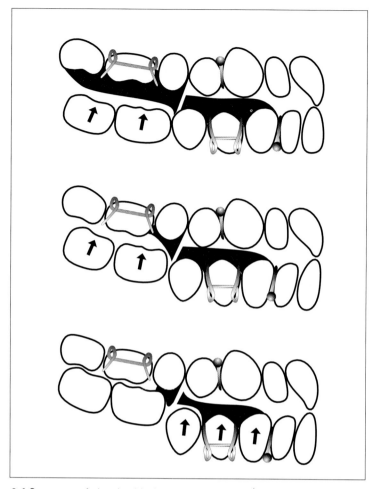

8.4 Sequence of trimming blocks to reduce overbite.

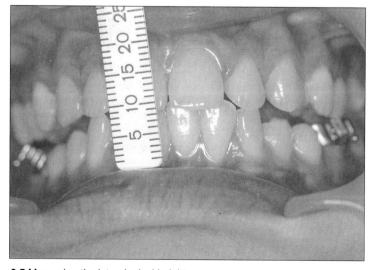

8.5 Measuring the intergingival height.

and to patients with an anterior open bite who have an increased intergingival height.

The intergingival height is a useful guideline to check progress and to establish the correct vertical dimension during treatment. Measurement of intergingival height is made by using a millimetre ruler or dividers with a vernier scale to measure the distance between the upper and lower gingival margins. To keep track of progress in opening or closing the bite, this measurement should be noted on the record card at every visit.

In Twin Block treatment the correct intergingival height is achieved with great consistency. Deep overbite may be overcorrected to an intergingival height of 20 mm to allow for a slight 'settling in' with a resultant increase in overbite after treatment. Overcorrection of deep overbite is advisable as a precaution against any tendency to relapse.

The intergingival height varies according to the patient's age and stage of development, and the height of the incisor crowns. It is smaller in a young patient whose incisors have recently erupted, and larger in an older patient with gingival recession. In the younger patient a range of 15–17 mm is normal and allowance should be made for the diminutive height of the clinical crowns.

SOFT TISSUE RESPONSE

Rapid changes occur in the craniofacial musculature in response to the altered muscle function that results from treatment of malocclusion by a full-time functional appliance. As a result of altered muscle balance, significant changes in facial appearance are seen within 2 or 3 weeks of starting treatment with Twin Blocks. The rapid improvement in muscle balance is very consistent and is observed on photographs as a more relaxed posture within minutes, hours or days of starting treatment.

The Twin Block appliance positions the mandible downwards and forwards, increasing the intermaxillary space. As a result it is difficult to form an anterior oral seal by contact between the tongue and the lower lip, and patients adopt a natural lip seal without instruction. As the appliance is worn full time, even during eating, rapid soft tissue adaptation occurs to assist the primary functions of mastication and swallowing, that necessitate an effective anterior oral seal. The patient adopts a lip seal when the overjet is eliminated in the most natural way possible, by eating and drinking with the appliance in the mouth. This encourages a good lip seal as a functional necessity to prevent food and liquid escaping from the mouth. A good lip seal is always achieved by normal function with Twin Blocks, without the need for lip exercises.

Case report: L.J. aged 10 years 9 months
This is an example of treatment of an uncrowded Class II division 1 malocclusion with good archform, deep overbite, a full unit distal occlusion and an 11 mm overjet. There is normally a good prognosis for correction of this type of occlusion (**8.6**).
Diagnosis, skeletal classification:
- Severe Class II.
- Facial type: mild brachyfacial.
- Maxilla: normal.
- Mandible: severe retrusion.
- Convexity = 7 mm.

Diagnosis, dental classification:
- Severe Class II division 1.
- Upper incisors: severe protrusion.
- Lower incisors: normal.
- No crowding.
- Overjet = 11 mm.
- Deep overbite.

Although cephalometric analysis indicates maxillary protrusion, clinical examination confirms that the profile improves when the patient postures the mandible downwards and forwards to a normal overjet with the lips closed. This is a simple diagnostic guideline which predicts the change in the facial profile as a result of functional therapy, and confirms the indication for functional correction.
Treatment plan. To improve the profile and correct to Class I occlusion with standard Twin Blocks followed by support and retention.
Bite registration. A construction bite with a blue exactobite registers an edge-to-edge occlusion with 2 mm interincisal clearance. This results in a vertical clearance in the first premolar region of 6 mm.

LJ

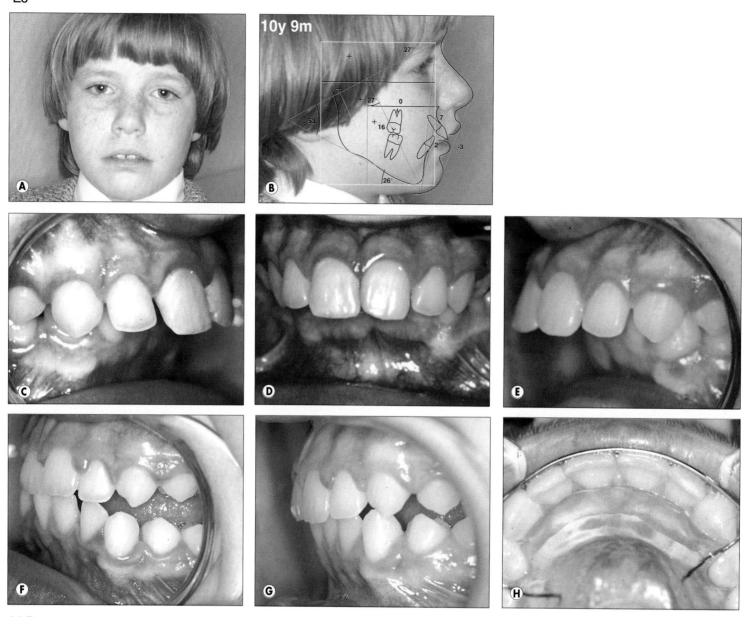

8.6 Treatment:

A, B Appearance before treatment at age 10 years 9 months.

C–E Occlusion before treatment: a narrow upper arch with a 10 mm overjet and lower incisors biting into the palate.

F After 6 months the overjet is corrected and a posterior open bite is present in the early stages of treatment. The upper block is trimmed to encourage lower molar eruption.

G After the lower molars have erupted into occlusion, the lower occlusal block is trimmed to allow the lateral open bite in the premolar region to reduce. The lower occlusal plane now begins to level, while the upper premolar height is maintained by the upper appliance. After 9 months' treatment the patient is ready to proceed to the support stage.

H An anterior inclined plane is fitted to support the corrected incisor relationship. The lower appliance is left out and the lower premolars and canines are free to erupt into occlusion.

LJ

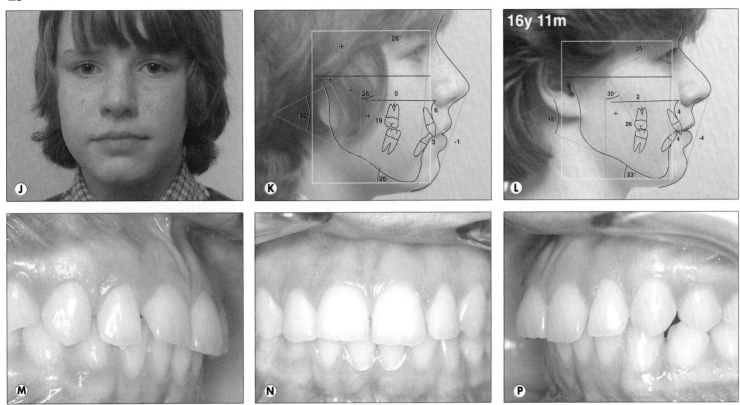

8.6 Treatment (cont.):
J, K Facial appearance after treatment.

L Profile 5 years out of retention.
M–P The occlusion 5 years out of retention

Adjustment:

- When the appliance is fitted at the insertion appointment, the patient is instructed to turn the midline screw one quarter turn per week, expanding the upper arch to assist in unlocking the mandible from distal occlusion.

- Correction of deep overbite is initiated at the start of treatment by trimming the upper bite block clear of the lower molars thereby stimulating molar eruption. It is important to leave only 1 or 2 mm occlusal clearance to encourage eruption, so that the tongue cannot spread between the teeth and delay vertical development. The leading edge of the inclined plane of the upper bite block remains intact to provide contact with the lower bite block. This contact is the key mechanism which provides the functional stimulus to growth by occlusion with the inclined plane on the lower appliance.

- To avoid gingival irritation in the initial stages of adaptation to the appliance, the fitting surface of the lower appliance is trimmed slightly in the area of the sulcus lingual to the lower incisors and canines.

After 3 months of treatment the overjet is reduced from 10 mm to 3 mm. The posterior teeth are still out of occlusion at this stage. Over the next 3 months the occlusal surface of the upper bite block is trimmed in a sequential fashion at each visit, still maintaining the leading edge of the inclined plane intact. This will eventually result in the removal of all the acrylic covering the upper molars. This allows the lower molars freedom to erupt fully into occlusion. The biting surface of the lower Twin Block is then trimmed slightly in the premolar region to allow eruption of the premolars carrying the lower appliance vertically with them as they erupt. This will then reduce the lateral open bite in the premolar region.

The open bite quickly resolves and after 6 weeks an upper support appliance is fitted with an anterior inclined plane and the lower Twin Block is left out. The occlusion settles without further adjustment. Full-time appliance wear continues for 4 months, followed by 4 months' night-time wear to retain the corrected occlusion.

Duration of treatment:

- Active phase: 7 months with Twin Blocks.
- Support phase: 4 months full time with an anterior inclined plane.
- Retention: 4 months anterior inclined plane at night only.
- Total treatment time: 15 months, including retention.
- Final records: 5 years out of retention.

LJ

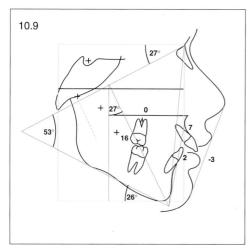

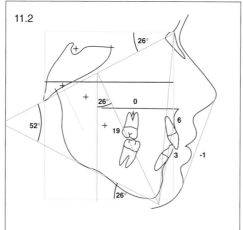

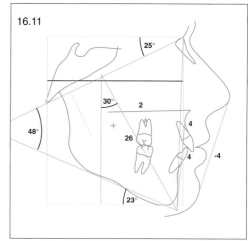

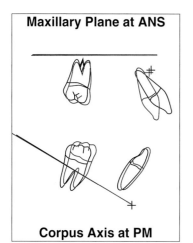

Maxillary Plane at ANS

Corpus Axis at PM

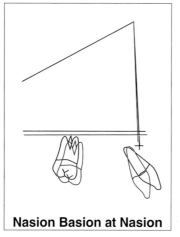

Nasion Basion at Nasion

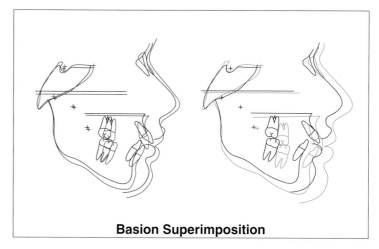

Basion Superimposition

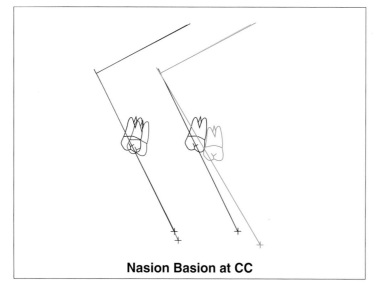

Nasion Basion at CC

L.J -	Age	10.9	11.2	16.11 (Yr.Mon)
Cranial Base Angle		27	26	25
Facial Axis Angle		27	26	30
F/M Plane Angle		26	26	23
Craniomandibular Angle		53	52	48
Maxillary Plane		0	0	2
Convexity		7	6	4
U/Incisor to Vertical		41	19	29
L/Incisor to Vertical		37	36	36
Interincisal Angle		102	125	115
6 to Pterygoid Vertical		16	19	26
L/Incisor to A/Po		2	3	4
L/Lip to Aesthetic Plane		–3	–1	–4

REACTIVATION OF TWIN BLOCKS

As indicated previously, an overjet of up to 10 mm in a patient who is growing well and has free protrusive movement may be corrected without reactivation of the Twin Blocks during treatment. If growth is less favourable, or in treatment of larger overjets, or when the protrusive path of the mandible is restricted, it is necessary to reactivate the inclined planes more gradually in progressive increments during treatment.

Reactivation is a simple procedure that is achieved by extending the anterior incline of the upper Twin Block mesially to increase the forward posture. Cold cure acrylic may be added at the chairside, inserting the appliance to record a new protrusive bite before the acrylic is fully set. Even in cases with an excessive overjet, a single reactivation of Twin Blocks is normally sufficient to correct most malocclusions (**8.7**).

It is important that no acrylic is added to the distal incline of the lower Twin Block, especially in the treatment of deep overbite. Extending occlusal acrylic of the lower block distally would prevent eruption of the lower first molar. It is necessary to leave the lower first molars free to erupt so that the overbite is reduced by increasing the vertical dimension.

If the patient's rate of growth is slow or the direction of growth is vertical rather than horizontal, it is advisable to advance the mandible more gradually over a longer period of time to allow compensatory mandibular growth to occur. This can be taken into account by reactivating Twin Blocks progressively to extend the inclined plane of the upper bite block mesially.

A preformed inclined wedge is being developed to simplify reactivation of Twin Block appliances. This allows progressive reactivation of 2, 3 or 5 mm increments using blocks which may be cold cured or light cured into place to advance the inclined plane on the upper appliance. This is designed for periodic activation in order to maximise the growth response (Petrovic & Stutzmann, 1977).

After extending the upper block forwards ,the contact of the upper block on the lower molar should be checked to make any necessary adjustment to clear the occlusion with the lower molar for correction of deep overbite.

PROGRESSIVE ACTIVATION OF TWIN BLOCKS

Progressive activation of the inclined planes is indicated as follows:

- If the overjet is greater than 10 mm it is advisable to step the mandible forwards, usually in two stages. The first activation is in the range of 7–10 mm. The second activation brings the incisors to an edge-to-edge occlusion.
- In any case where full correction of arch relationships is not achieved after the initial activation, an additional activation is necessary.
- If the direction of growth is vertical rather than horizontal, the mandible may be advanced more gradually to allow adequate time for compensatory mandibular growth to occur.
- Phased activation is recommended in adult treatment, where the muscles and ligaments are less responsive to a sudden large displacement of the mandible (see Chapter 21).
- In the treatment of temporomandibular joint dysfunction, care must be exercised so as not to introduce activation that is beyond the level of tolerance of injured tissue. It is best to be conservative and advance the mandible slowly to a position that is comfortable and will allow the patient to rest and function without discomfort.

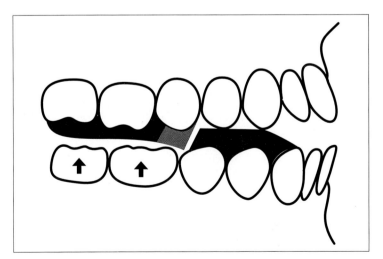

8.7 Addition of acrylic to the anterior incline of the upper inclined plane to reactivate Twin Blocks. It is incorrect to reactivate by addition to the lower Twin Block.

PK

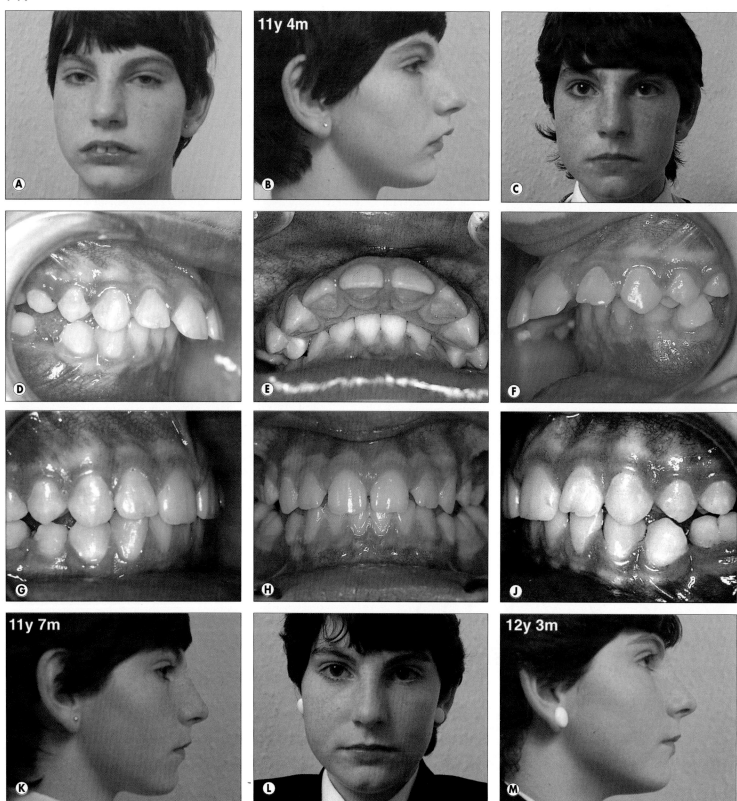

PK

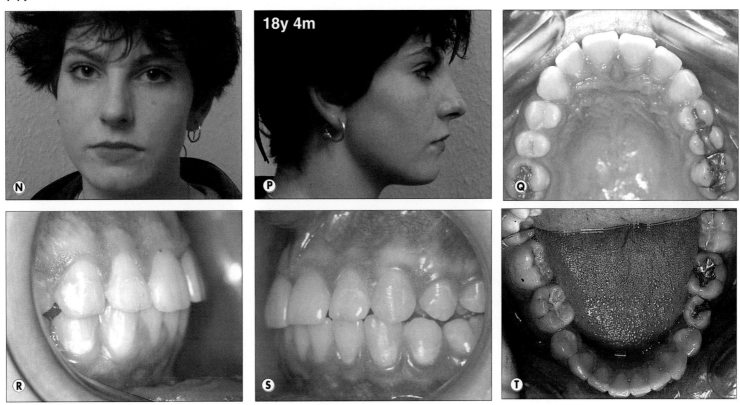

18y 4m

8.8 Treatment:

A, B Facial appearance before treatment at age 11 years 4 months.

C Facial change after 3 months treatment, showing marked physiological improvement.

D–F Occlusion before treatment: overjet = 17 mm.

G–J Occlusal change after 11 months.

K Profile at age 11 years 7 months showing rapid change after 3 months of treatment.

L, M Facial change after 11 months of treatment.

N, P Facial appearance at 18 years 4 months.

Q Upper occlusal view after treatment.

R, S Occlusion at age 18 years 7 months.

T Lower occlusal view after treatment, note congenital absence of ⎺5|.

Case report: P.K. aged 11 years 4 months

This girl presents a severe Class II division 1 malocclusion with an overjet of 17 mm that is a result of a combination of maxillary protrusion and mandibular retrusion. This case was complicated by the congenital absence of |5⎺, resulting in displacement of the lower centre line to the left (**8.8 A–T**).

Diagnosis, skeletal classification:
- Severe Class II.
- Facial type: mild brachyfacial.
- Maxilla: mild prognathic.
- Mandible: mild retrognathic.
- Convexity = 9 mm.

Diagnosis, dental classification:
- Severe Class II division 1.
- Upper incisors: severe protrusion.
- Lower incisors: moderate retrusion.
- Overjet = 17 mm.
- Excessive overbite.
- Congenitally absent: |5⎺.
- Upper pharyngeal space = 5 mm.

Treatment plan. To retract the maxilla and advance the mandible. The dental asymmetry would be difficult to eliminate in view of the absence of |5⎺. An orthodontic phase of treatment was planned to complete treatment.

PK

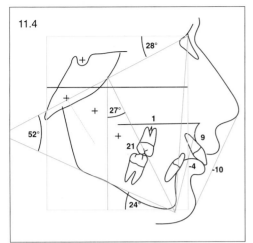

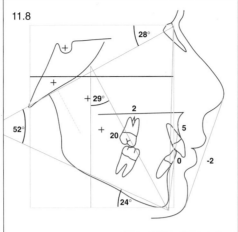

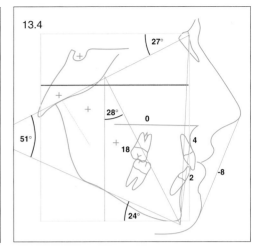

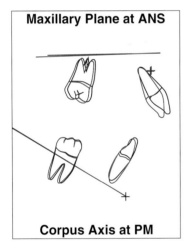

Corpus Axis at PM

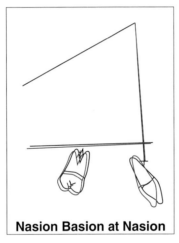

Nasion Basion at Nasion

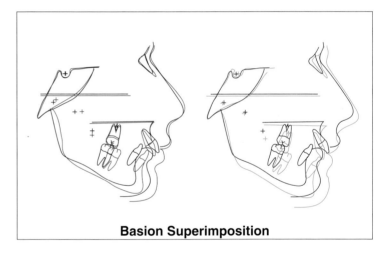

Basion Superimposition

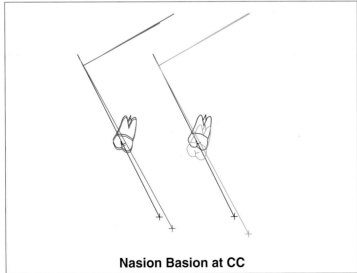

Nasion Basion at CC

P.K.. -	Age	11.4	11.8	13.4 (Yr.Mon)
Cranial Base Angle		28	28	27
Facial Axis Angle		27	29	28
F/M Plane Angle		24	24	24
Craniomandibular Angle		52	52	51
Maxillary Plane		1	2	0
Convexity		9	5	4
U/Incisor to Vertical		35	27	19
L/Incisor to Vertical		33	24	25
Interincisal Angle		112	129	136
6 to Pterygoid Vertical		21	20	18
L/Incisor to A/Po		−4	0	2
L/Lip to Aesthetic Plane		−10	−2	−8

Appliances:
- Standard Twin Blocks.
- Support phase with an anterior inclined plane.
- Fixed appliances to complete the treatment.

Adjustment. The registration bite reduced the overjet from 15 mm to 8 mm on the initial activation. This correction was achieved in 8 weeks, when the inclined planes were reactivated to an edge-to-edge incisor occlusion by adding cold cure acrylic to the mesial of the upper inclined plane. The normal adjustments were made to reduce the overbite by trimming the occlusal surface of the upper bite blocks to allow eruption of the lower molars.

Twin Blocks were effective in quickly reducing the overjet from 17 mm to 2 mm in 6 months. After 8 months of treatment the lower appliance was left out and an anterior inclined plane was fitted to retain the position as the remaining posterior open bite resolved and the buccal teeth settled into occlusion. The space was closed with a simple fixed appliance, and the slight displacement of the centre line was accepted. This was followed by an orthodontic phase to complete treatment.

Duration of treatment:
- Active phase: Twin Blocks for 7 months.
- Support phase: 6 months full-time wear.
- Orthodontic phase: 12 months.

Summary. Facial photographs before treatment show the listless appearance that is typical of many severe Class II division 1 malocclusions. This has been described as 'adenoidal facies' and is evident in the dull appearance of the eyes and poor skin tone. A distal occlusion is associated frequently with a backward tongue position, which may reduce airway efficiency. A consistent feature of functional appliance therapy in the early stages of treatment is the improvement in facial appearance. The patient appears more alert and there is a marked improvement in the eyes and the complexion. These changes are evident in the first few months of treatment. The upper pharyngeal space increased from 5 mm before treatment to 20 mm after treatment.

A functional approach achieved a rapid improvement in the profile and simplified the orthodontic treatment. It was necessary to accept some asymmetry due to the absence of the lower left second premolar.

SUMMARY: ADJUSTMENT AND CLINICAL MANAGEMENT

Stage 1: active phase
Appliance fitting

It is first necessary to check that the patient bites comfortably in a protrusive bite with the inclined planes occluding correctly. To avoid irritation as the appliance is driven home by the occlusion during the first few days of wear, it is important to relieve the lower appliance slightly over the gingivae lingual to the lower incisors. The clasps are adjusted to hold the appliance securely in position without impinging on the gingival margin. If a labial bow is present, it should be out of contact with the upper incisors.

Initial adjustment – after 10 days

The patient should now be wearing the appliances comfortably and eating with them in position. The initial discomfort of a new appliance should have resolved and the patient should be biting consistently in the protrusive bite. Patient motivation is reinforced by offering encouragement for their success on becoming accustomed to the appliance so quickly, and reassurance on any difficulties.

The patient should now be turning the upper midline screw one quarter turn per week. In the treatment of deep overbite the upper bite block should be trimmed clear of the lower molars leaving a clearance of 1–2 mm to allow these to erupt.

At this stage, it is important to detect if the patient is failing to posture forwards consistently to occlude correctly on the inclined planes. This would indicate that the appliance has been activated beyond the level of tolerance of the patient's musculature. It would then be appropriate to reduce the activation by trimming the inclined planes, to reduce the forward mandibular displacement until the patient closes comfortably on the appliances. The angulation of the inclined planes may be reduced to 45° if the patient is failing to posture consistently forwards to occlude the blocks correctly.

This may be an early sign that progress will be slower than normal, due to weakness in the patient's musculature reducing the functional response. This response is more likely in the patient who has a vertical growth pattern. Mandibular advancement will then be more gradual, usually requiring incremental activation of the occlusal inclined planes.

Adjustment visit – after 4 weeks

At the first monthly visit positive progress should already be evident with respect to better facial balance. Photographs demonstrate this very clearly, and may be repeated at this stage to record progress.

Progress can be confirmed also by noting the amount of reduction in overjet, as measured intraorally with the mandible fully retracted. To monitor progress, the overjet should be measured and noted on the record card at each visit. This allows any lapse in progress or cooperation to be detected readily. There should be a steady and consistent reduction of overjet and correction of distal occlusion. If cooperation is suspect it is advisable to fix the appliance in place in the mouth to exert immediate control and restore full-time appliance wear.

Apart from monitoring progress, only minor adjustment is required at this stage. Check that the screw is operating correctly, and adjust the clasps if necessary to improve retention. If the appliance includes a labial bow, adjust it so as to be out of contact with the upper incisors.

In the treatment of deep overbite ensure that the lower molars are not in contact with the upper block. The upper block is trimmed occlusodistally to clear the occlusion, using a probe (explorer) to confirm that the lower molars do not contact the upper block.

Routine adjustment – time interval 6 weeks
A similar pattern of adjustment continues with steady correction of distal occlusion and reduction of overjet. The upper archwidth is checked at each visit, until the expansion is sufficient to accommodate the lower arch in its corrected position and no further turns of the screw are required.

Trimming of the upper block continues until all the occlusal cover is removed from the upper molars to allow the lower molars to erupt completely into occlusion.

The overjet, overbite and distal occlusion should be fully corrected by the end of the Twin Block phase. A slight open bite in the buccal segments should be limited to the premolar region. It is now appropriate to proceed to the support phase.

Stage 2: support phase

Anteroposterior and vertical control remain equally important in the support phase to maintain the correction achieved in the active phase.

The purpose of the support phase is to maintain the corrected incisor relationship until the buccal segment occlusion is fully established. To achieve this objective, an upper removable appliance is fitted with an anterior inclined plane to engage the lower incisors and canines.

The lower appliance is left out at this stage and removal of the posterior bite blocks allows the posterior teeth to erupt into occlusion. The anterior inclined plane extends distally to engage all six lower anterior teeth and the patient must not be able to occlude lingual to the inclined plane. It must be adequate to retain the incisor relationship effectively, but at the same time should be neat and unobtrusive so as not to interfere with speech.

Many anterior inclined planes are mistakenly made too large and bulky which causes discomfort for the patient, who may then be discouraged from wearing such an appliance. There is no necessity for the anterior inclined plane to extend much beyond the level of the incisal tips of the upper incisors, provided it also extends far enough distally to engage the canines.

The patient must understand the importance of wearing the support appliance full time to prevent relapse at this critical stage of treatment. An appliance that is comfortable and carefully designed is more readily accepted by the patient.

Vertical control is essential during the support phase after reduc-tion of overbite. To maintain the corrected vertical dimension, a flat occlusal stop of acrylic extends forwards from the inclined plane to engage the lower incisors. The occlusal stop is an important addition to maintain the corrected intergingival height as the posterior teeth erupt into occlusion. The upper and lower buccal teeth should normally settle into occlusion within 2–6 months, depending on the depth of the overbite.

Retention

Treatment is followed by a normal period of retention. As the buccal segments settle in fully, full-time wear of the support appliance allows time for internal bony remodelling to support the corrected occlusion. A good buccal segment occlusion is the cornerstone of stability after correction of arch-to-arch relationships. Appliance wear is reduced to night-time only when the occlusion is fully established.

If treatment is carried out in the mixed dentition, retention may continue with an anterior inclined plane to support the occlusion during the transition to the permanent dentition. In early treatment of severe skeletal discrepancies a night-time functional appliance of the monobloc type may be used as a retainer. This gives additional functional support and may be activated to enhance the orthopaedic response to treatment during the transitional dentition.

Advantages of Twin Blocks

The Twin Block is the most comfortable, the most aesthetic and the most efficient of all the functional appliances. Twin Blocks have many advantages compared to other functional appliances:

- *Comfort.* Patients wear Twin Blocks 24 hours per day and can eat comfortably with the appliances in place.
- *Aesthetics.* Twin Blocks can be designed with no visible anterior wires without losing efficiency in correction of arch relationships.
- *Function.* The occlusal inclined plane is the most natural of all the functional mechanisms. There is less interference with normal function because the mandible can move freely in anterior and lateral excursion without being restricted by a bulky one-piece appliance.
- *Patient compliance.* Twin Blocks may be fixed to the teeth temporarily or permanently to guarantee patient compliance. Removable Twin Blocks can be fixed in the mouth for the first week or 10 days of treatment to ensure that the patient adapts fully to wearing them 24 hours per day.
- *Facial appearance.* From the moment Twin Blocks are fitted the appearance is noticeably improved. The absence of lip, cheek or tongue pads, as used in some other appliances, places no restriction on normal function, and does not distort the patient's facial appearance during treatment. Improvements in facial balance are seen progressively in the first 3 months of treatment.

- *Speech.* Patients can learn to speak normally with Twin Blocks. In comparison with other functional appliances, Twin Blocks do not distort speech by restricting movement of the tongue, lips or mandible.

- *Clinical management.* Adjustment and activation is simple. The appliances are robust and not prone to breakage. Chairside time is reduced in achieving major orthopaedic correction.

- *Arch development.* Twin Blocks allow independent control of upper and lower archwidth. Appliance design is easily modified for transverse and sagittal arch development.

- *Mandibular repositioning.* Full-time wear consistently achieve rapid mandibular repositioning that remains stable out of retention.

- *Vertical control.* Twin Blocks achieve excellent control of the vertical dimension in treatment of deep overbite and anterior open bite. Vertical control is significantly improved by full-time wear.

- *Facial asymmetry.* Asymmetrical activation corrects facial and dental asymmetry in the growing child.

- *Safety.* Twin Blocks can be worn during sports activies with the exception of swimming and violent contact sports, when they may be removed for safety.

- *Efficiency.* Twin Blocks achieve more rapid correction of mal-occlusion compared to one-piece functional appliances because they are worn full time. This benefits patients in all age groups.

- *Age of treatment.* Arch relationships can be corrected from early childhood to adulthood. However, treatment is slower in adults and the response is less predictable.

- *Integration with fixed appliances.* Integration with conventional fixed appliances is simpler than with any other functional appliance. In combined techniques, Twin Blocks can be used to maximise the skeletal correction while fixed appliances are used to detail the occlusion. Because Twin Blocks need have no anterior wires, brackets can be placed on the anterior teeth to correct tooth alignment simultaneously with correction of arch relationships during the orthopaedic phase. During the support phase an easy transition can be made to fixed appliances.

- *Treatment of temporomandibular joint dysfunction.* The Twin Block may at times also be used as an effective splint in treatment of patients who present temporomandibular joint dysfunction due to displacement of the condyle distal to the articular disc. Full-time wear allows the disc to be recaptured, when disc reduction is possible in early stage TMJ problems, and at the same time sagittal, vertical and transverse arch development proceeds to eliminate unfavourable occlusal contacts (see Chapter 21.)

CHAPTER
9

Treatment in Mixed Dentition

Treatment of skeletal discrepancies should not be delayed until the permanent dentition has been established. Interceptive treatment is indicated frequently in the mixed dentition to restore normal function and correct arch relationships by means of functional appliance therapy.

Prominent upper incisors are vulnerable to accidental trauma and breakage, and early treatment is advisable to avoid fracture or damage by placing the incisors within the protection of the lips. Early treatment of crowded dentitions can combine arch development with correction of arch relationships.

The principles of treatment are unchanged in the mixed dentition although the response to treatment may prove to be slower depending on the patient's rate of growth. Bite registration follows the same procedures as described for treatment in the permanent dentition.

APPLIANCE DESIGN

Appliance design may be modified to meet the requirements of the mixed dentition, when retention may be limited by deciduous teeth that are unfavourably shaped with respect to adequately accepting retention clasps of removable appliances.

Standard Twin Block appliance design for Class II division 1 malocclusion in the mixed dentition is similar to appliance design for the permanent dentition. Delta clasps may be fitted on lower first or second deciduous molars if they are suitably shaped for retention.

Alternatively, C-clasps may be used for retention on deciduous molars. The C-clasp is well suited to this stage of development of the dentition and there are several ways to improve retention even if the teeth are unfavourably shaped (**9.1 A, B**)

The simplest method of improving retention on deciduous teeth is to bond composite on to the buccal surfaces of these teeth to create an additional undercut. Both cooperation and retention can be improved by bonding C-clasps directly to deciduous molars for the first week or 10 days before freeing the clasps and rounding the edges of the composite that remains attached to the teeth to improve retention.

It is also possible to grind retention grooves into the buccal surfaces of deciduous teeth to improve undercuts, for example, gingival to the line of a C-clasp. Alternatively, a round bur may be used to grind a concavity to accommodate a ball clasp. Sealant can then be applied to protect the tooth and a ready-made undercut has been created to improve retention.

Synthetic crown contours (Truax), which are preformed plastic pads, may be bonded to the buccal surfaces of deciduous cuspids and molars to reshape these teeth with additional undercuts. This will then improve the retention of clasps (**9.2**).

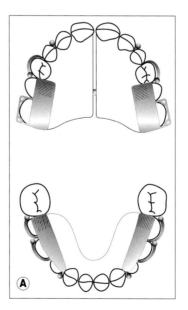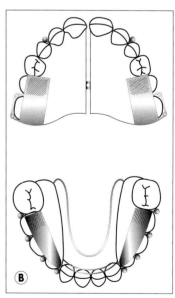

9.1 A, B Typical appliance design for mixed dentition.

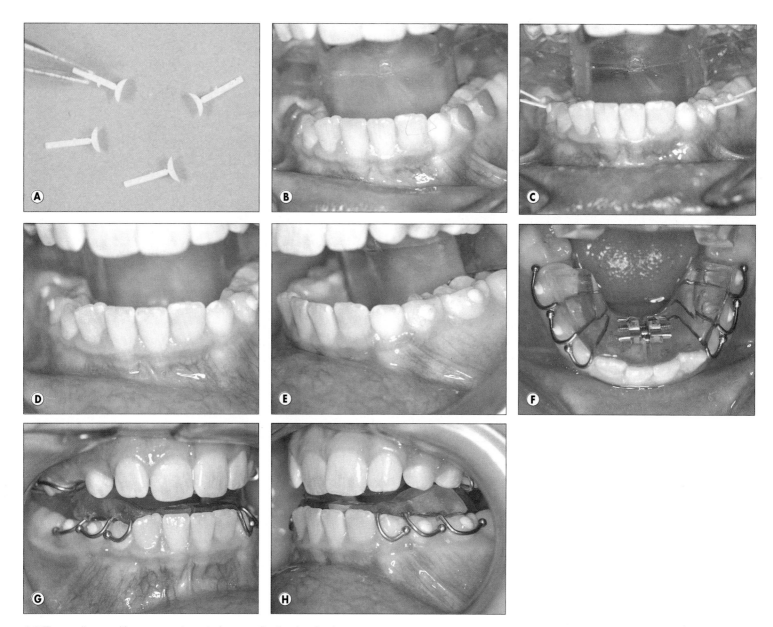

9.2 The appliance with crown contours to improve fixation in mixed dentition:

A Crown contours.

B Etching deciduous molars with paper pads soaked in etching fluid.

C The crown contours bonded to the teeth.

D, E After cutting off the sprues, the impression is taken to make the appliance.

F–H The C-clasps are shaped to gain retention from the crown contours.

FD

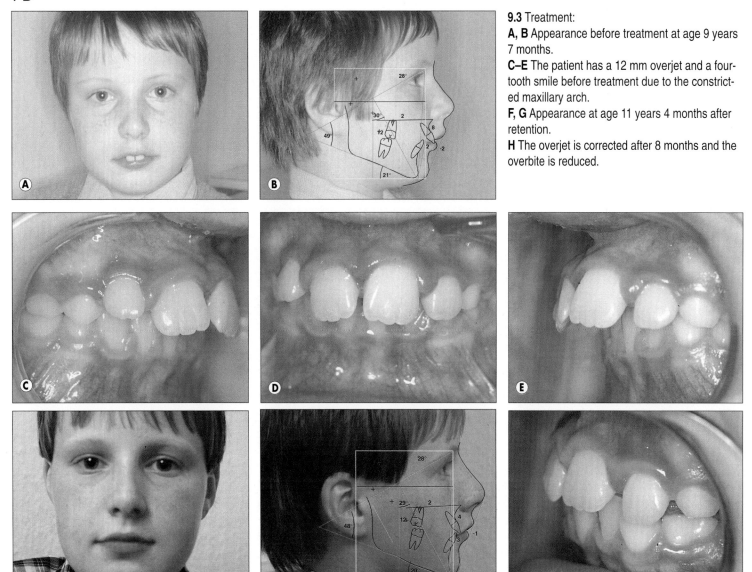

9.3 Treatment:

A, B Appearance before treatment at age 9 years 7 months.

C–E The patient has a 12 mm overjet and a four-tooth smile before treatment due to the constricted maxillary arch.

F, G Appearance at age 11 years 4 months after retention.

H The overjet is corrected after 8 months and the overbite is reduced.

Case report: F.D. aged 9 years 7 months

This is a typical example of a young boy in mixed dentition who has a severe Class II dental relationship with the lower lip trapped under a large overjet of 12 mm. Early treatment is indicated for many reasons, not least of which is to protect the upper incisors from injury by placing them inside the protective envelope of the lips (**9.3**).

Diagnosis, skeletal classification:
*   Severe Class II.
*   Facial type: severe brachyfacial.
*   Severe maxillary protrusion.
*   Mandible normal.
*   Convexity = 9 mm.

Diagnosis, dental classification:
*   Severe Class II division 1.
*   Upper incisors: severe protrusion.
*   Lower incisors: mild retrusion.
*   Overjet = 12 mm.
*   Overbite = 3 mm with lower incisors biting in the palate.
*   Full unit distal occlusion.
*   No crowding.
*   Upper pharyngeal airway = 8 mm.

On clinical examination the profile improves when the mandible postures forwards with the lips closed together. This is a fundamental diagnostic criterion for functional therapy, and takes precedence over

FD

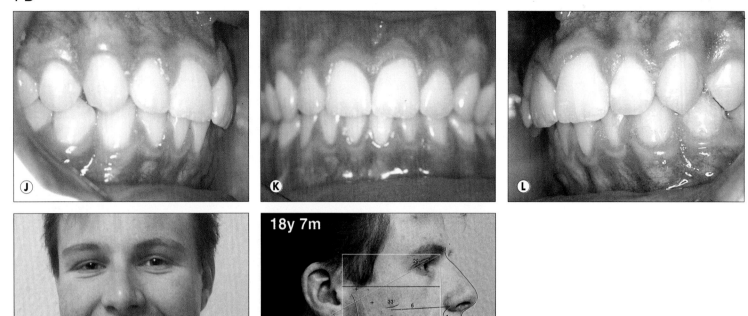

9.3 Treatment (cont.):
J–L Occlusion at age 18 years. No further treatment was required after support and retention.
M Appearance at age 16 years 7 months.
N Profile at age 18 years 7 months.

other factors in analysis. Although cephalometric analysis confirms severe maxillary protrusion, correction is planned by mandibular advancement to compensate for the forward position of the maxilla.

Treatment plan. To expand the upper arch, reduce the overjet and correct the distal occlusion. Reciprocal functional forces aim to correct arch relationships by a combination of maxillary retraction and mandibular advancement to improve the skeletal discrepancy between maxillary and mandibular development.

Appliances:
- Standard Twin Blocks for functional correction, designed to open the bite by increasing the vertical dimension.
- Anterior inclined plane to support the vertical and anteroposterior correction as the buccal teeth erupt fully into occlusion.
- Retain during the transition to permanent dentition.

Bite registration. The construction bite is registered with a blue exactobite gauge to reduce the overjet by 8 mm on the first activation with 2 mm interincisal clearance. A second activation of the Twin Blocks is planned during treatment for anteroposterior correction because the overjet is too large to reduce by a single activation.

Adjustment. The midline screw is turned one quarter turn per week for 4 months to expand the upper arch. In the early stages of treatment the upper blocks are trimmed horizontally in the molar region to encourage eruption of lower molars for overbite reduction. The initial construction bite reduces the overjet from 12 mm to 4 mm.

After 6 months the Twin Blocks are reactivated to an edge-to-edge incisor relationship by addition of acrylic to the mesial of the inclined plane of the upper blocks. It is important to remember that this activation is made by adjustment to the upper Twin Block, as addition to the lower bite blocks would obstruct lower molar eruption and would interfere with reduction of the overbite.

Duration of treatment:
- Active phase: 1 year with Twin Blocks.
- Support phase: 6 months full-time with an upper anterior inclined plane.
- Retention: 2 years of night-time wear with an anterior inclined plane until the occlusion is fully established in the permanent dentition.

After treatment in the mixed dentition there is diminished occlusal support during the transition to the permanent dentition. A night-time functional appliance may be selected as a retention appliance to provide a positive functional stimulus to growth during the transition from mixed to permanent dentition. For example, the occluso-guide is a simple preformed appliance, resembling a mini-positioner, which can be worn at night to retain the incisor and molar relationship, while

FD

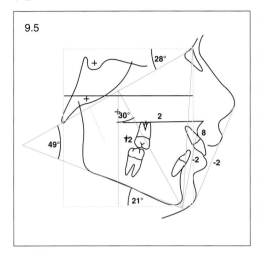

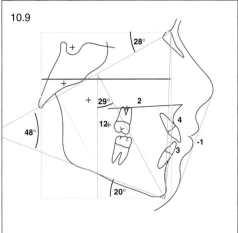

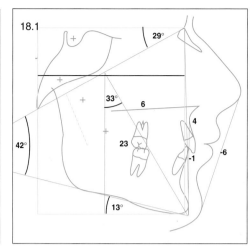

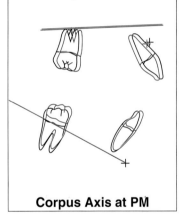

Maxillary Plane at ANS

Corpus Axis at PM

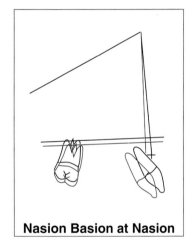

Nasion Basion at Nasion

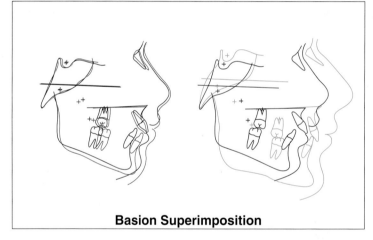

Basion Superimposition

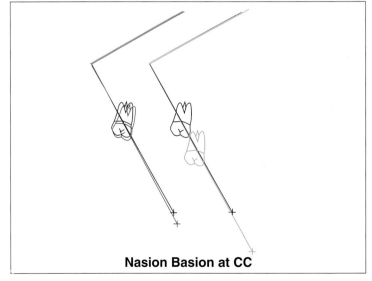

Nasion Basion at CC

F.D. -	Age	9.5	10.9	18.1	(Yr.Mon)
Cranial Base Angle		28	28	29	
Facial Axis Angle		30	29	33	
F/M Plane Angle		21	20	13	
Craniomandibular Angle		49	48	42	
Maxillary Plane		2	2	6	
Convexity		8	4	4	
U/Incisor to Vertical		35	35	24	
L/Incisor to Vertical		35	34	24	
Interincisal Angle		110	111	132	
6 to Pterygoid Vertical		12	12	23	
L/Incisor to A/Po		–2	3	–1	
L/Lip to Aesthetic Plane		–2	–1	–6	

maintaining space for eruption of premolars and canines.

Final records. Five years out of retention at age 18 years, when the occlusion has settled satisfactorily without further treatment.

Growth change. The upper pharyngeal airway increased from 8 to 11 mm during the Twin Block stage of treatment. Facial convexity reduced from 9 to 4 mm during treatment as a result of horizontal mandibular growth. Post-treatment change shows a further reduction of convexity to 3 mm at the age of 18. Although maxillary growth continued in the middle and late teens, compensatory mandibular growth maintained the improvement achieved during functional correction by the Twin Blocks in the mixed dentition. No further treatment was carried out and the occlusion is stable 5 years out of retention at the age of 18 years.

TRANSVERSE DEVELOPMENT

Twin Blocks for Arch Development

Case report: A.G. aged 9 years 6 months

This boy has a mild Class II division 1 malocclusion in the mixed dentition and a normal skeletal base relationship with a straight facial profile. The maxilla is narrow and there is crowding in the lower labial segment. The profile dictates nonextraction therapy and expansion is indicated in both arches. The orthopaedic phase of treatment was initiated before the growth spurt during a period of slow growth, to minimise the skeletal change. No labial bow is used in order to maintain the labial position of the upper incisors. This case illustrates the use of upper and lower Schwarz Twin Blocks for expansion in both arches in mixed dentition (**9.4, 9.5 A–S**).

Diagnosis, skeletal classification:
* Class I.
* Facial type: severe brachyfacial.
* Maxilla: mild retrognathic – contracted laterally.
* Mandible: normal.
* Convexity = 1 mm.

Diagnosis, dental classification:
* Moderate Class II division 1.
* Upper incisors: protrusive.
* Lower incisors: normal.
* Overjet = 8mm.
* Deep overbite.
* Full unit distal occlusion.
* Lower incisor crowding = 7 mm.
* Airway: normal.

Treatment plan:
* Orthopaedic phase: correct to Class I occlusion and expand the upper and lower arches laterally to develop the archform. Also increase the vertical dimension by controlled eruption of posterior teeth.

* Support phase: maintain the corrected occlusion and continue to support and establish the vertical dimension.
* Orthodontic phase: align the lower labial segment and detail the occlusion.

Appliances:
* Twin Blocks to expand both arches and advance the mandible.
* Anterior inclined plane with a flat occlusal stop to maintain the vertical dimension. Wilson lower lingual arch to maintain the archform.
* Lower fixed appliance to align and detail the occlusion.
* Positioner to retain.

Duration of treatment:
* Orthopaedic phase: the overjet and distal occlusion were corrected in 4 months. The active phase continued for an additional 8 months to allow for vertical development.
* Support phase: night-time appliance wear continued until premolars and canines erupted.
* Orthodontic phase: 6 months to complete.
* Retention: 1 year.

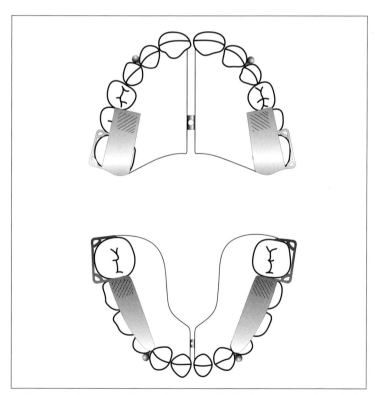

9.4 The use of upper and lower Schwarz Twin Blocks for expansion in both arches in mixed dentition.

AG

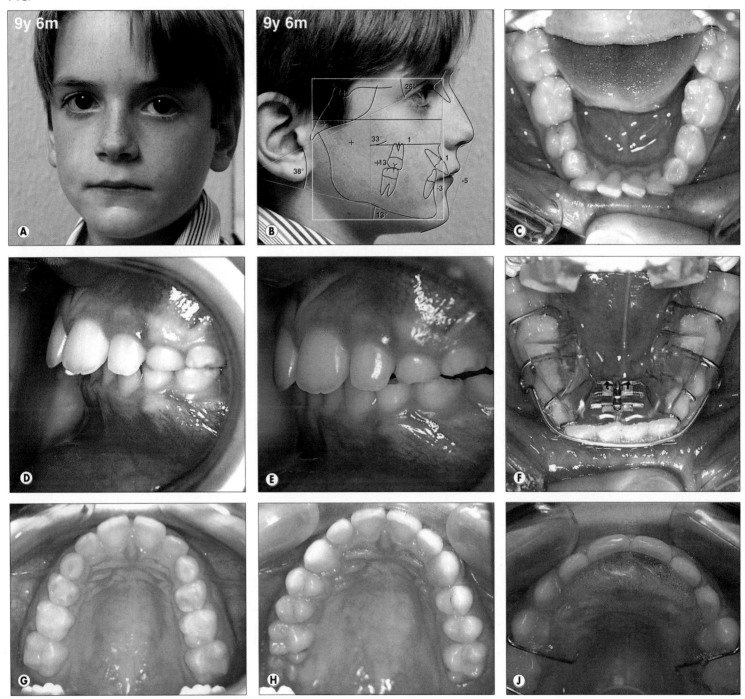

9.5 Treatment:

A, B Facial appearance at age 9 years 6 months.

C Lower arch before treatment.

D, E Overjet correction after 4 months of treatment.

F The lower Twin Block has a midline screw for expansion.

G, H Expansion achieved in the upper arch.

J The anterior inclined plane with occlusal stops to control the vertical dimension.

AG

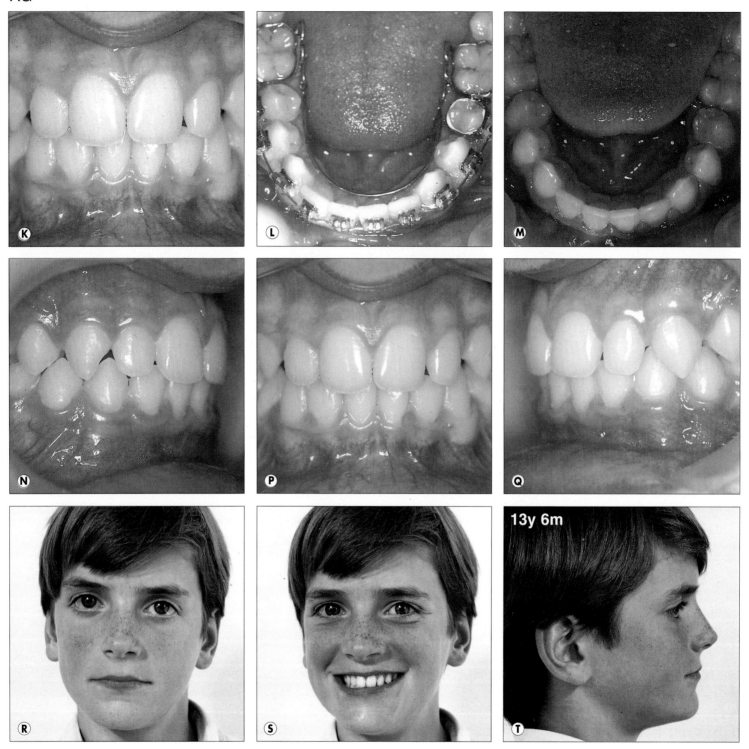

9.5 Treatment (cont.)
K Retention continued until the premolars and canines erupted.
L, M Because of the lower arch crowding a lower fixed appliance with three-dimensional control is necessary to correct the labial segment.

N–Q Occlusion at age 13 years 6 months.
R–T Appearance at age 13 years 6 months.

AG

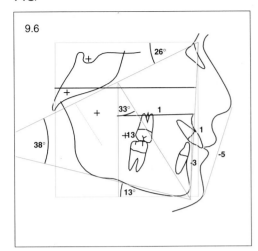

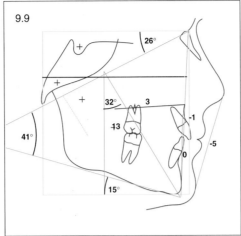

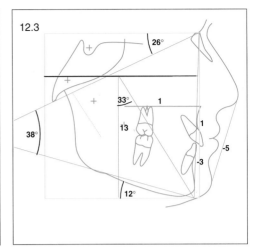

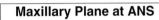

Maxillary Plane at ANS

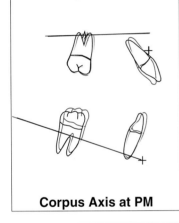

Corpus Axis at PM

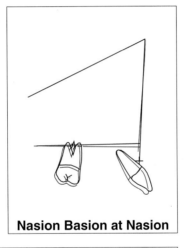

Nasion Basion at Nasion

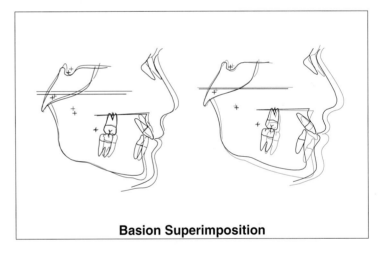

Basion Superimposition

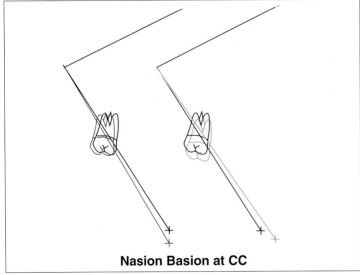

Nasion Basion at CC

A.G. -	Age	9.6	9.9	12.3	(Yr.Mon)
Cranial Base Angle		26	26	26	
Facial Axis Angle		33	32	33	
F/M Plane Angle		13	15	12	
Craniomandibular Angle		38	41	38	
Maxillary Plane		1	3	1	
Convexity		1	−1	1	
U/Incisor to Vertical		42	32	31	
L/Incisor to Vertical		18	22	21	
Interincisal Angle		120	126	128	
6 to Pterygoid Vertical		13	13	13	
L/Incisor to A/Po		−3	0	−3	
L/Lip to Aesthetic Plane		−5	−5	−5	

TWO-PHASE TREATMENT IN MIXED AND PERMANENT DENTITION

Case report: J.C. aged 8 years 9 months

This boy presents a disfiguring malocclusion in the early mixed dentition with the upper incisors extremely vulnerable to trauma, resting completely outside the lower lip. The lower lip is trapped under an overjet of 15 mm. The lower incisors are biting into the soft tissue of the palate 5 mm lingual to the upper incisors. Early treatment is essential in this type of malocclusion to place the upper incisors safely under lip control. The maxilla is typically narrow with a full unit distal occlusion. A 'gummy' smile necessitates intrusion of the upper incisors during treatment to improve the position of the upper lip relative to the incisors. This will improve to some extent when the patient develops a lip seal during the Twin Block phase, but a further stage may be necessary to intrude the upper incisors (**9.6 A–Z**).

Diagnosis, skeletal classification:
- Severe Class II.
- Facial type: mesofacial, brachyfacial tendency
- Maxilla: normal.
- Mandible: retrognathic.
- Convexity = 9 mm.

Diagnosis, dental classification:
- Severe Class II division 1.
- Upper incisors: severe protrusion.
- Lower incisors: slight retrusion.
- Overjet = 15 mm.
- Deep overbite.
- Full unit distal occlusion.
- Upper pharyngeal space = 7 mm.

Cephalometric analysis. In this case the A-point is close to the nasion vertical, which confirms that the maxilla is related correctly to the anterior cranial base. The chin point, pogonion, is set back from the nasion vertical, confirming that severe mandibular retrusion is the underlying cause of the malocclusion.

In this case, mandibular retrusion is due to horizontal flexion of the cranial base to the Frankfort plane, which results in a high distal position of the temporomandibular joint. This is confirmed by a reduced cranial base angle of 25° (the ideal is 29°). As a result, the gradient of chin growth is vertical. The facial axis angle is 25° (the ideal is 29°).

Treatment plan. The objective of the first stage of treatment is to expand the maxilla laterally and to advance the mandible to improve the mandibular retrusion, followed by support and retention in the transition from mixed to permanent dentition. A final orthodontic phase of treatment is planned in the permanent dentition with fixed appliances to detail the occlusion and improve the 'gummy' smile.

Appliances:
- Active phase: Twin Blocks for functional correction.
- Support and retention: an upper removable appliance with an anterior inclined plane during the transition to the permanent dentition.
- Orthodontic phase: bioprogressive technique with utility arches to intrude the upper and lower incisors to overcorrect the overbite and improve the smile line.

Bite registration. Functional correction is planned in two steps to reduce the excessive overjet of 15 mm. The Twin Blocks are constructed to a registration bite that reduces the overjet initially by 8 mm, planning to reactivate the blocks during treatment to complete reduction of the overjet.

Appliance design. In order to reduce the overbite it is essential to leave the lower molars free of any obstruction that would inhibit vertical development. The lower Twin Block is designed so as not to extend distally over the first permanent molar region. It is retained by clasps on the second deciduous molars with the addition of three ball-ended clasps in the lower incisor region.

Adjustment. The midline screw expands the maxilla to accommodate the forward positioning of the lower dental arch. The occlusion is checked at each visit to monitor expansion and to coordinate arch width. In this case upper arch expansion is complete after 4 months, operating the midline screw one quarter turn per week.

Vertical development to reduce the overbite is effected by trimming the upper bite block to encourage eruption of the lower molars. The upper Twin Block is trimmed occluso-distally to clear bite block acrylic from over the lower molars when the Twin Blocks are first fitted and also at subsequent visits to allow the lower molars to erupt continuously into occlusion. An occlusal clearance of 1–2 mm is maintained to allow the lower molars to erupt. This amount of clearance does not allow the tongue to spread laterally between the teeth, which might delay eruption.

After 4 months, the occlusion has corrected by 8 mm to the position of initial activation of the occlusal inclined planes and the Twin Block is now reactivated by the addition of acrylic to the mesial incline of the upper appliance. This adjustment is made at the chairside to bring the mandible forwards to an edge-to-edge incisor relationship to complete correction of the overjet.

Duration of treatment:
- Active phase: mixed dentition – Twin Blocks were worn for 14 months to achieve full correction to a Class I occlusion.
- Support and retention: the anterior inclined plane was worn full time for 6 months, followed by night-time retention in transition to the permanent dentition.
- Orthodontic phase: orthopaedic correction to a Class I occlusion was followed in the permanent dentition by a short period of orthodontic treatment during which time fixed appliances were worn for a year to detail the occlusion. A utility arch was used to intrude the upper incisors to improve the 'gummy' smile.

JC

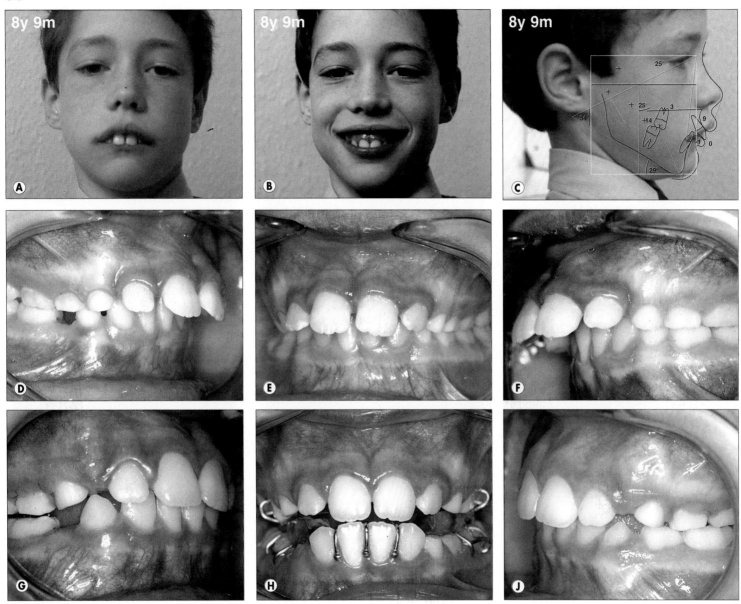

9.6 Treatment:

A–C Appearance before treatment at age 8 years 9 months. Note the 'gummy' smile.

D–F Occlusion before treatment.

G–J Twin Blocks were worn for 14 months.
Occlusion after 8 months of treatment.

JC

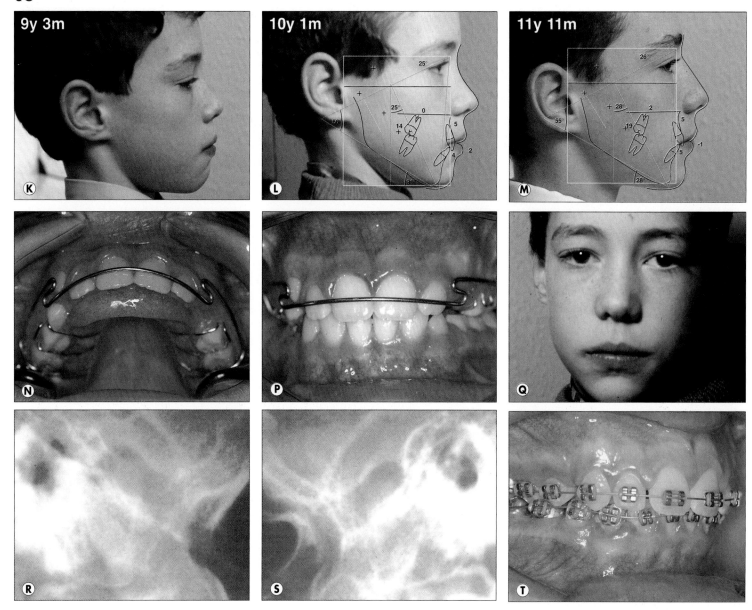

9y 3m

K

10y 1m

25°

25°   0

14

50

5

L

11y 11m

26

28   2

19   5

55

5

-1

28

M

N

P

Q

R

S

T

9.6 Treatment (cont.):
K Profile afer 6 months of treatment.
L Profile after treatment at age 10 years 1 months.
M Profile at age 11 years 11 months – before the fixed appliances.
N, P Upper retainer with an anterior inclined plane.

Q After treatment at age 10 years 1 months.
R, S Radiographs in occlusion confirm the good relationship of the condyles in the glenoid fossae at age 13 years 6 months.
T Orthodontic phase – the fixed appliances.

JC

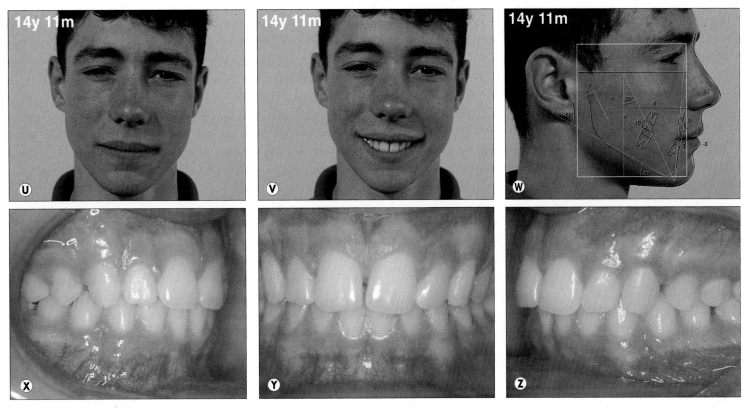

9.6 Treatment (cont.):
U–W Facial views 1 year out of retention at age 14 years 11 months.
X–Z Occlusion 1 year out of retention at age 14 years 11 months.

Response to treatment. The upper pharyngeal space increased from 7–11 mm after 1 year's treatment, then to 14 mm 2 years later and, finally, to 21 mm after 6 years.

Radiographic examination of the temporomandibular joints confirm that the condyles are in good position in the articular fossa at the age of 11 years 11 months, 3 years after the start of treatment.

The mandibular length, measured from the articular to the gnathion, increased by 16 mm during 16 months of Twin Block treatment, and by 6 mm in the subsequent 22 months of retention. This represents 22 mm over a period of 3 years, during the Twin Block phase of treatment and subsequent retention in the transition to permanent dentition. The average annual growth increment of boys in this age group is 2.4 mm, equivalent to 7.2 mm in 3 years.

In cephalometric analysis, we are accustomed to assessing growth increments in two dimensions on a cephalometric film in 'norma lateralis'. It is important to take into account that growth occurs in three dimensions and, therefore, the increase in mandibular size, in this case from condyle-to-condyle, totals 44 mm in 3 years, compared to a mean increase of 14.4 mm in the control. The gain in mandibular length compared to average growth, expressed in control values, is 29.6 mm.

In comparing values before the Twin Block stage of treatment and after an interval of 3 years, angular change does not appear to be significant, whereas linear analysis shows an exceptional growth response.

Differing interpretations of the results of functional therapy may be related to the method of analysis. This case demonstrates the divergence of views that can result from angular and linear interpretation. Angular changes can be misleading, especially if the direction of growth is along a vertical facial axis, as in this case. Significant linear growth does not register a significant angular change if the direction of growth is on a vertical axis.

JC

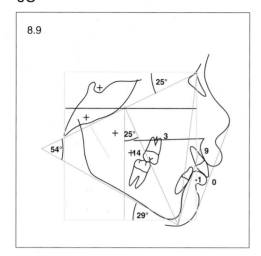

8.9

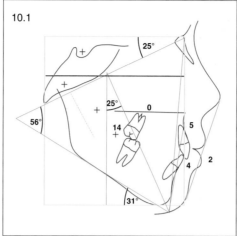

10.1

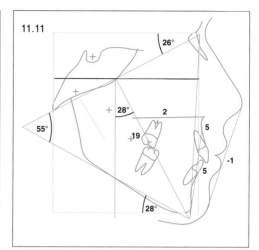

11.11

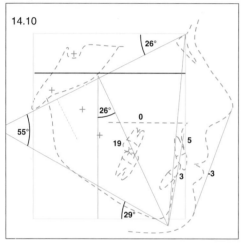

14.10

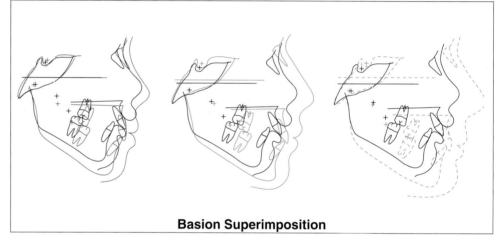

Basion Superimposition

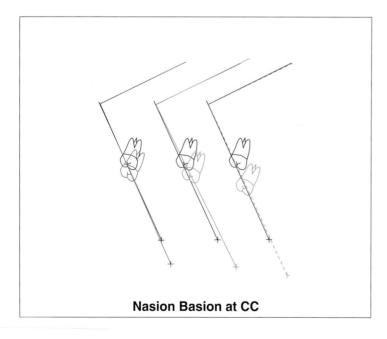

Nasion Basion at CC

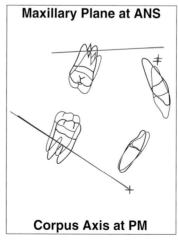

Maxillary Plane at ANS

Corpus Axis at PM

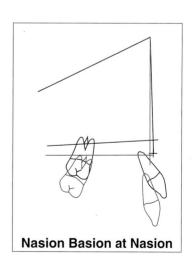

Nasion Basion at Nasion

J.C. - Age (Yr.Mon)	8.9	10.1	11.11	14.10
Cranial Base Angle	25	25	26	26
Facial Axis Angle	25	25	28	26
F/M Plane Angle	29	31	28	29
Craniomandibular Angle	54	56	55	55
Maxillary Plane	3	0	2	0
Convexity	9	5	5	5
U/Incisor to Vertical	30	12	23	14
L/Incisor to Vertical	32	41	40	41
Interincisal Angle	118	127	117	125
6 to Pterygoid Vertical	14	14	19	19
L/Incisor to A/Po	−1	4	5	3
L/Lip to Aesthetic Plane	0	2	−1	−3

Case report: J.B. aged 9 years 11 months

This girl presents a Class II division 1 malocclusion with a prognathic facial profile. A tongue thrust is associated with an incomplete overbite and incompetent lip behaviour. Treatment was initiated in mixed dentition and completed in permanent dentition (**9.7A–T**).

Diagnosis, skeletal classification:
- Mild Class II.
- Facial type: severe brachyfacial.
- Maxilla: severe prognathic.
- Mandible: mild protrusion.
- Convexity = 5 mm.

Diagnosis, dental classification:
- Severe Class II division 1.
- Upper incisors: mild protrusion.
- Lower incisors: normal.
- Overjet = 7 mm.
- Anterior open bite due to tongue thrust.
- No crowding.
- Upper pharyngeal airway = 7 mm.

Although cephalometric analysis shows a prognathic tendency, the profile improves when the mandible postures forwards. This confirms that functional therapy will improve the profile in spite of the prognathic growth pattern. Clinical assessment takes precedence over cephalometric norms in predicting the response to a functional approach to treatment.

Appliances:
- Twin Blocks in mixed dentition.
- Anterior inclined plane for support and retention.
- Detailing by fixed appliances in permanent dentition.
- For a short period Twin Blocks were integrated with fixed appliances to improve the profile.

Adjustment. The upper arch was expanded to accommodate advancement of the lower arch. The edge-to-edge construction bite produced a rapid response to initial correction. The overjet corrected from 9 mm to 4 mm in 6 weeks and the incisors were in edge-to-edge occlusion in 3 months. The upper pharyngeal airway increased from 7 to 9 mm during treatment.

A new upper appliance was fitted with a tongue guard formed from heavy gauge wire, which also served as an anterior inclined plane to retain the corrected incisor relationship. This appliance was effective in retaining the advanced mandibular position through the transition into permanent dentition.

After 18 months of treatment with functional appliances, upper and lower fixed appliances were fitted to complete the treatment.

Growth during support and retention resulted in a slight return of convexity in the profile. Twin Blocks were integrated with fixed appliances for 3 months to improve the facial result before detailing the occlusion with fixed appliances. The additional short orthopaedic phase was successful in improving the profile.

JB

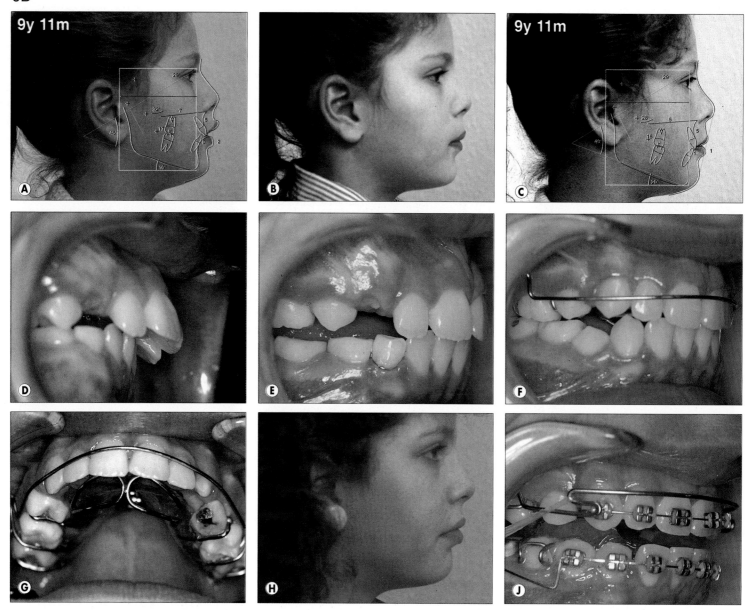

9.7 Treatment:
A–C Profile before treatment, after 6 weeks and after 9 months.
D–F Occlusion before treatment, after 6 weeks and after 1 year.
G The recurved lingual tongue guard acts as an inclined plane.
H Profile before orthodontic phase at age 11 years 11 months.
J Phase 2: Twin Blocks combined with fixed appliance.

Case report: J.B. aged 9 years 11 months

This girl presents a Class II division 1 malocclusion with a prognathic facial profile. A tongue thrust is associated with an incomplete overbite and incompetent lip behaviour. Treatment was initiated in mixed dentition and completed in permanent dentition (**9.7A–T**).

Diagnosis, skeletal classification:

- Mild Class II.
- Facial type: severe brachyfacial.
- Maxilla: severe prognathic.
- Mandible: mild protrusion.
- Convexity = 5 mm.

JB

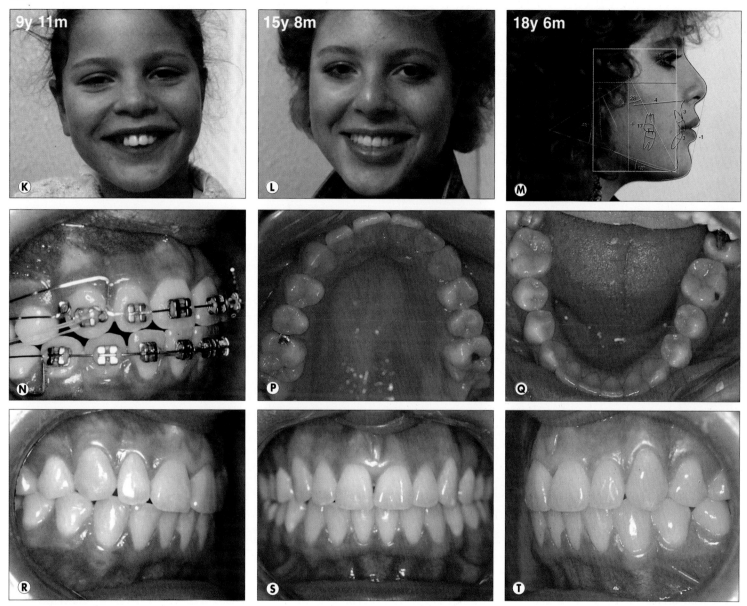

9.7 Treatment (cont.):

K, L Facial appearance at age 9 years 11 months and 15 years 8 months.

M Profile at age 18 years 6 months.

N Fixed appliance to finish.

P, Q Occlusal views after treatment.

R–T Occlusion at age 18 years 6 months.

JB

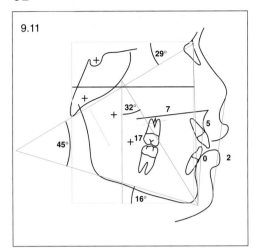

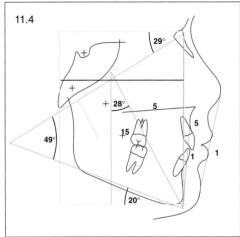

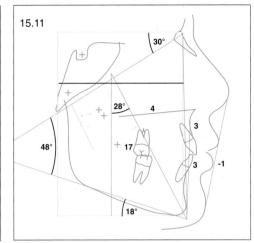

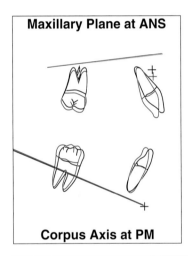

Maxillary Plane at ANS

Corpus Axis at PM

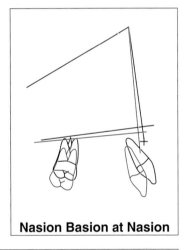

Nasion Basion at Nasion

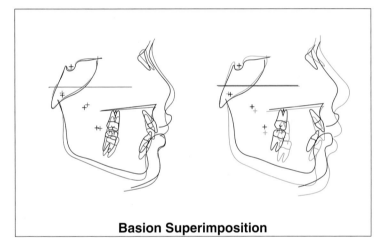

Basion Superimposition

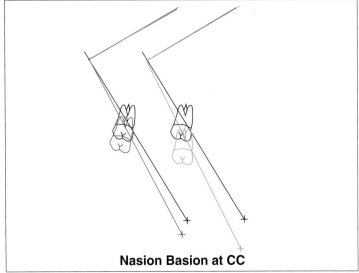

Nasion Basion at CC

J.B.. -	Age 9.11	11.4	15.11 (Yr.Mon)
Cranial Base Angle	29	29	30
Facial Axis Angle	32	28	28
F/M Plane Angle	16	20	18
Craniomandibular Angle	45	49	48
Maxillary Plane	7	5	4
Convexity	5	5	3
U/Incisor to Vertical	33	20	27
L/Incisor to Vertical	30	28	31
Interincisal Angle	117	132	122
6 to Pterygoid Vertical	17	15	17
L/Incisor to A/Po	0	1	3
L/Lip to Aesthetic Plane	2	1	−1

Case report: C.M. aged 7 years 10 months

This patient presents in the early mixed dentition with upper incisors proclined and flared. The patient also exhibits a reduced anterior facial height. Treatment ias accomplished in two stages: first with interceptive functional treatment to correct to Class I occlusion in the mixed dentition (followed by support and retention); and, secondly, with a finishing stage of orthodontic treatment in the permanent dentition (**9.8A–X**).

Diagnosis, skeletal classification:
* Mild Class II.
* Facial type: severe brachyfacial Class II division 1.
* Maxilla: moderate prognathic.
* Mandible: mild prognathic.
* Convexity = 5 mm.

Diagnosis, dental classification:
* Severe Class II division 1.
* Upper incisors: severe protrusion.
* Lower incisors: mild retrusion.
* Overjet = 11 mm.
* Deep overbite.
* Full unit distal occlusion.
* No crowding.
* Upper pharyngeal airway = 8 mm.

Although the growth pattern is prognathic on cephalometric analysis, the profile improves when the mandible postures downwards and forwards. This confirms that the profile will improve with functional correction. Clinical assessment takes precedence over cephalometric analysis in evaluating the change anticipated in the profile.

Treatment plan:
* Orthopaedic phase: early functional correction is indicated in view of the proclined upper incisors that are vulnerable to trauma.
* Support phase: in the transition from deciduous to permanent dentition.
* Orthodontic phase: to detail the occlusion in permanent dentition.

Bite registration. An edge-to-edge construction bite was registered with 2 mm interincisal clearance.

Appliances:
* Standard Twin Blocks in mixed dentition.
* Anterior inclined plane to support and retain.
* Straightwire technique in permanent dentition.

Clinical management. The active Twin Block phase reduced the overjet from 11 to 2 mm in 4 months. The upper Twin Block was trimmed occluso-distally to encourage eruption of the lower molars to reduce the overbite. To encourage vertical development, Twin Blocks continued to be worn full time for 2 months after the overjet had been reduced and before discarding the lower appliance and fitting an upper anterior inclined plane. It had an occlusal stop on the incisors to retain the reduction in overbite and overjet. The upper pharyngeal airway increased from 8 to 10 mm during treatment.

The anterior inclined plane was worn full time for 7 months to support the corrected occlusion, and was then worn at night only as a retainer during the transition to permanent dentition. At the age of 11 years, the orthodontic phase commenced after eruption of the permanant teeth and was completed in 7 months.

Duration of treatment:
* Active phase: 6 months with Twin Blocks.
* Support phase: 7 months with an anterior inclined plane.
* Transition to permanent dentition: 15 months night-time retention; 10 months with no appliance.
* Orthodontic phase: 7 months straightwire technique.
* Retention: 1 year.

CM

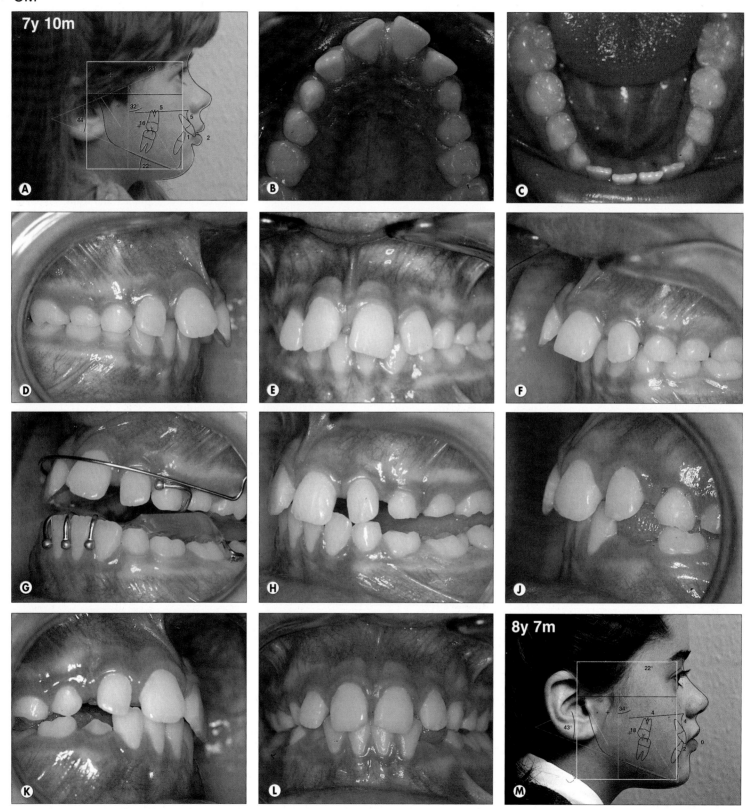

CM

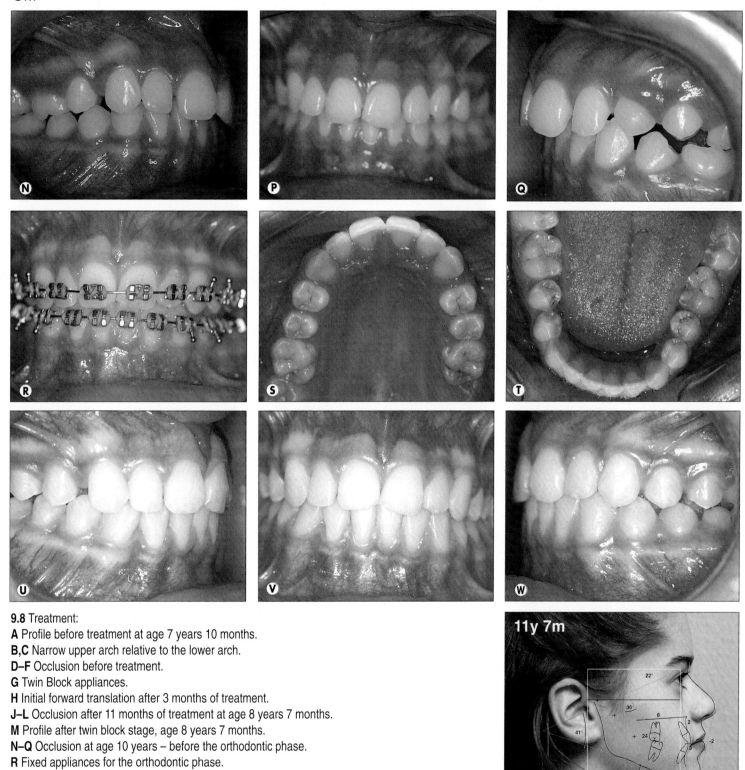

9.8 Treatment:

A Profile before treatment at age 7 years 10 months.

B,C Narrow upper arch relative to the lower arch.

D–F Occlusion before treatment.

G Twin Block appliances.

H Initial forward translation after 3 months of treatment.

J–L Occlusion after 11 months of treatment at age 8 years 7 months.

M Profile after twin block stage, age 8 years 7 months.

N–Q Occlusion at age 10 years – before the orthodontic phase.

R Fixed appliances for the orthodontic phase.

S, T Upper and lower archforms after treatment.

U–W Occlusion after treatment at age 11 years 7 months.

X Profile after treatment.

CM

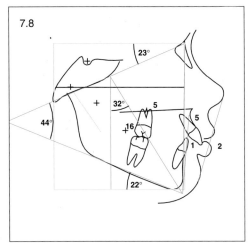

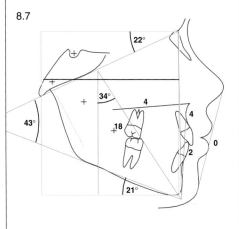

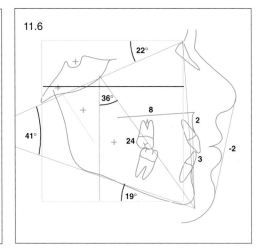

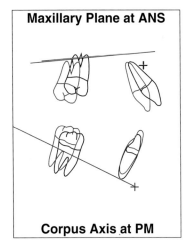

Maxillary Plane at ANS

Corpus Axis at PM

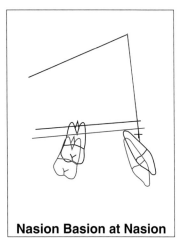

Nasion Basion at Nasion

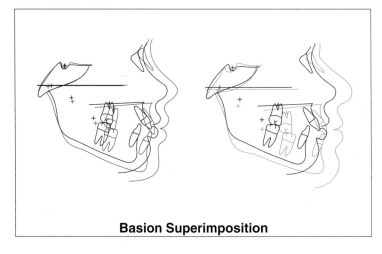

Basion Superimposition

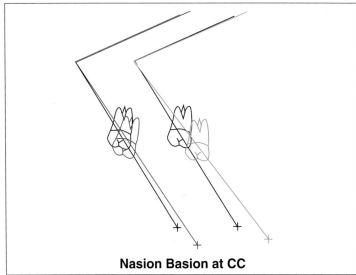

Nasion Basion at CC

C.M.-	Age	7.8	8.7	11.6	(Yr.Mon)
Cranial Base Angle		23	22	22	
Facial Axis Angle		32	34	36	
F/M Plane Angle		22	21	19	
Craniomandibular Angle		44	43	41	
Maxillary Plane		5	4	8	
Convexity		5	4	2	
U/Incisor to Vertical		37	25	24	
L/Incisor to Vertical		24	27	24	
Interincisal Angle		119	128	124	
6 to Pterygoid Vertical		16	18	24	
L/Incisor to A/Po		1	2	3	
L/Lip to Aesthetic Plane		2	0	−2	

CHAPTER
10

Combination Therapy – Permanent Dentition

Case report: C.D. aged 11 years 1 month

This is a typical example of treatment of a girl in the early permanent dentition, using Twin Blocks for initial functional correction, followed by fixed appliances to detail the occlusion (**10.1 A–Q**).

Diagnosis, skeletal classification:
- Moderate Class II.
- Facial type: severe brachyfacial.
- Maxilla: normal position – contracted laterally.
- Mandible: mild retrusion.
- Convexity = 6 mm.

Diagnosis, dental classification:
- Severe Class II division 1.
- Upper incisors: severe protrusion.
- Lower incisors: normal.
- Overjet = 10 mm.
- Deep overbite.
- Full unit distal occlusion.
- No crowding.

Treatment plan:
- Orthopaedic phase: mandibular advancement to improve mandibular retrusion and correct to Class I occlusion.
- Support phase: allow the occlusion to settle.
- Orthodontic phase: detail the occlusion with fixed appliances.
- Retention.

Appliances:
- Standard Twin Blocks.
- Anterior inclined plane.
- Simple upper and lower fixed appliances to complete the treatment.

Bite registration. The construction bite is registered with a blue exactobite bite gauge to an edge-to-edge occlusion with 2 mm interincisal clearance for full correction of arch relationships on the first activation.

Clinical management. The upper arch is expanded by a midline screw for the first 3 months of treatment. The upper bite blocks are progressively trimmed over the lower molars to encourage molar erup-tion to reduce the overbite, taking care to maintain the leading edge of the inclined plane intact as the functional mechanism. Brackets are added to align the upper anterior teeth during the Twin Block phase. The overjet is fully reduced and the distal occlusion corrected after 5 months. By this time the overbite is also reduced and the molars are in occlusion.

At this stage a lateral open bite remains in the premolar region and the height of the lower bite block may be reduced gradually to resolve this, again being careful not to lose the guidance of the inclined planes. Before making the transition to fixed appliances, Twin Blocks continue to be worn for 3 months to support the position.

Duration of treatment:
- Orthopaedic phase: 5 months with Twin Blocks.
- Support phase: 3 months to stabilise the corrected occlusion.
- Orthodontic phase: 1 year with fixed appliances.
- Retention: 1 year with a positioner.

Final records. 18 years 8 months; 5 years out of retention.

Growth change. Facial convexity reduced from 6 to 3 mm during treatment by a combination of maxillary retraction and mandibular advancement. This improvement was maintained by good post-treatment growth which further reduced convexity to 2 mm by compensatory mandibular growth after the occlusion had been corrected. The dental and facial improvement was maintained at the age of 18 years 8 months, when third molars erupted into good occlusion.

Summary. The integration of Twin Blocks and fixed appliances combines the benefits of fixed and functional therapy. Contrary to many other forms of cosmetic treatment, the benefits of combined dental orthopaedic and orthodontic therapy are not temporary, but permanent. These techniques improve facial development and are of benefit as the patient grows from childhood into maturity. Interceptive treatment in the growing child by an orthopaedic approach can enhance facial growth. In many cases it helps to avoid surgical correction at a later stage of development. When required, orthopaedic correction is followed by an orthodontic phase of treatment to detail the occlusion.

CD

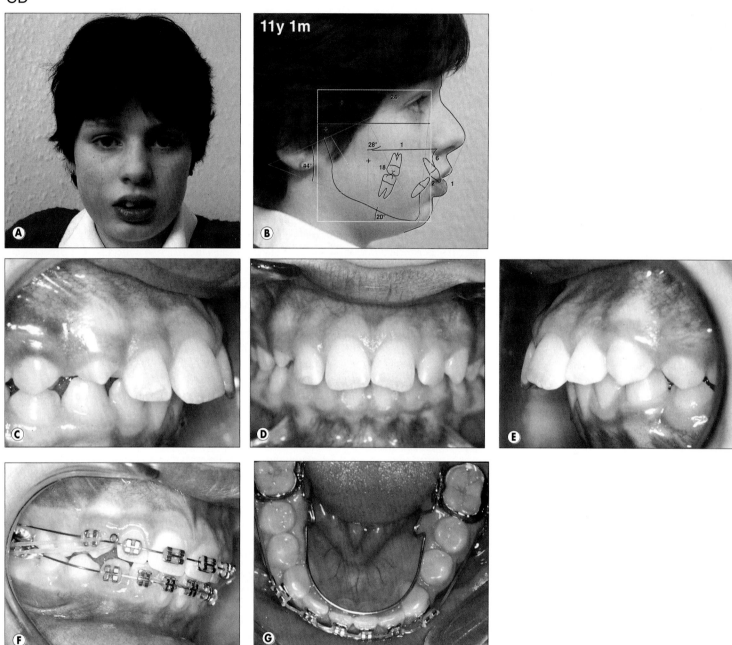

10.1 Treatment:
A, B Appearance before treatment at age 11 years 1 month.
C–E Occlusion before treatment.
F, G Appliances in the orthodontic phase.

CD

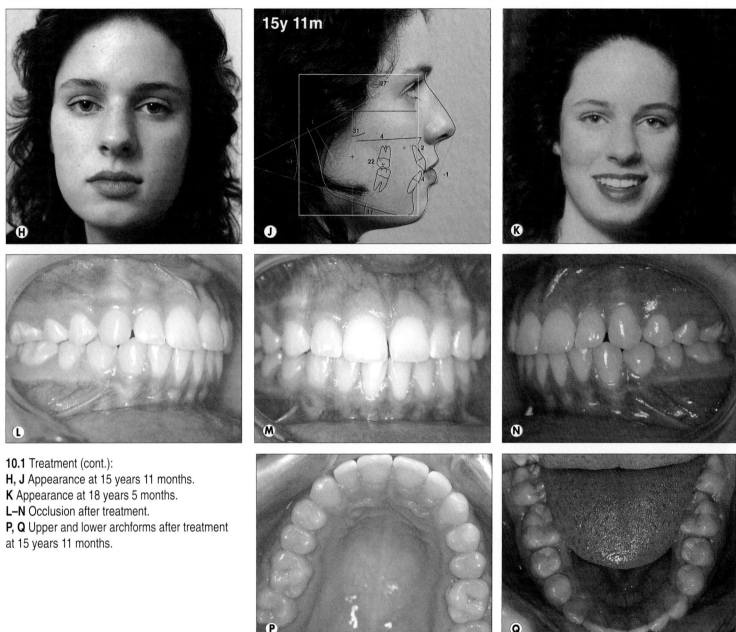

10.1 Treatment (cont.):
H, J Appearance at 15 years 11 months.
K Appearance at 18 years 5 months.
L–N Occlusion after treatment.
P, Q Upper and lower archforms after treatment
at 15 years 11 months.

CD

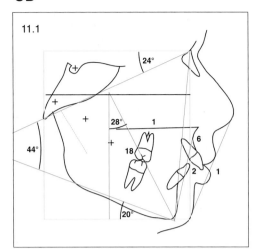

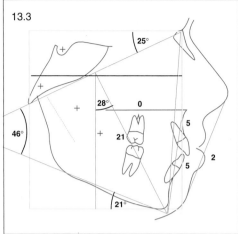

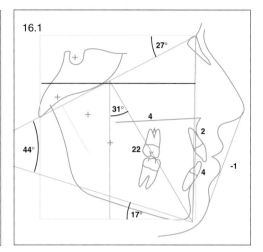

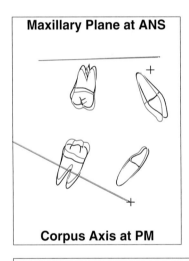

Maxillary Plane at ANS

Corpus Axis at PM

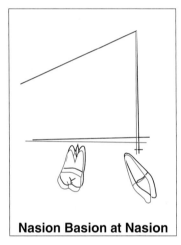

Nasion Basion at Nasion

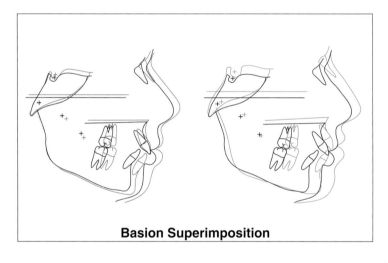

Basion Superimposition

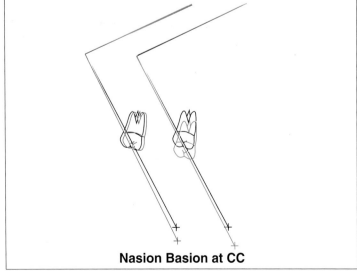

Nasion Basion at CC

C.D. -	Age	11.1	13.3	16.1	(Yr.Mon)
Cranial Base Angle		24	25	27	
Facial Axis Angle		28	28	31	
F/M Plane Angle		20	21	17	
Craniomandibular Angle		44	46	44	
Maxillary Plane		1	0	4	
Convexity		6	5	2	
U/Incisor to Vertical		35	27	26	
L/Incisor to Vertical		41	34	31	
Interincisal Angle		104	119	123	
6 to Pterygoid Vertical		18	21	22	
L/Incisor to A/Po		2	5	4	
L/Lip to Aesthetic Plane		1	2	−1	

Case report: J.S. aged 10 years 3 months

This girl presents a mild Class II division 1 malocclusion on a Class I skeletal base treated in permanent dentition in two stages with Twin Blocks and straightwire technique(**10.2A–U**).

Diagnosis, skeletal classification:
- Class I: mild retrognathic.
- Facial type: mesofacial with dolichofacial tendency.
- Maxilla: mild retrognathic.
- Mandible: mild retrognathic.

Diagnosis, dental classification:
- Severe Class II division 1.
- Overjet = 7 mm.
- Overbite incomplete due to tongue thrust.
- Full unit distal occlusion.

Treatment plan. Functional correction to Class I occlusion followed by detailed finishing with fixed appliances.

Bite registration. The blue exactobite was used to record an edge-to-edge bite with 2 mm interincisal clearance.

Appliances:
- Standard Twin Blocks to expand the upper arch and advance the lower arch.
- Straightwire appliance to detail the occlusion.

Clinical management. The upper arch was expanded for the first 3 months with a midline screw until the archwidth was sufficient to accommodate the lower arch in correct occlusion. The overjet was overcorrected to an edge-to-edge incisor relationship in 7 months. The lower appliance was left out and an anterior inclined plane was fitted, set back slightly to allow the lower incisors to settle to a normal overjet and overbite. After 1 year the position was retained at night only.

Upper and lower second molars were extracted on eruption to resolve potential crowding of the third molars. Although the mandibular position after Twin Block treatment was aesthetically acceptable, it was decided to proceed with an orthodontic phase to detail the occlusion and to correct the torque and angulation of tooth positions to ideal values by the straightwire technique. This stage was completed in 9 months.

Duration of treatment
- Orthopaedic phase: 7 months with Twin Blocks to correct the occlusion.
- Support phase: 4 months.
- Orthodontic phase: 9 months.
- Retention: 1 year.

This case illustrates controlled functional correction of a Class II division 1 malocclusion on a Class I skeletal base to improve the profile without excessive mandibular advancement. It also demonstrates the improvement resulting from detailing the occlusion with a finishing stage of orthodontic treatment.

JS

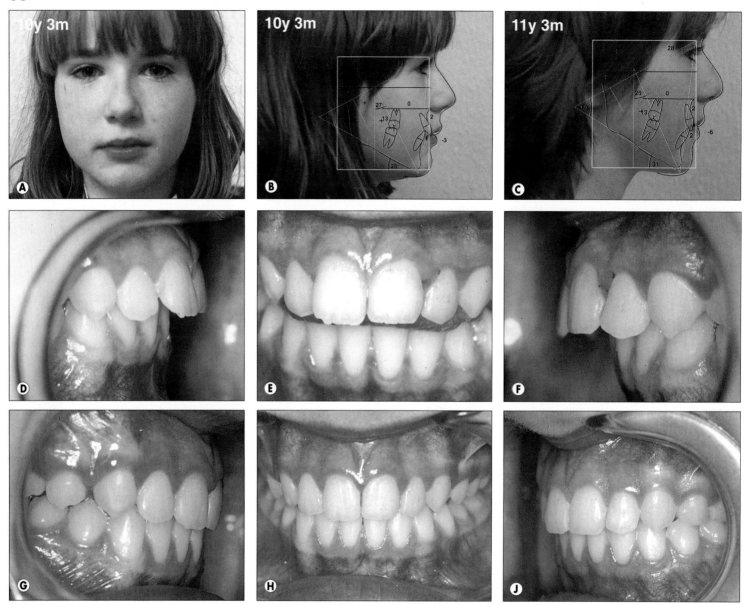

10.2 Treatment:

A, B Appearance before treatment at age 10 years 3 months.

C Profile after the Twin Blocks phase at age 11 years 3 months.

D–F Occlusion before treatment; the anterior view shows the tongue thrust.

G–J After 11 months of treatment.

JS

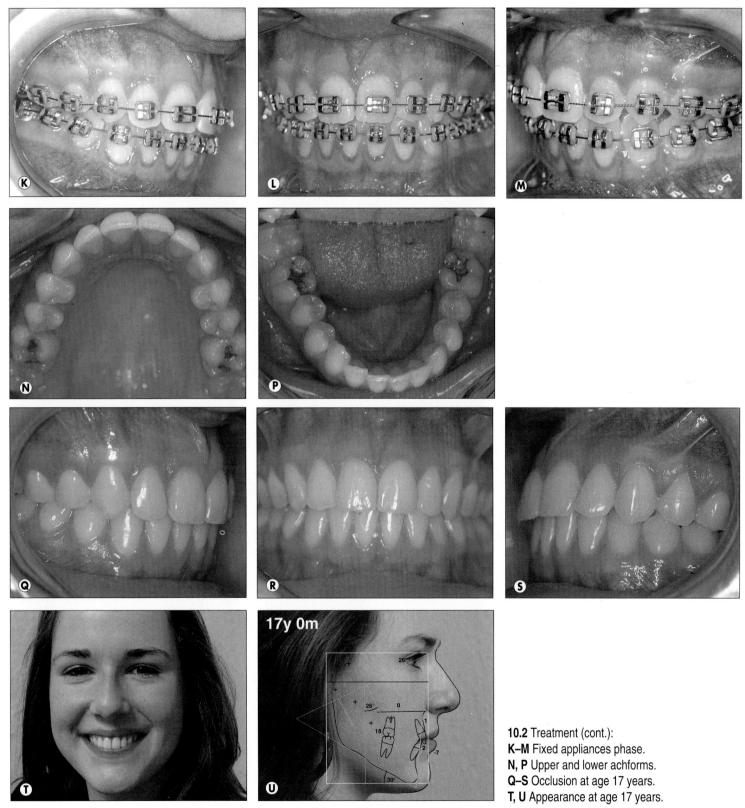

17y 0m

10.2 Treatment (cont.):
K–M Fixed appliances phase.
N, P Upper and lower achforms.
Q–S Occlusion at age 17 years.
T, U Appearance at age 17 years.

JS

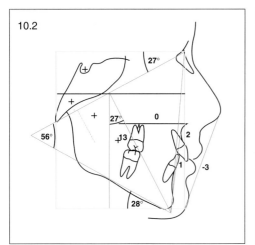

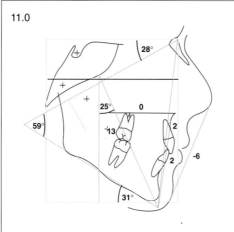

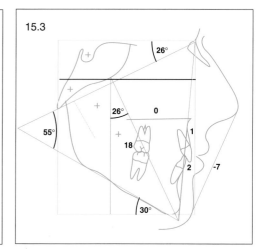

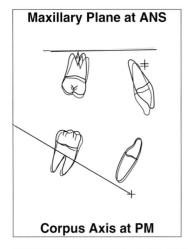

Maxillary Plane at ANS

Corpus Axis at PM

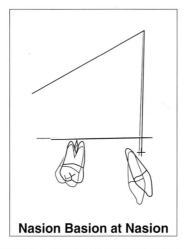

Nasion Basion at Nasion

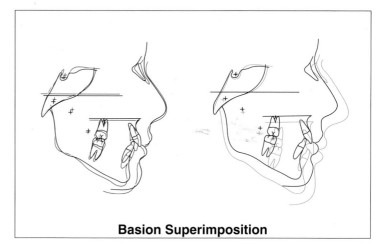

Basion Superimposition

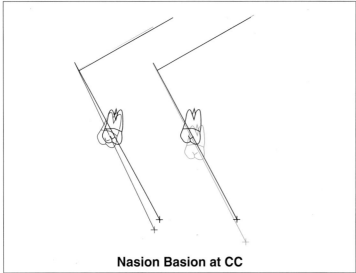

Nasion Basion at CC

J.S. -	Age	10.2	11.0	15.3	(Yr.Mon)
Cranial Base Angle		27	28	26	
Facial Axis Angle		27	25	26	
F/M Plane Angle		28	31	30	
Craniomandibular Angle		56	59	55	
Maxillary Plane		0	0	0	
Convexity		2	2	1	
U/Incisor to Vertical		20	12	14	
L/Incisor to Vertical		31	32	32	
Interincisal Angle		129	136	134	
6 to Pterygoid Vertical		13	13	18	
L/Incisor to A/Po		1	2	2	
L/Lip to Aesthetic Plane		−3	−6	−7	

The Twin Block Traction Technique

ORTHOPAEDIC TRACTION

In most cases, full functional correction of occlusal relationships can be achieved with Twin Blocks without the addition of any orthopaedic or traction forces. Where the response to functional correction is poor, the addition of orthopaedic traction force may be considered.

In the early stages of development of the Twin Block technique a method was devised to combine functional therapy with orthopaedic traction. This approach should be limited to treatment of severe malocclusion, where growth is unfavourable for conventional fixed or functional therapy. Functional therapy combined with traction achieves rapid correction of malocclusion.

The indications are confined to a minority of cases with growth patterns where maxillary retraction is the treatment of choice. For example:

- In the treatment of severe maxillary protrusion.
- To control a vertical growth pattern by the addition of vertical traction to intrude the upper posterior teeth.
- In adult treatment where mandibular growth cannot assist the correction of a severe malocclusion.

The Concorde facebow

Before Twin Blocks were developed, the author used extraoral traction with removable appliances as a means of anchorage to retract upper buccal segments to correct Class II malocclusion (Cousins & Clark, 1965). In the early years using Twin Blocks, tubes were added to clasps for extraoral traction on the upper appliance to be worn at night so as to reinforce the functional component for correction of a Class II buccal segment relationship.

A method was developed to combine extraoral and intermaxillary traction by adding a labial hook to a conventional facebow and extending an elastic back to attach to the lower appliance in the incisor region (Clark, 1982). This development was based on previous experience of functional appliances that were worn part time and were slow and unpredictable in correcting arch relationships.

The Concorde facebow is a new means of applying intermaxillary and extraoral traction to restrict maxillary growth and, at the same

time, to encourage mandibular growth in combination with functional mandibular protrusion. A conventional facebow is adapted by soldering a recurved labial hook to extend forwards to rest outside the lips as an anchor point to combine intermaxillary and extraoral traction. Patient comfort and acceptance is similar to a conventional facebow. Intermaxillary traction was added to the appliance system to ensure that if the patient postured out of the appliance during the night, the intermaxillary traction force would increase. This ensured that the appliance was effective 24 hours per day (**11.1 A–C**)

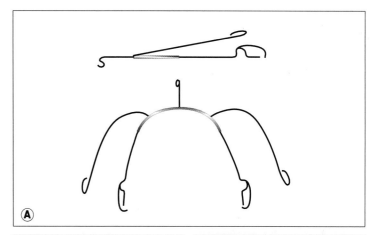

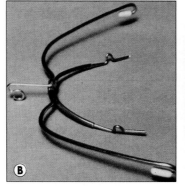
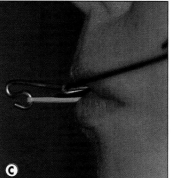

11.1 A–C Concorde facebow.

The labial hook is positioned extraorally, 1 cm clear of the lips in the midline. This enables an elastic back to pass intraorally to attach anteriorly to the lower appliance to apply intermaxillary traction as a horizontal force vector. This has the advantage of eliminating the unfavourable upward component of force in conventional intermaxillary elastic traction, which can extrude lower molars and cause tipping of the occlusal plane.

When distal extraoral traction is applied to a removable appliance, the outer bow of the facebow should be adjusted to lie slightly above the inner bow in order to apply a slight upward component of force to help retain the upper appliance. Fixation of the appliance must be excellent before any orthopaedic force is applied to a removable appliance, and poor fixation contraindicates the addition of traction, except to a fixed attachment.

The traction components are worn at night only to reinforce the action of the occlusal inclined plane. If the patient fails to posture the mandible to the corrected occlusal position during the night, the intermaxillary traction force is automatically increased to compensate and to ensure that favourable intermaxillary forces are applied continuously. The aim is to make the appliances active 24 hours per day to maximise the orthopaedic response.

Careful case selection is essential before using a combination of Twin Blocks with orthopaedic traction. This is a very powerful mechanism for maxillary retraction and, as the majority of Class II malocclusions are due to mandibular retrusion, it is contraindicated in most cases. The headgear effect tends to tip the occlusal plane and palatal plane down anteriorly and to retrocline the upper incisors, which may cause unfavourable autorotation of the mandible. Extraoral traction should be used selectively, bearing in mind that most patients respond to treatment without the addition of traction components.

Later experience in using Twin Blocks confirmed that the addition of a traction component was not necessary to achieve correction of the buccal segment relationship, and extraoral traction is no longer used to reinforce the action of the inclined planes. Study of early cases showed that the headgear effect caused unneccessary maxillary retraction.

Occasionally (Orton, 1990), high pull traction may be indicated to intrude the upper posterior teeth in cases with a severe vertical growth pattern, in an effort to achieve a forward mandibular rotation by intruding upper molars. The same objective can be achieved more simply by using vertical intraoral elastics to intrude the posterior teeth.

TWIN BLOCKS COMBINED WITH ORTHOPAEDIC TRACTION

Treatment of maxillary protrusion

Case report: K.A. aged 9 years 6 months

Diagnosis, skeletal classification:
- Severe Class II.
- Facial type: mild brachyfacial.
- Maxilla: mild prognathic.
- Mandible: normal.
- Convexity = 6 mm.

Diagnosis, dental classification:
- Severe Class II division 1.
- Overjet = 14 mm.
- Anterior open bite associated with thumbsucking.
- Upper incisors: moderate protrusion.
- Lower incisors: severe retrusion.
- No crowding.
- Upper pharyngeal space = 3 mm (restricted).

Treatment plan. Standard Twin Blocks with the Concorde facebow to be worn at night for maxillary retraction in addition to mandibular advancement (**11.2 A–E**).

Duration of treatment
- Orthopaedic phase: 8 months with Twin Blocks.
- Retention: 6 months with an anterior inclined plane.

The response to treatment in this case was achieved with spasmodic appliance wear. Twin Blocks were reactivated midway through treatment by addition of cold cure acrylic to the inclined plane of the upper bite block. The upper pharyngeal space increased from 3 to 6 mm.

KA

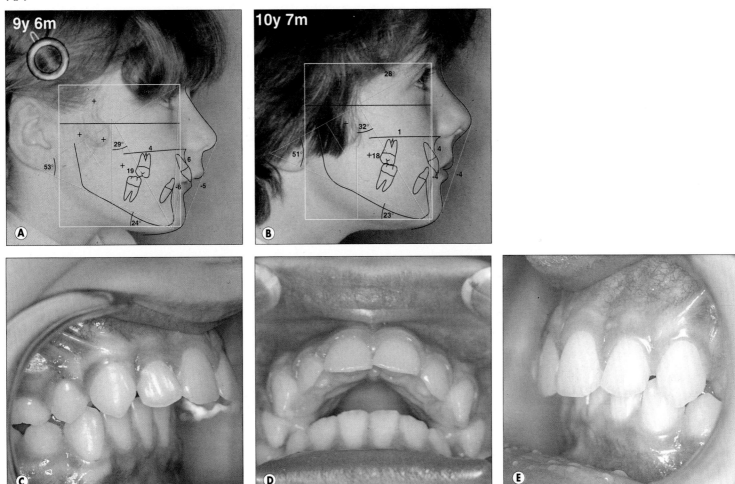

11.2 Treatment:

A Profile before treatment at age 9 years 6 months

B Profile after 8 months of treatment.

C, D Occlusion before treatment at age 9 years 6 months (note the anterior open bite).

E Occlusion after 8 months of treatment.

KA

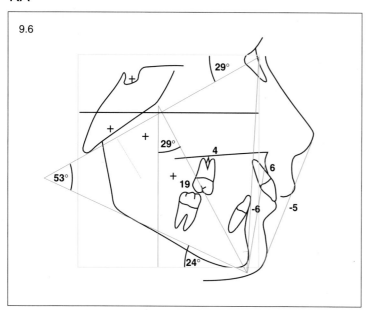

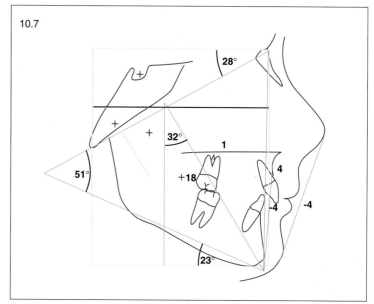

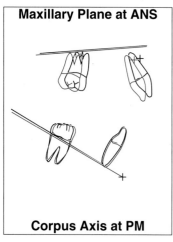

Maxillary Plane at ANS

Corpus Axis at PM

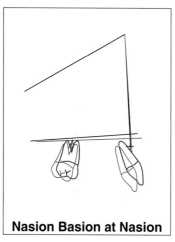

Nasion Basion at Nasion

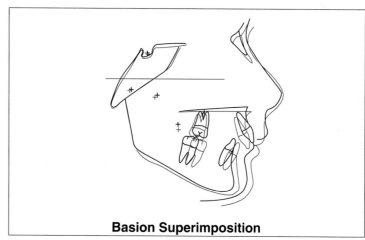

Basion Superimposition

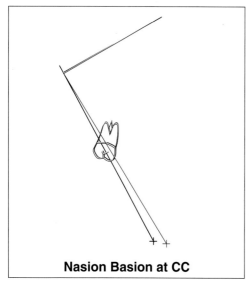

Nasion Basion at CC

K.A.-	Age 9.6	10.7 (Yr.Mon)
Cranial Base Angle	29	28
Facial Axis Angle	29	32
F/M Plane Angle	24	23
Craniomandibular Angle	53	51
Maxillary Plane	4	1
Convexity	6	4
U/Incisor to Vertical	27	24
L/Incisor to Vertical	29	28
Interincisal Angle	124	128
6 to Pterygoid Vertical	19	18
L/Incisor to A/Po	−6	−4
L/Lip to Aesthetic Plane	−5	−4

WF

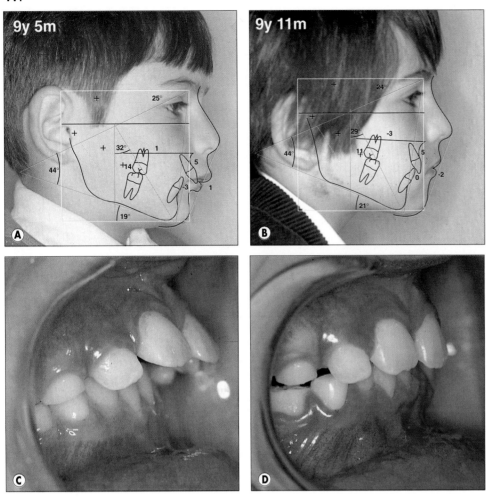

11.3 Treatment:
A, B Profile before and after treatment.
C, D Occlusion after 5 months of treatment at age 9 years 11 months.

Case report: W.F. aged 9 years 5 months

Diagnosis, skeletal classification:
- Moderate Class II.
- Facial type: severe brachyfacial.
- Maxilla: normal, contracted laterally.
- Mandible: mild retrognathic.
- Convexity = 5 mm.

Diagnosis, dental classification:
- Severe Class II division 1.
- Upper incisors: protrusive.
- Lower incisors: protrusive.
- Overjet = 12 mm.
- Deep overbite.
- Full unit distal occlusion.
- No crowding.
- Upper pharyngeal space = 11 mm (within normal range).

In addition to mandibular advancement, light extraoral traction was added at night to retract the maxillary dentition (**11.3 A–D**).

Duration of treatment:
- Orthopaedic phase: 9 months.
- Support and retention: 9 months.

WF

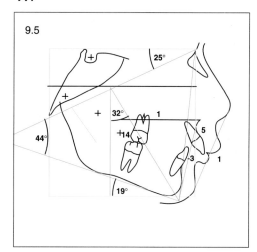

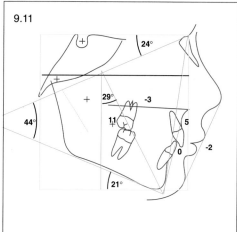

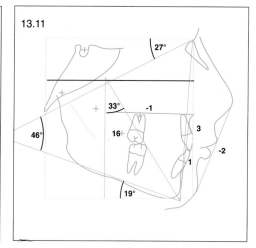

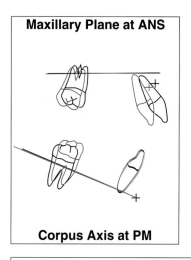

Maxillary Plane at ANS

Corpus Axis at PM

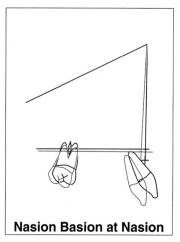

Nasion Basion at Nasion

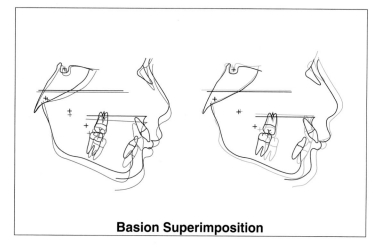

Basion Superimposition

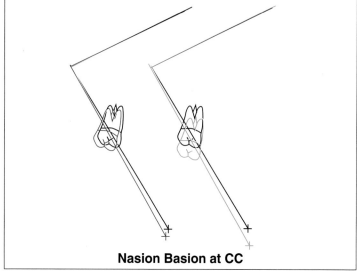

Nasion Basion at CC

W.F. -	Age	9.5	9.11	13.11 (Yr.Mon)
Cranial Base Angle		25	24	27
Facial Axis Angle		32	29	33
F/M Plane Angle		19	21	19
Craniomandibular Angle		44	44	46
Maxillary Plane		1	−3	−1
Convexity		5	5	3
U/Incisor to Vertical		32	18	16
L/Incisor to Vertical		30	34	39
Interincisal Angle		118	128	125
6 to Pterygoid Vertical		14	11	16
L/Incisor to A/Po		−3	0	1
L/Lip to Aesthetic Plane		1	−2	−2

KS

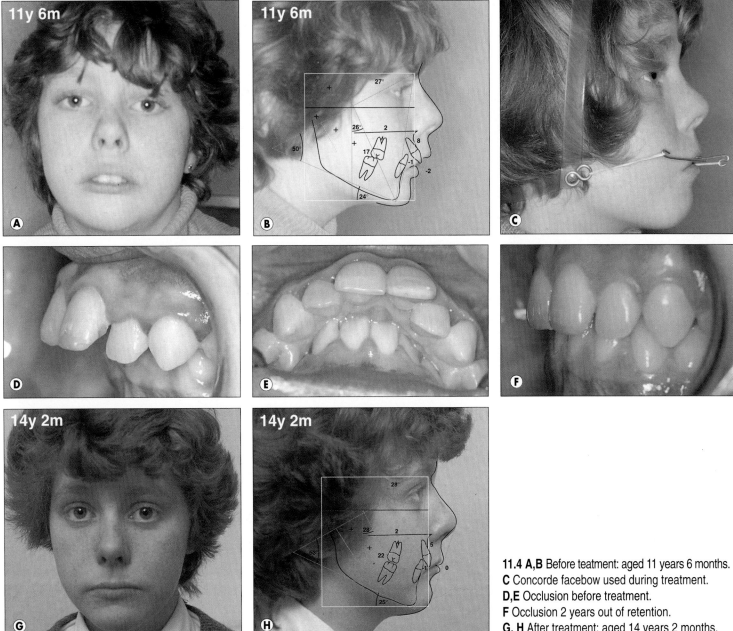

11.4 A,B Before teatment: aged 11 years 6 months.
C Concorde facebow used during treatment.
D,E Occlusion before treatment.
F Occlusion 2 years out of retention.
G, H After treatment: aged 14 years 2 months.

Case Report : K.S. aged 11 years 6 months

Diagnosis, skeletal classification:
- Severe Class II.
- Facial type: mild brachyfacial.
- Maxilla: normal.
- Mandible: severe retrognathic.
- Convexity = 8 mm.

Diagnosis, dental classification:
- Severe Class II division I.
- Upper incisors: severe protrusion.
- Overjet = 12 mm.
- Overbite = 9 mm (excessive)

An early example of Twin Block treatment for a girl with a severe Class II division I malocclusion with excessive overbite. The case was complicated by previous loss of $\overline{6|}$, and was treated by extraction of $\underline{4|4}$ and $\overline{4|}$ to achieve better symmetry (**11.4 A–H**).

Treatment was effective in reducing the overjet and overbite. A Concorde facebow was used in this case and maxillary retraction resulted in flattening of the profile.

The combination of extraction and extraoral traction is not normally indicated and should be avoided because of the excessive retraction force applied to the maxilla.

KS

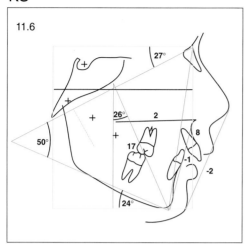

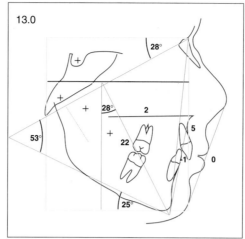

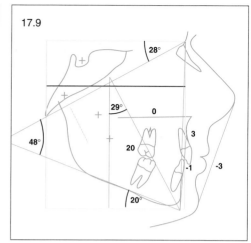

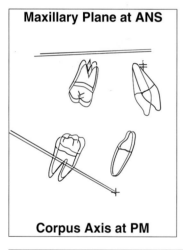

Maxillary Plane at ANS

Corpus Axis at PM

Nasion Basion at Nasion

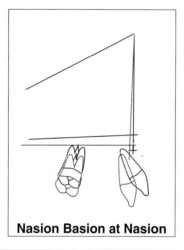

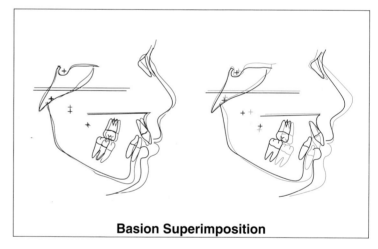

Basion Superimposition

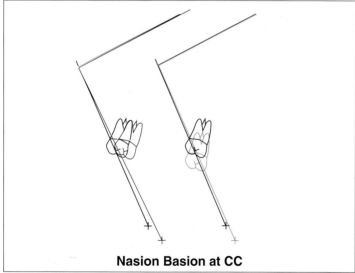

Nasion Basion at CC

K.S. -	Age	11.6	13.0	17.9	(Yr.Mon)
Cranial Base Angle		27	28	28	
Facial Axis Angle		26	28	29	
F/M Plane Angle		24	25	20	
Craniomandibular Angle		50	53	48	
Maxillary Plane		2	2	0	
Convexity		8	5	3	
U/Incisor to Vertical		32	14	17	
L/Incisor to Vertical		26	20	17	
Interincisal Angle		122	146	146	
6 to Pterygoid Vertical		17	22	20	
L/Incisor to A/Po		−1	−1	−1	
L/Lip to Aesthetic Plane		−2	0	−3	

DIRECTIONAL CONTROL OF ORTHOPAEDIC FORCE

Additional orthopaedic forces may help to control vertical growth by applying an intrusive orthopaedic force to the upper posterior teeth. A high pull headgear is used to apply an intrusive force to the upper molars to resist the vertical component of growth and to reduce the anterior open bite. The Concorde facebow is a unique method of delivering an intrusive force to upper molars and, at the same time, a protrusive force to the mandible and the lower dentition.

The direction of extraoral force is especially important in the treatment of patients with a vertical growth pattern. A vertical orthopaedic force to the upper appliance applies an intrusive force to the upper posterior teeth and palate, and limits downward maxillary growth.

Intrusion of the upper posterior teeth allows the bite to close by a favourable forward rotation of the mandible, and facilitates correction of mandibular retrusion in vertical growth discrepancies.

Case report: L.G. aged 9 years 1 month

Diagnosis, skeletal classification:
- Severe Class II.
- Facial type: mild brachyfacial.
- Maxilla: mild prognathic.
- Mandible: moderate retrognathic.
- Convexity = 10 mm.

Diagnosis, dental classification:
- Severe Class II division 1.
- Upper incisors: severe protrusion.
- Lower incisors: normal.
- Overjet = 10 mm.
- Reduced overbite: tongue thrust and tooth apart swallow.
- No crowding.
- Upper pharyngeal space = 3 mm.

The lower incisors normally erupt into contact with the upper incisors or the soft tissue of the palate, unless they are prevented from doing so by intervening soft tissues or by a thumb- or finger-sucking habit. Reduced overbite may present as a small separation of the lower incisors from the palate. This is due to an atypical swallowing pattern as the tongue thrusts between the teeth to contact the lower lip to form an anterior oral seal in a 'tooth apart' swallow. The soft-tissue pattern improves when the mandible postures forwards and an anterior seal is formed by closing the lips together over the teeth. The soft tissues adapt quickly to full-time appliance wear as the patient eats with the appliance in the mouth. This will produce an effective oral seal.

Treatment plan. Retract the maxilla and advance the mandible. Intrude the upper posterior teeth to reduce the anterior open bite.

Appliances. Twin Blocks to close the bite with occlusal contact of the bite blocks on all posterior teeth supported by high pull extraoral traction at night.

Clinical management. The overjet reduced from 10 to 2 mm in 3 months. During this period a slight posterior open bite developed. To maintain an intrusive occlusal force on the posterior teeth, Twin Blocks continued to be worn full time without reducing the occlusal

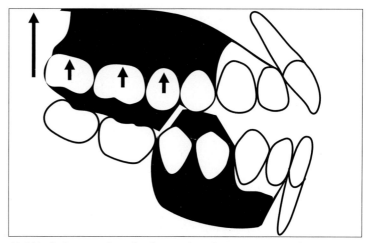

11.5 Vertical extraoral traction force to intrude upper posterior teeth.

blocks. This helps to resolve an anterior open bite. The Concorde facebow was worn at night for the first 6 months of treatment.

An anterior inclined plane was designed for retention without an occlusal stop to allow the lower incisors to occlude on the cingulae of the upper incisors, and to allow the buccal teeth to settle into occlusion. The upper pharyngeal space increased from 3–10 mm after 4 months of treatment.

Duration of treatment:
- Active phase: 4 months.
- Support phase: 6 months.
- Retention: 4 months.
- Total treatment time: 14 months including retention.

Final records. 6 years 9 months out of retention.

The addition of traction is optional in reduced overbite cases, and many cases respond well to treatment without traction. Traction is indicated in severe discrepanies of vertical growth that are unfavourable for functional correction. A vertical component of traction force is particularly effective in controlling this type of malocclusion. The Concorde facebow is adjusted so that it lies just below the level of the upper lip at rest, with the ends of the outer bow sloping slightly upwards above the level of the inner bow. The resulting extraoral traction applies an upward component of force that helps to retain the upper appliance (**11.5, 11.6 A–S**).

REFERENCES

Clark, W.J. (1982). The twin-block traction technique. *Eur. J. Orthod.,* **4**: 129–38.

Cousins, A.J.P. & Clark, W.J. (1965). Extra-oral traction. Theoretical considerations and the development of the removable appliance system. *Trans BSSO*, 29–38.

Orton, H.S. (1990). *Functional Appliances in Orthodontic Treatment.* London, Quintessence.

FURTHER READING

Clark, W.J. (1988). The twin-block technique. *Am. J. Orthod. & Dentofacial Orthoped.,,* **93**: 1–18.

LG

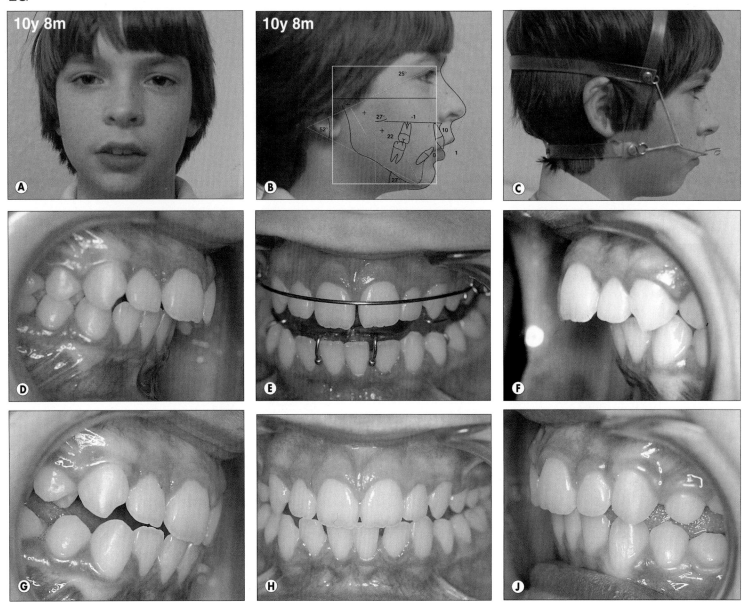

11.6 Treatment:

A, B Appearance before treatment at age 10 years 8 months.

C Concorde facebow and combination headgear with high pull.

D Occlusion before treatment.

E Twin Blocks.

F Occlusion before treatment.

G–J Occlusion after 3 months of treatment.

LG

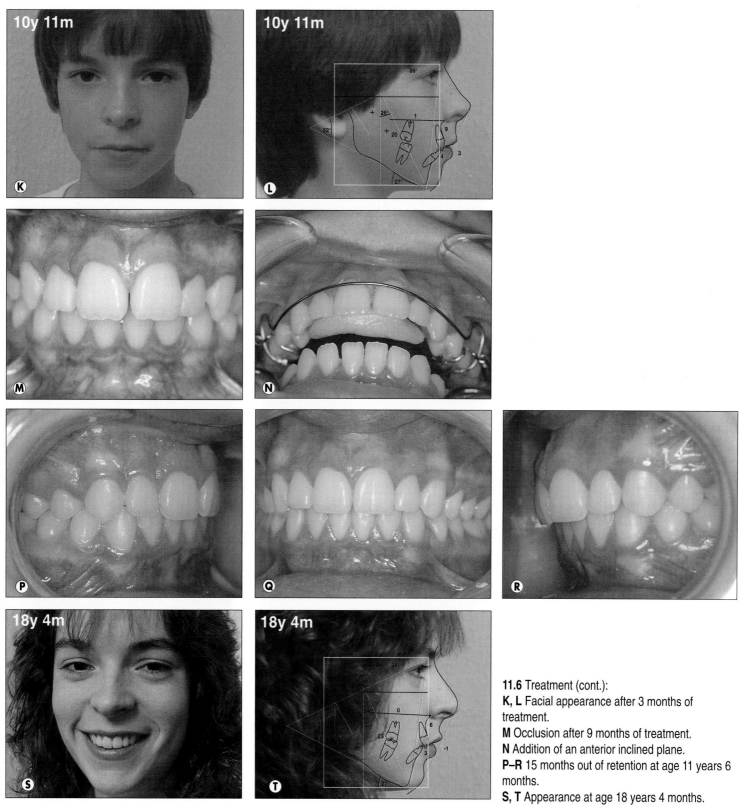

11.6 Treatment (cont.):
K, L Facial appearance after 3 months of treatment.
M Occlusion after 9 months of treatment.
N Addition of an anterior inclined plane.
P–R 15 months out of retention at age 11 years 6 months.
S, T Appearance at age 18 years 4 months.

LG

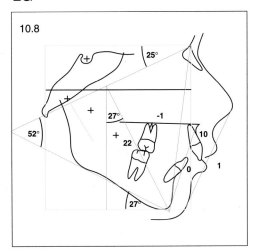

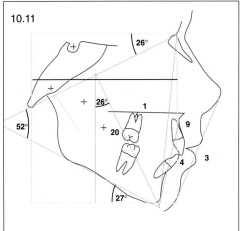

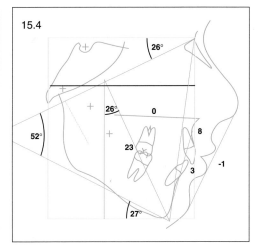

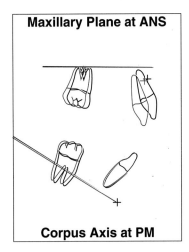

Maxillary Plane at ANS

Corpus Axis at PM

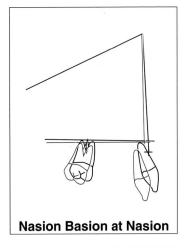

Nasion Basion at Nasion

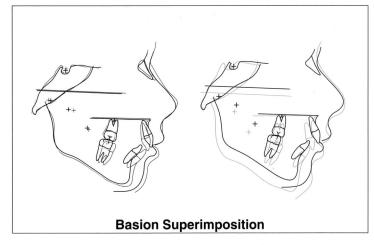

Basion Superimposition

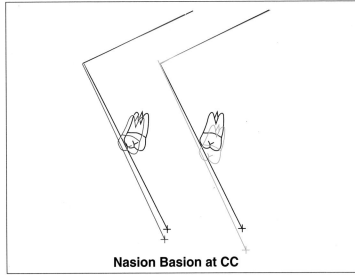

Nasion Basion at CC

L.G. -	Age	10.8	10.11	15.4 (Yr.Mon)
Cranial Base Angle		25	26	26
Facial Axis Angle		27	26	26
F/M Plane Angle		27	27	27
Craniomandibular Angle		52	52	52
Maxillary Plane		−1	1	0
Convexity		10	9	8
U/Incisor to Vertical		19	18	17
L/Incisor to Vertical		46	47	41
Interincisal Angle		115	115	122
6 to Pterygoid Vertical		22	20	23
L/Incisor to A/Po		0	4	3
L/Lip to Aesthetic Plane		1	3	−1

CHAPTER
12
Treatment of Anterior Open Bite

The anterior open bite is frequently due to a combination of skeletal and soft tissue factors. A full clinical and cephalometric diagnosis is necessary to establish the aetiology of the problem. This includes evaluation of the airway, which is a factor in achieving lip competence after treatment.

Airway obstruction may be due to enlargement of tonsils or adenoids and should be referred for evaluation or treatment when required. The upper pharyngeal airway is measured from the posterior pharyngeal wall to the outline of the upper half of the soft palate. An upper airway of 12 mm is typical in the mixed dentition. This increases with age to a mean of 17.4 mm in the adult (McNamara & Brudon, 1993). Narrowing of the pharyngeal airway appears to be improved by mandibular advancement during the first few months of Twin Block treatment. Long-term observation after treatment confirms that the increase in upper pharyngeal width is maintained and lip competence is also achieved consistently during Twin Block treatment.

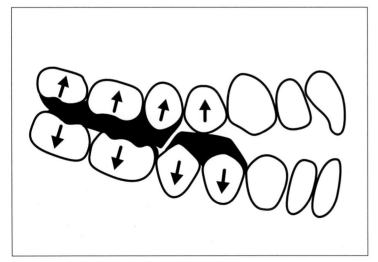

12.1 A Maintain occlusal contact to intrude posterior teeth.

The prognosis for correction of anterior open bite depends on the degree of skeletal and soft tissue imbalance. In addition, assessment of the direction of facial growth to identify a horizontal or vertical growth tendency helps to establish the prognosis for treatment.

Early treatment is frequently effective in controlling the functional imbalance associated with adverse soft-tissue behaviour patterns. Tongue thrust is often a necessary functional adaptation required to form an effective anterior oral seal by means of tongue contact with a trapped lower lip. This type of tongue thrust is usually adaptive after expanding the maxilla and correcting arch relationships. Learning to eat with Twin Blocks in the mouth encourages the formation of a good lip seal. When the overjet is reduced, a lip seal can be formed more efficiently without the support of the tongue. The oral musculature then adapts accordingly.

A more persistent anterior open bite is related occasionally to a tongue thrust which does not adapt to corrective treatment and can be one of the most difficult orthodontic problems to resolve. This condition is related frequently to a lisp and a habitual forward tongue position, causing a bimaxillary protrusion. Some patients have a pernicious habit of licking the lips, which is associated with a tongue thrust and may be difficult to resolve.

Reduced overbite or anterior open bite is often related to unfavourable vertical growth and requires careful management. Throughout treatment, all posterior teeth must remain in occlusal contact with the opposing bite blocks to prevent overeruption. It is important to avoid overeruption of posterior teeth, as this would accentuate the vertical growth tendency and tend to open the bite even more. Intrusion of posterior teeth helps reduce anterior open bite and encourages a favourable mandibular rotation to close the mandibular plane angle (**Fig 12.1 A**).

PITFALLS IN TREATMENT OF ANTERIOR OPEN BITE

The worst complications of Twin Block treatment of anterior open bite arise from careless management of the occlusal blocks, by allowing eruption of posterior teeth. This results in an increase in the anterior open bite. Two common mistakes are therefore to be avoided.

First, it is necessary to be attentive to avoid overeruption of second molars behind the appliance (**12.1B**). It is all too easy to make this mistake by failing to check for eruption of second molars at every visit. If the patient attends once every 6 weeks, a lapse of concentration at one visit can allow the second molars to erupt unimpeded for 3 months. Prevention is better than cure for this problem. Attention to appliance design is effective, and if second molars are likely to erupt during treatment it is appropriate to include occlusal rests, even before these teeth erupt, in order to control their eruption.

The second complication is equally damaging. If the upper block is trimmed occlusally in treatment of anterior open bite this will allow the lower molars to erupt, again propping the bite open and increasing the anterior open bite (**12.1C**). Fortunately, anterior open bite cases are in the minority, but as a result it is easy to become accustomed to trimming the upper block as a matter of routine. To avoid the problem it is strongly suggested that a clear note or colour code is placed on the patient's record card to draw attention to the anterior open bite and as a reminder not to trim the blocks at any stage during treatment.

Patients with anterior open bite and a vertical growth pattern tend to have weak musculature and may have difficulty in consistently maintaining a forward posture to engage the occlusal inclined planes of the bite blocks. They are prone to posture out of the appliance, which reduces the effectiveness in correcting both sagittal and vertical discrepancies. These patients may benefit from phased progressive activation to allow the muscles to adapt more gradually to mandibular advancement. Vertical elastics or attracting magnets can help overcome this problem (see case reports below).

BITE REGISTRATION

It is important to relate the degree of activation to the freedom of movement of the mandible by measuring the protrusive path. The overjet is measured with the mandible retruded and in the position of maximum protrusion. The activation must not exceed 70% of the total protrusive path. It is especially important in vertical growth patterns to ensure that the patient can maintain comfortably the protrusive position and, if necessary, to settle for a lesser amount of initial activation.

The yellow projet or exactobite is designed to register a 4 mm interincisal clearance, resulting in approximately 5 mm clearance between the cusps of the first premolars or deciduous molars. It is necessary to accommodate blocks of sufficient thickness between the posterior teeth to open the bite beyond the free-way space so as to intrude the posterior teeth. The objective is to make it difficult for the patient to disengage the blocks. The process of bite registration is similar in other respects to the method described for treatment of deep overbite.

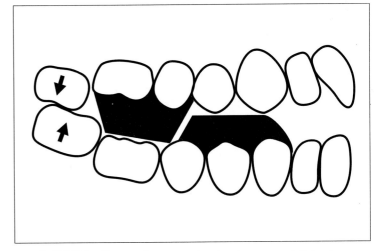

12.1 B PITFALL – Do not allow second molars to overerupt. Extend occlusal cover or occlusal rests distally to second molars.

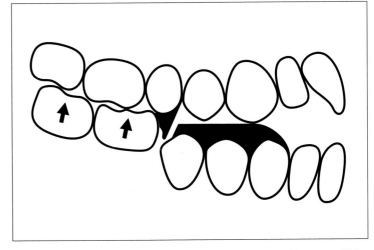

12.1 C PITFALL – Do not trim upper block in reduced overbite cases. This increases the anterior open bite.

Appliance design: Twin Blocks to close the bite

Appliance design is modified to achieve vertical control and close the anterior open bite. The lower appliance extends distally to the lower molar region with clasps on the lower first molars and occlusal rests on the second molars to prevent their eruption. It is not necessary to extend acrylic to contact the upper and lower anterior teeth so that they are free to erupt to reduce the anterior open bite (**12.1 D–F**).

A palatal spinner may be added to the upper appliance to help control an anterior tongue thrust. The spinner is an acrylic bead that is free to rotate round a transpalatal wire positioned in the palate. The objective is to encourage the tongue to curl upwards and backwards instead of thrusting forwards. This is especially effective in younger patients and the spinner should be used as early as possible to control tongue thrust.

A spinner may be incorporated in an upper appliance with a midline screw without interfering with the action of the midline screw to expand the arch. The spinner may be mounted on a piece of steel tubing supported by wires extending from either side of the midline. Alternatively, the spinner may be attached by a wire that extends towards the midline from one side, and is then recurved on itself to retain the spinner in position (**12.2 A, B**).

Young children respond to the suggestion that the spinner is a toy for the tongue to play with. They learn first to spin it with the finger, then with the tongue. Anything that moves in the mouth is irresistible to the tongue. This is a very positive mechanism for controlling tongue thrust by retraining the tongue to move up into the palate rather than thrusting forwards between the teeth.

A tongue guard is a more passive obstruction to discourage the tongue from thrusting forwards against the lingual surfaces of the upper incisors. It is in the form of a recurved wire extending from the premolar region towards the midline and is recurved to its point of attachment. This wire lies in the vertical plane and is clear of the lingual surface of the upper incisors to allow them to settle lingually.

A labial bow may be added to retract the upper incisors if they have been significantly proclined by tongue and lip action.

In the treatment of reduced overbite it is essential that no trimming is done on the blocks, and that occlusal contact of the posterior teeth is maintained on the blocks throughout treatment.

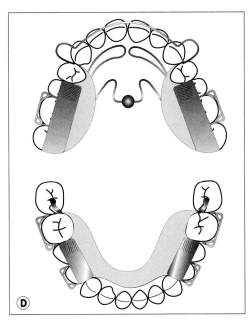
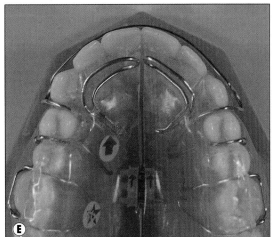
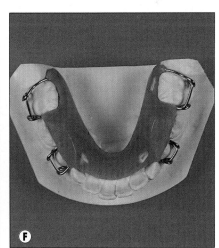

12.1 D Appliance design with spinner.
12.1 E Upper appliance with palatal spinner.
12.1 F Lower appliance with clasps extended to lower molars.

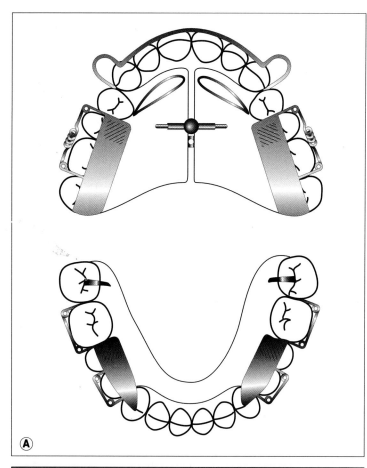

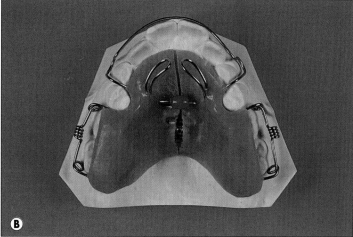

12.2 A, B Spinner on tubing.

Case report: D.P. aged 10 years 10 months

This boy had a history of thumbsucking and presented an anterior open bite associated with a tongue thrust (**12.3 A–M**).

Diagnosis, skeletal classification:
- Mild Class II.
- Facial type: severe brachyfacial.
- Maxilla: normal.
- Mandible: mild retrusion.
- Convexity = 5 mm.

Diagnosis, dental classification:
- Severe Class II division 1.
- Overjet = 10 mm.
- Tongue thrust and anterior open bite.
- History of thumbsucking.
- Full unit distal occlusion.
- Upper pharyngeal space = 6 mm.

Treatment plan. Mandibular advancement to correct the distal occlusion and improve the profile, followed by support and retention.

Bite registration. This patient had weak musculature and did not easily posture forwards to maintain an edge-to-edge incisor occlusion. The bite was registered with a yellow exactobite to reduce the overjet by 5 mm on the first activation, with 4 mm interincisal clearance.

Appliances. Twin Blocks were designed to close the anterior open bite. A labial bow was included for slight retraction of the upper incisors, and clasps were extended to the lower molars as these teeth should be prevented from erupting during treatment.

Clinical management. The overjet reduced from 8 to 4 mm after 3 months of treatment; at this stage the Twin Blocks were reactivated by the addition of cold cure acrylic to the anterior aspect of the inclined planes on the upper Twin Block. During the course of treatment the occlusal bite blocks were not trimmed, but were maintained in occlusal contact with all the posterior teeth. This had the effect of intruding the posterior teeth to produce a slight posterior open bite that allowed a positive overbite to develop anteriorly. The overjet was fully reduced after 10 months and an anterior inclined plane was fitted to support the corrected occlusion. Support and retention continued for a year after treatment. The upper pharyngeal space increased from 6 to 10 mm.

Duration of treatment:
- Active phase: 10 months with Twin Blocks.
- Support and retention: 1 year.

DP

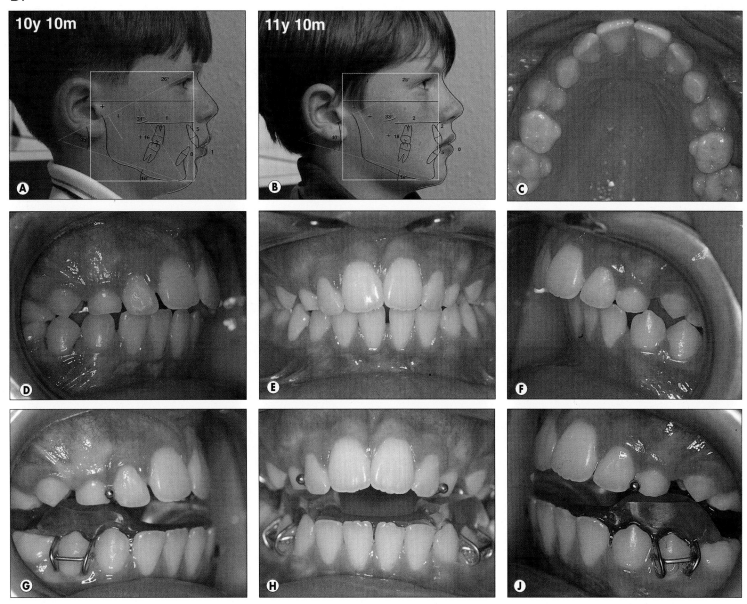

12.3 Treatment:
A Profile before treatment at age 10 years 10 months.
B Profile after 12 months of treatment at age 11 years 10 months.
C Contracted upper arch due to thumbsucking.
D–F Occlusion before treatment.
G–J Twin Blocks.

DP

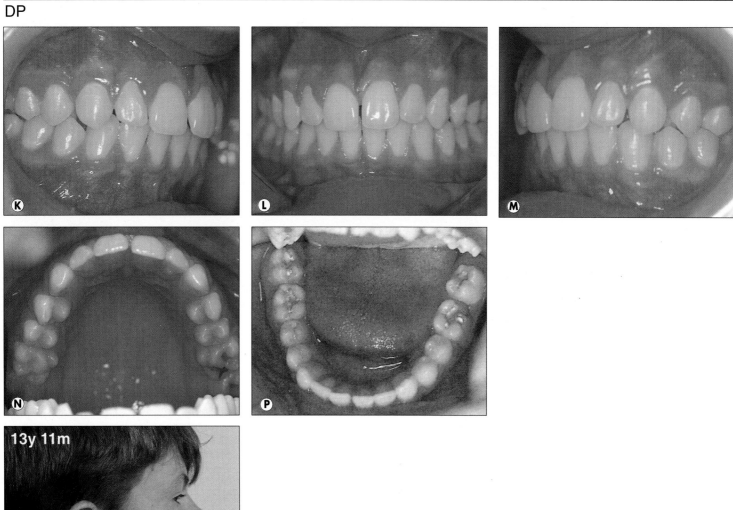

12.3 Treatment (cont.):
K–M Occlusion at age 13 years 11 months.
N, P Upper and lower archforms after treatment.
Q Profile at age 13 years 11 months.

DP

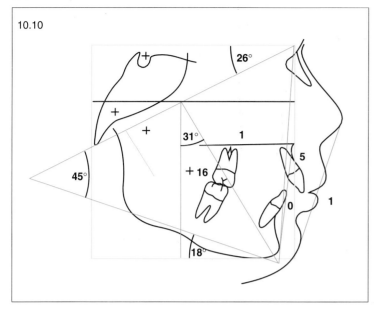

10.10

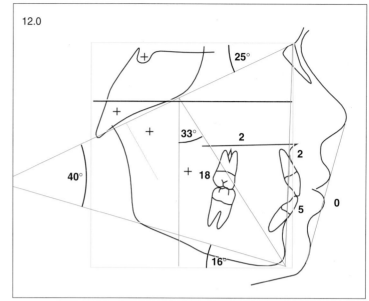

12.0

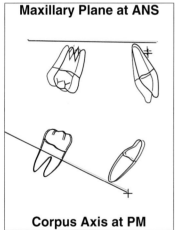

Maxillary Plane at ANS

Corpus Axis at PM

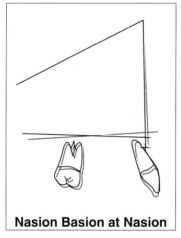

Nasion Basion at Nasion

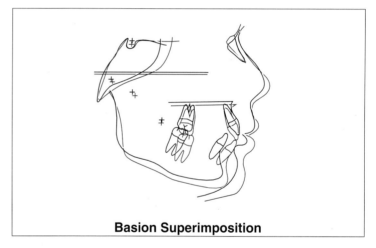

Basion Superimposition

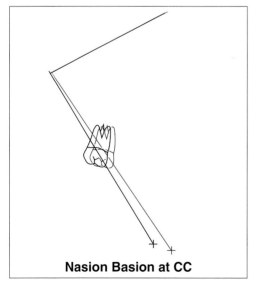

Nasion Basion at CC

D.P.-	Age	10.10	12.0	(Yr.Mon)
Cranial Base Angle		26	25	
Facial Axis Angle		31	33	
F/M Plane Angle		18	16	
Craniomandibular Angle		45	40	
Maxillary Plane		1	2	
Convexity		5	2	
U/Incisor to Vertical		27	23	
L/Incisor to Vertical		37	40	
Interincisal Angle		116	117	
6 to Pterygoid Vertical		16	18	
L/Incisor to A/Po		0	5	
L/Lip to Aesthetic Plane		1	0	

Case report: S.S. aged 14 years 1 month

This patient presented a Class II division 1 malocclusion in the permanent dentition with vertical growth, and an anterior open bite with increased lower facial height. Vertical control was achieved by the Twin Block in the active phase, followed by retention with a bionator to close the bite (**12.4**).

Diagnosis, skeletal classification:
- Severe Class II
- Facial type: severe dolichofacial; vertical growth.
- Maxilla: normal.
- Mandible: severe retrognathic.
- Convexity = 11 mm.

Diagnosis, dental classification:
- Severe Class II division 1.
- Upper incisors: normal.
- Lower incisors: normal.
- Full unit distal occlusion.
- Anterior open bite.
- High mandibular plane angle.
- Low facial axis angle.
- Narrow upper arch.
- Upper pharyngeal space = 9 mm (not restricted).

Treatment plan:
- Mandibular advancement.
- Close anterior open bite.

Appliances:
- Twin Blocks with full occlusal cover to expand the upper arch and intrude the posterior teeth.
- Bionator to retain.

Bite registration. The construction bite was registered with a yellow exactobite in an edge-to-edge incisor relationship with 4 mm interincisal clearance to give sufficient space between the molars for the bite blocks to extend distally between the molars, to exert an intrusive force on the opposing posterior teeth.

Appliance design: In the treatment of an anterior open bite, occlusal contact must be maintained on all posterior teeth to prevent eruption.

Clinical management:
- It is important that no trimming is done on the bite blocks over the posterior teeth. This principle applies throughout the treatment of an anterior open bite. The overjet reduced from 10 to 2 mm in 5 months, and the buccal segment corrected to Class I occlusion. As the mandible translated forwards, an open bite of 2 mm remained between the upper and lower incisors. The occlusion was then edge-to-edge with an interincisal clearance of 2 mm.
- A bionator to close the bite was used during support and retention in preference to an anterior inclined plane to maintain the functional correction. There was full cover over all posterior teeth and a lingual shelf to restrict forward tongue thrust. The appliance was kept clear of the lingual surfaces of the upper and lower incisors. After 4 months the anterior open bite had closed and the incisor relationship was satisfactory. Appliance wear was then reduced to night only to retain the position.

Duration of treatment:
- Active phase: 5 months with Twin Blocks.
- Support phase: 4 months with the bionator for day and night-time wear.
- Retention: 12 months of night-time wear.
- Total period of treatment: 1 year 9 months.

Final records. 2 years 3 months out of retention at age 18 years.

Summary. The combination of Twin Block and bionator appliance treatment is the best of both worlds in the control of an anterior open bite in Class II division 1 malocclusion with a vertical growth pattern.

The Twin Block achieves a more rapid response in the active phase to correct the anteroposterior arch relationships. During this period the patient enjoys the freedom of wearing a less restricting two-piece appliance, with better speech and less interference with normal function.

This is followed by a short period of day- and night-time wear of the bionator, to encourage closure of the anterior open bite by preventing the tongue from resting between the teeth. The bionator continues as a retainer with a favourable functional component. This approach observes the principle of using a retainer that supports the objectives of treatment. The upper pharyngeal space increased from 9 mm before treatment to 14 mm 4 years later.

SS

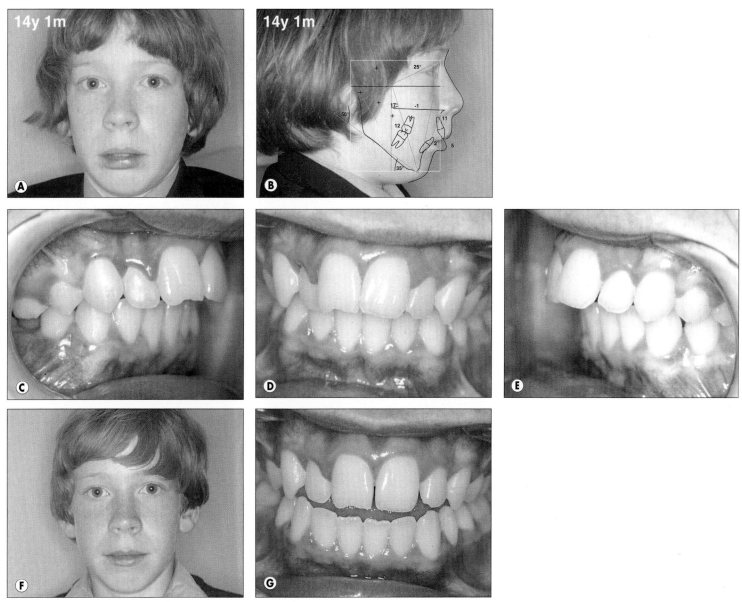

12.4 Treatment:

A, B Appearance before treatment at age 14years 1 month.

C–E Occlusion before treatment.

F, G Appearance and occlusion after 4 months of treatment at age 14 years 5 months.

SS

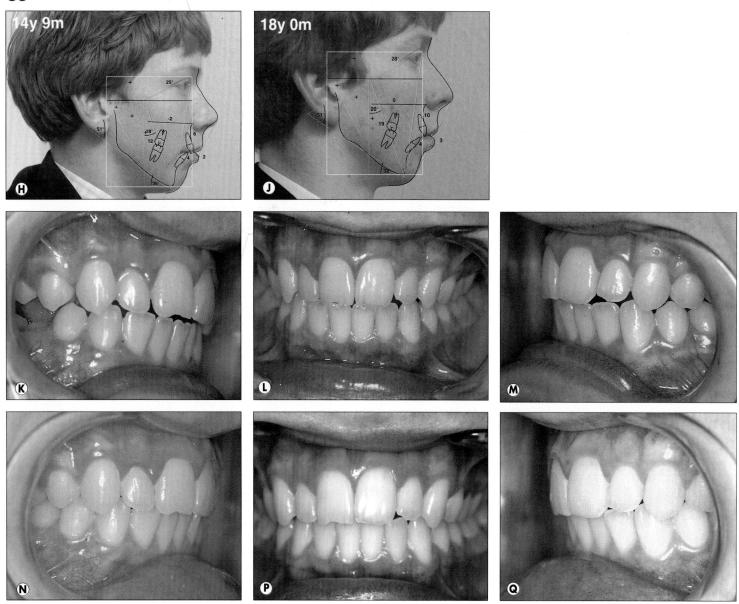

12.4 Treatment (cont.):
H Profile after 8 months of treatment at age 14 years 9 months.
J Profile out of retention at age 18 years.
K–M Occlusion after 8 months of treatment at age 14 years 9 months.
N–Q Occlusion out of retention at age 18 years.

SS

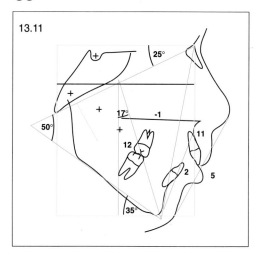

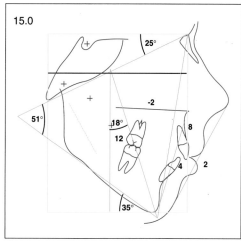

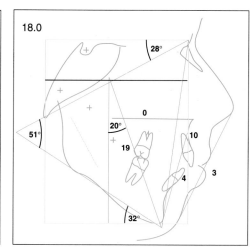

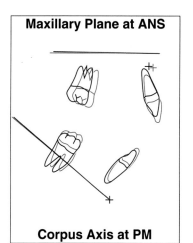

Maxillary Plane at ANS

Corpus Axis at PM

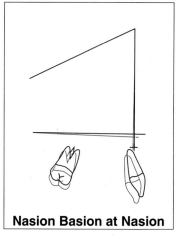

Nasion Basion at Nasion

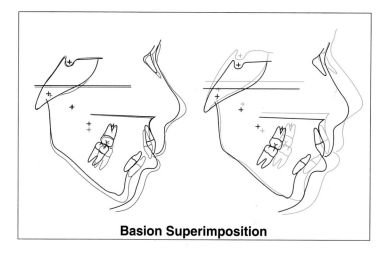

Basion Superimposition

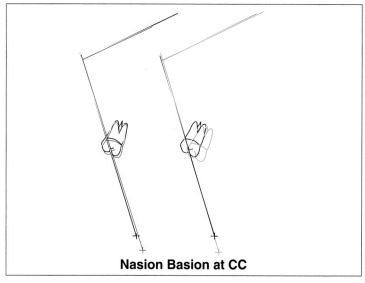

Nasion Basion at CC

S.S. -	Age	13.11	15.0	18.0	(Yr.Mon)
Cranial Base Angle		25	25	28	
Facial Axis Angle		17	18	20	
F/M Plane Angle		35	35	32	
Craniomandibular Angle		50	51	51	
Maxillary Plane		−1	−2	0	
Convexity		11	8	10	
U/Incisor to Vertical		16	13	16	
L/Incisor to Vertical		43	42	45	
Interincisal Angle		121	125	119	
6 to Pterygoid Vertical		12	12	19	
L/Incisor to A/Po		2	4	4	
L/Lip to Aesthetic Plane		5	2	3	

INTRAORAL TRACTION TO CLOSE ANTERIOR OPEN BITE

Intraoral elastics may be used to accelerate bite closure as an efficient alternative to high-pull extraoral traction. This simple mechanism is very effective in closing anterior open bites. The method was brought to the author's attention by Dr Christine Mills who first used the system in orthodontic practice in Vancouver. Vertical elastics were first applied to help patients maintain occlusal contact on the appliances overnight. The author observed at a study group in Vancouver that the elastics had the additional benefit of closing the bite (**12.5**).

The intrusive effect of the bite blocks is reinforced by running a vertical elastic between upper and lower teeth on both sides. Elastics may be attached directly to the upper and lower appliances or to brackets or bands with gingival hooks. An effective vector is produced by passing an elastic from between the brackets on the upper first deciduous molar and lower second deciduous molar (or the upper first and lower second premolars). The elastics are worn at night to maintain occlusal contact of the posterior teeth on the bite blocks to intrude posterior teeth. All posterior teeth must contact the occlusal blocks to prevent eruption and to deliver intrusive forces.

To maximise the effects of elastic traction, the elastics may be worn full time. It is important that the construction bite should open the bite beyond the rest position to ensure that the patient cannot comfortably posture out of the blocks.

Intraoral vertical elastics have the additional advantage of increasing occlusal contact on the inclined planes. This is an important factor in patients who have weak musculature and do not occlude positively on the occlusal inclined planes. These are generally patients with a vertical growth pattern who do not respond well to functional therapy, because their potential for horizontal growth is poor. The addition of a mechanical component of elastic traction is effective in improving the response to treatment by assisting muscle action in maintaining contact on the occlusal inclined planes. This helps by intruding the posterior teeth and also accelerates the correction of distal occlusion (**12.6, 12.7 A,B**).

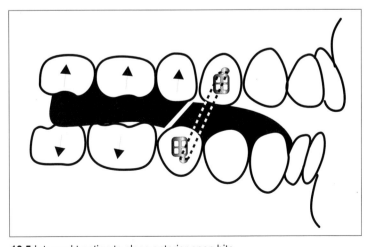

12.5 Intraoral traction to close anterior open bite.

Magnetic force

Magnetic force is an alternative method of increasing forces for intrusion of opposing posterior teeth by incorporating magnets in the inclined planes on the posterior bite blocks. Either attracting or repelling magnets may be used and both are effective. Repelling magnets increase the opposing forces in the occlusal bite blocks to intrude opposing teeth. This principle has been investigated by Dellinger (1986).

Attracting magnets increase the frequency of occlusal contacts on the inclined planes. Occlusal forces are the activating mechanism of Twin Blocks and increasing the forces of occlusion is effective in accelerating both anteroposterior and vertical correction. The application of magnets in Twin Block treatment is discussed further in Chapter 19.

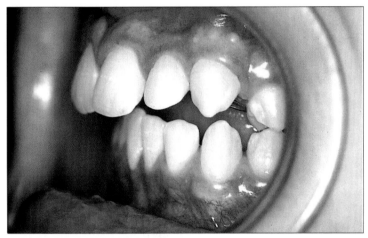

12.6 Treatment in this case was slow, and an anterior open bite persisted because the patient did not close consistently into the blocks.

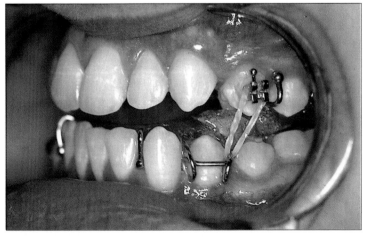

12.7 A Intraoral vertical elastics to intrude posterior teeth. When vertical elastics were added an immediate improvement in response was noted.

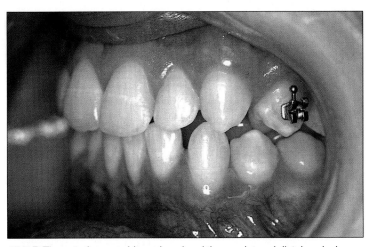

12.7 B The anterior open bite reduced and the overjet and distal occlusion corrected.

TREATMENT OF VERTICAL GROWTH PATTERNS

Case report: H.D. aged 12 years 2 months

This patient presented a vertical growth pattern and was past the adolescent or pubertal growth spurt at the start of treatment. As a result the response to treatment was slower than normal due to a limited growth response combined with the vertical direction of growth (**12.8 A–F**).

Diagnosis, skeletal classification:
- Severe Class II.
- Facial type: severe dolichofacial, vertical growth.
- Maxilla: normal.
- Mandible: severe retrognathic.
- Convexity = 9 mm.
- Mandibular plane angle = 29°.

Diagnosis, dental classification:
- Severe Class II division 1.
- Upper incisors: normal.
- Lower incisors: moderate retrusion – 1 to A–Po = –4 mm.
- Overjet = 14 mm.
- Excessive overbite.
- Narrow upper arch, molar crossbite, right side.
- Lower arch mild buccal crowding, ALD = 4 mm.
- Upper pharyngeal space: no obstruction.

Treatment plan:
- Mandibular advancement to improve the mandibular retrusion. Orthopaedic traction with the Concorde facebow as the patient was past the ideal growth stage.
- Support the corrected occlusion with an anterior inclined plane.

Appliances:
- Standard Twin Blocks with the Concorde facebow for combined intermaxillary and extraoral traction.
- Anterior inclined plane in the support phase.

Clinical management. The Twin Blocks were made with occlusal contact on all posterior teeth to apply an intrusive force to minimise vertical growth. The Concorde facebow was worn intermittently at night for the first 5 months to maintain a forward component of force on the mandible via the horizontal labial elastic.

The overjet and distal occlusion corrected within 4 months from 14 to 5 mm and after 10 months of treatment down to 4 mm. No trimming was done on the bite blocks and there was still a posterior open bite at this stage. In this case, the posterior open bite was larger than normal because of the excessive overbite, and therefore was slower to resolve.

In view of the severe skeletal discrepancy, a second set of Twin Blocks was worn for another year to continue active correction, this time trimming the bite blocks to allow eruption to resolve the posterior open bite. Support and retention by an anterior inclined plane continued for a year.

Duration of treatment:
- Active phase: 12 months with each set of Twin Blocks.
- Support phase: 6 months full time with an anterior inclined plane.
- Retention: 6 months night-time retention.

All second molars were extracted to accommodate the third molars.

Post-treatment records. 2 years out of retention.

Discussion

An alternative approach when a deep overbite is associated with a vertical growth pattern would be an initial stage of arch development to level and align the lower arch before the Twin Block stage. This may reduce the vertical component of growth during treatment, as the mandible may then be advanced with a smaller vertical component of activation.

HD

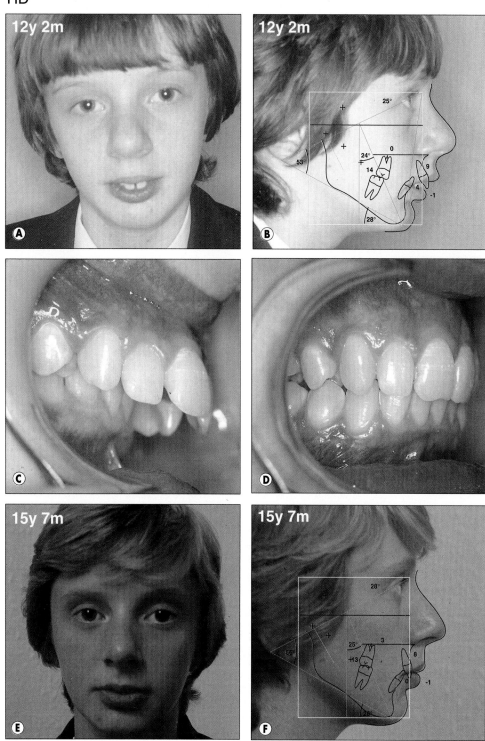

12.8 Treatment:
A, B Appearance before treatment at age 12 years 2 months.
C, D Occlusal change at age 12 years 2 months and 15 years 1 month.
E, F Appearance at age 15 years 7 months.

HD

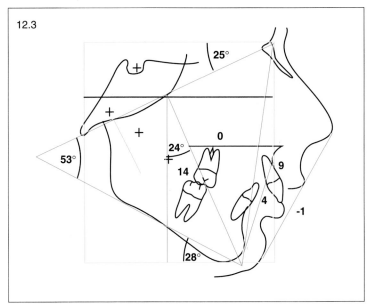

12.3

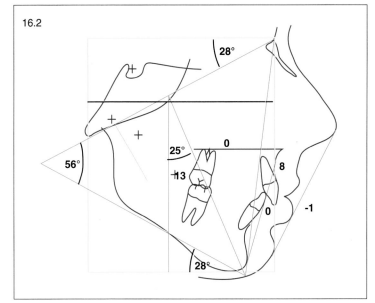

16.2

Maxillary Plane at ANS

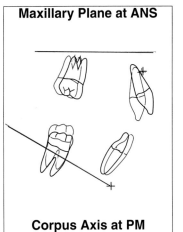

Corpus Axis at PM

Nasion Basion at Nasion

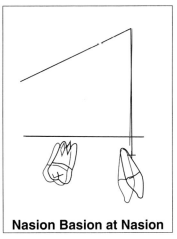

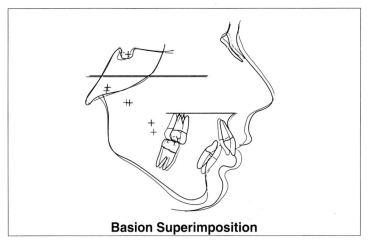

Basion Superimposition

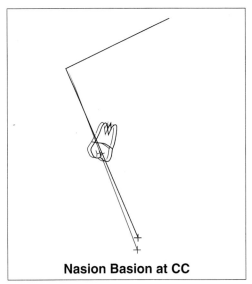

Nasion Basion at CC

H.D.-	Age	12.3	16.2 (Yr.Mon)
Cranial Base Angle		25	28
Facial Axis Angle		24	25
F/M Plane Angle		28	28
Craniomandibular Angle		53	56
Maxillary Plane		0	0
Convexity		9	8
U/Incisor to Vertical		22	8
L/Incisor to Vertical		24	36
Interincisal Angle		134	134
6 to Pterygoid Vertical		14	13
L/Incisor to A/Po		4	0
L/Lip to Aesthetic Plane		−1	−1

Case report: L.J. aged 9 years 10 months

This is an example of the response to treatment in a girl with a severe vertical growth pattern (**12.9**).

Diagnosis, skeletal classification:
- Severe Class II.
- Facial type: severe dolichofacial.
- Vertical growth axis.
- Maxilla: moderate prognathia.
- Mandible: moderate retrognathic.
- Convexity = 8 mm.
- High maxillo-mandibular plane angle.

Diagnosis, dental classification:
- Severe Class II division 1.
- Upper incisors: severe protrusion.
- Lower incisors: mild retrusion.
- Overjet = 11 mm.
- No crowding.
- Upper pharyngeal space = 7 mm.

Treatment plan:
- Mandibular advancement to attempt to improve the mandibular retrusion. An addition of high pull traction to the upper posterior teeth to reduce downward and forward maxillary growth.
- Support the corrected occlusion with an anterior inclined plane.

Appliances:
- Standard Twin Blocks with the Concorde facebow for combined intermaxillary and extraoral traction.
- Anterior inclined plane in the support phase.

Clinical management. The Twin Blocks were made with occlusal contact on all posterior teeth to apply an intrusive force to minimise vertical growth. The response to treatment was slow in this case, because the patient did not appear to posture her mandible consistently forward on the inclined planes. This was probably related to weak musculature associated with vertical growth.

The overjet reduced over a period of 12 months using the Concorde facebow. The facebow was worn at night only to maintain a forward component of force on the mandible via the horizontal labial elastic.

The overjet and distal occlusion were corrected within a year and support and retention were by an anterior inclined plane. The upper pharyngeal space increased from 7 to 9 mm during treatment.

Duration of treatment:
- Active phase: 12 months with Twin Blocks.
- Support phase: 3 months full time with an anterior inclined plane.
- Retention: 1 year.

REFERENCES

McNamara, Jr, J.A. & Brudon, W.L. (1993). *Orthodontic and Orthopedic Treatment in the Mixed Dentition*. Needham Press.

Dellinger, E.L. (1986). A clinical assessment of the active vertical corrector, a non-surgical alternative for skeletal open bite treatment. *Am. J. Orthod.*, **89** (5): 428–36.

LJ

12.9 Treatment:
A Profile before treatment.
B Profile 1 year 10 months out of retention.
C Profile at age 16 years 10 months.
D, E, F Occlusion before treatment.
G, H, J Occlusion 5 years out of retention.
K, L Facial appearance before and after treatment.

LJ

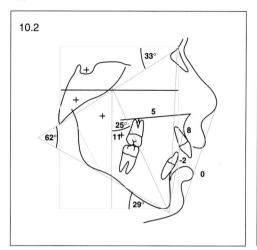

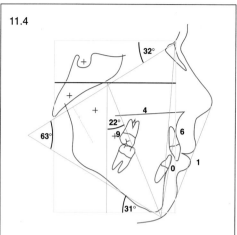

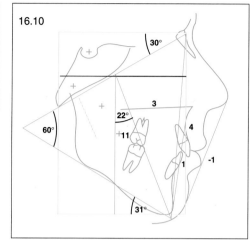

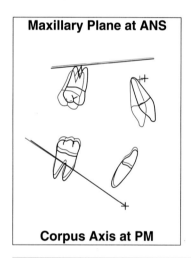

Maxillary Plane at ANS

Corpus Axis at PM

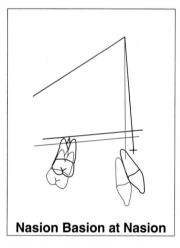

Nasion Basion at Nasion

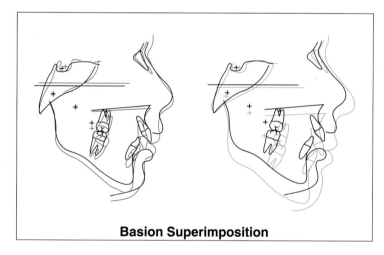

Basion Superimposition

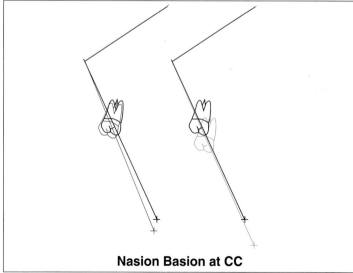

Nasion Basion at CC

L.J. -	Age	10.2	11.4	16.10 (Yr.Mon)
Cranial Base Angle		33	32	30
Facial Axis Angle		25	22	22
F/M Plane Angle		29	31	31
Craniomandibular Angle		62	63	60
Maxillary Plane		5	4	3
Convexity		8	6	4
U/Incisor to Vertical		28	11	23
L/Incisor to Vertical		31	30	32
Interincisal Angle		121	139	123
6 to Pterygoid Vertical		11	9	11
L/Incisor to A/Po		–2	0	1
L/Lip to Aesthetic Plane		0	1	–1

Treatment of Class II Division 2 Malocclusion

Retroclined upper incisors are responsible for holding the mandible in a distal position in Angle's Class II division 2 malocclusion. Twin Blocks have the effect of unlocking the malocclusion by releasing the mandible from an entrapped position of distal occlusion and thereby encouraging a rapid transition to Class I arch relationship.

Correction of Class II division 2 malocclusion is achieved by releasing the mandible downwards and forwards and encouraging the lower molars to erupt. At the same time, the upper incisors are advanced to achieve a normal upper-to-lower incisor relationship that is cleared far enough forwards to accommodate the progressively advancing mandibular arc of closure (**13.1**).

BITE REGISTRATION

The construction bite in Class II division 2 malocclusion is registered with the incisors in edge-to-edge occlusion. When the overbite is excessive, the clearance between the posterior teeth is correspondingly increased. These patients require more vertical development, so that the occlusal bite blocks tend to be thicker in the premolar region to allow clearance of the upper and lower incisors.

The amount of mandibular advancement is limited in Class II division 2 malocclusion as this malocclusion is normally associated with a mild Class II skeletal relationship with a horizontal growth pattern and a well-developed chin. It is important in treating this malocclusion not to overcorrect the mandibular position, which would result in a 'dished in' or Class III profile.

The easiest way to register the construction bite with the blue exactobite is first to record an edge-to-edge incisor relationship with 2 mm clearance between the upper and lower incisors when the patient occludes into the bite gauge. The handle is then cut off the bite gauge using Mauns cutters before softening the wax so that the patient can now close edge-to-edge with the incisors in contact (**13.2**).

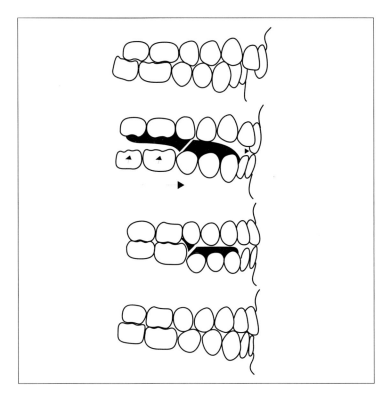

13.1 Management of Class II division 2.

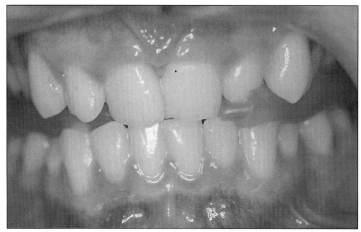

13.2 Registering an edge-to-edge construction bite.

APPLIANCE DESIGN: TWIN BLOCK SAGITTAL APPLIANCE

Sagittal development

In the treatment of Class II division 2 malocclusion, sagittal arch development is necessary to increase arch length and to advance retroclined incisors.

Sagittal appliances were formerly used in anteroposterior development of archform (Witzig & Spahl, 1987) as an initial stage of treatment to improve archform before functional correction of arch-to-arch relationships. The distalisation of the posterior quadrants is about 20–25% of the total arch development; the other 75–80% of the movement is exhibited by the anteriors as they tip forwards. This 20–80% ratio of posterior movement to anterior movement is a product of the anchorage of the second molars (Spahl, 1993).

Functional correction may now proceed simultaneously with sagittal arch development by adding sagittal screws to upper and lower Twin Blocks to combine the features of Twin Block and sagittal appliances.

The design of the upper Twin Block is modified by the addition of two sagittal screws set in the palate for anteroposterior arch development. The screws expand the arch by advancing the upper incisors and, at the same time, drive the upper buccal segments distally and buccally along the line of the arch (**13.3 A,B**).

In appliance construction it is important that the screws are positioned in the horizontal plane and angled along the line of the buccal segments to achieve the desired expansion. If the screws are angled downwards anteriorly, the appliance tends to ride down off the upper incisors as the screws are opened.

The sagittal design is suitable for both upper and lower arches to increase arch length. In the lower arch there is a choice of positioning the screws forwards in the canine region, when small curved screws may be used, or in the premolar region, when straight screws may be used to open premolar spaces.

Combined transverse and sagittal development

Many patients with malocclusion present archforms that are restricted in both transverse and anteroposterior dimensions. The Class II division II malocclusion and variations often require a combination of transverse and anteroposterior arch development in order to free the mandible from a distal occlusion.

Examination of the occlusion and study models in such cases shows retroclined upper and lower incisors. Deficient archwidth is associated with distal occlusion, and crowding is present in the upper incisor or canine region. Sometimes all four upper incisors are retroclined and the upper canines are crowded buccally. The upper anterior teeth cause interference when the lower model is advanced and it is not possible to engage the molars in Class I occlusion because of occlusal interference. Appliances must be designed to improve archform in order to free the mandible from distal occlusion (see case report T.S. in Chapter 16, **16.4**). It was formerly necessary to complete separate stages of treatment to improve archform before proceeding to functional correction.

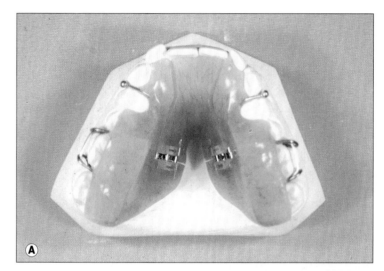

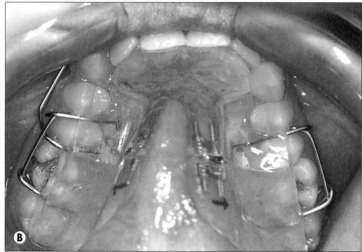

13.3 A, B Sagittal Twin Blocks for correction of Class II division 2.

The triple-screw sagittal Twin Block appliance is designed to improve archform in anteroposterior and transverse dimensions and simultaneously correct arch relationships for patients presenting complex problems of arch development. This appliance is a very powerful mechanism for interceptive treatment and arch development (**13.4 A–C**).

Alternatively, the three-way screw combines transverse and sagittal arch development. This incorporates two screws housed in a single unit and operated independently to expand in the transverse and sagittal dimensions. The three-way screw must be positioned in the midline behind the anterior teeth. It has the disadvantage of being bulky to accommodate comfortably in this area, but it is effective if the patient will tolerate the bulk in the anterior part of the palate (**13.5 A, B**).

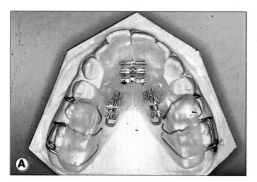

13.4 A A triple screw sagittal Twin Block appliance.

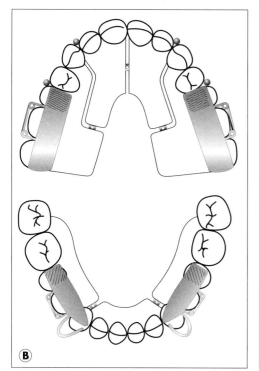

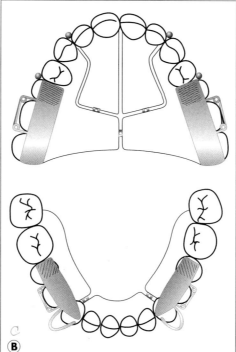

13.4 B, C Triple screw sagittal appliance.

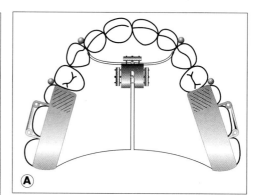

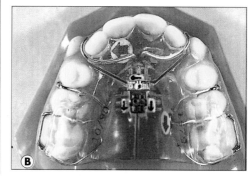

13.5 A, B Three-way screw for combined transverse and anteroposterior arch development.

THE TWIN BLOCK SAGITTAL APPLIANCE

Case report: H.McL. aged 14 years 5 months

In this typical Class II division 2 malocclusion in the permanent dentition, the major correction of arch relationships was achieved in 6 months with Twin Blocks. Brackets were fitted to improve alignment of the upper anterior teeth during this stage, before progressing to a simple fixed appliance to complete treatment. This case illustrates the clinical management of the Twin Block sagittal appliance in treatment of Class II division 2 malocclusion.

Clinical management. Both palatal screws are opened by two quarter turns per week, once in midweek and once at the weekend. This maintains contact of the appliance on the lingual of the upper incisors, and is effective in advancing these teeth to release the mandible from its retrusive position, locked in distal occlusion. The palatal acrylic adjacent to the attached gingiva and rugae of the premaxillary area may need slight reduction to allow the plate to abut against the lingual surfaces of the crowns of the upper anteriors.

The same sequence of trimming the occlusal blocks applies in the management of deep overbite in treatment of Class II division 2 as in that of Class II division 1 malocclusion (**13.6**). The upper bite block is progressively trimmed posteriorly to clear the occlusion for molar eruption in the early stages (**13.7**). When the molars are in occlusion, the lower appliance is gradually trimmed occlusally to allow lower premolar eruption to reduce the lateral open bite.

After 5 months of treatment, brackets were placed on the upper anterior teeth to initiate alignment at the end of the Twin Block phase. At the next visit, the lower appliance was left out and a Wilson lingual arch was fitted to hold the position in the lower arch. An anterior inclined plane with an occlusal stop for the lower incisors was worn for 6 months to maintain the vertical correction and allow the buccal teeth to settle fully into occlusion. The removable appliance was then discarded and treatment was completed in 6 months with a simple upper fixed appliance, followed by retention (**13.8 A–L**).

Discussion

The main advantage of using a Twin Block sagittal appliance in the management of Class II division 2 malocclusion is that the major correction of arch relationships is achieved quickly and consistently. There is the additional advantage of controlling the vertical dimension to increase lower facial height. Subsequent fixed appliance treatment to complete orthodontic correction is then greatly simplified.

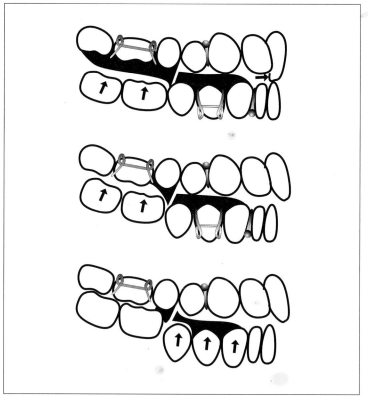

13.6 Sequence of trimming blocks for Class II division 2.

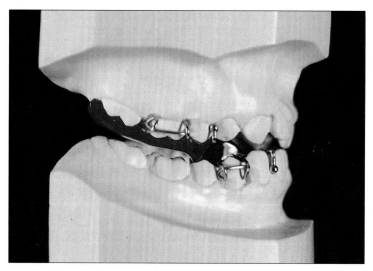

13.7 Occlusion cleared for molar eruption.

HMcL

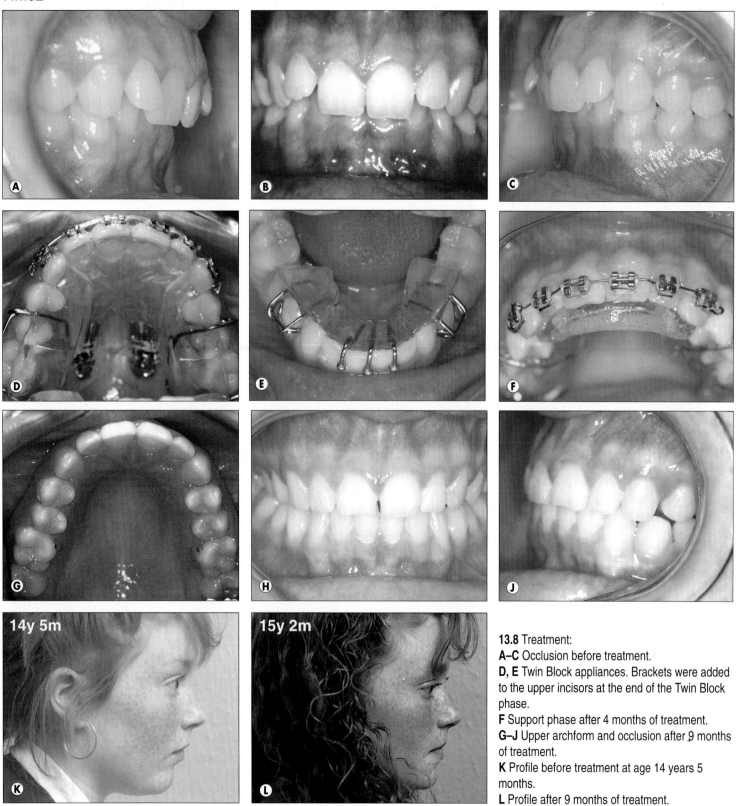

13.8 Treatment:
A–C Occlusion before treatment.
D, E Twin Block appliances. Brackets were added to the upper incisors at the end of the Twin Block phase.
F Support phase after 4 months of treatment.
G–J Upper archform and occlusion after 9 months of treatment.
K Profile before treatment at age 14 years 5 months.
L Profile after 9 months of treatment.

167

Case report: H.K. aged 14 years 6 months

Diagnosis, skeletal classification:
- Class I – mild class II tendency.
- Facial type: severe brachyfacial, horizontal growth.
- Maxilla: normal.
- Mandible: normal.
- Convexity = 2 mm.

Diagnosis, dental classification:
- Class II division 2.
- 1|1 retroclined and 2|2 proclined.
- Lower incisors: slight retrusion.
- Full unit distal occlusion.
- Deep overbite.
- Minimal crowding in lower arch.

Treatment plan:
- Functional correction to open the bite and correct the distal occlusion. Initiate fixed appliance treatment during the Twin Block stage.

- An anterior inclined plane to support the vertical dimension and to allow the buccal segment occlusion to settle. Correct the lower archform with a lower lingual arch.
- Complete the treatment with an upper fixed appliance (**13.9 A–S**).

Appliances:
- Upper sagittal/lower standard Twin Blocks. Sectional fixed appliance to align 321|123.
- Anterior inclined plane/Wilson lower lingual arch.
- Simple upper fixed appliance to complete the alignment.

Duration of treatment:
- Functional phase: 5 months with Twin Blocks.
- Support phase: 6 months for the occlusion to settle and to develop the archform.
- Orthodontic phase: 6 months to complete.
- Retention: 1 year.
- Total treatment time: 2 years 5 months, including retention,

Final records. 1 year out of retention.

HK

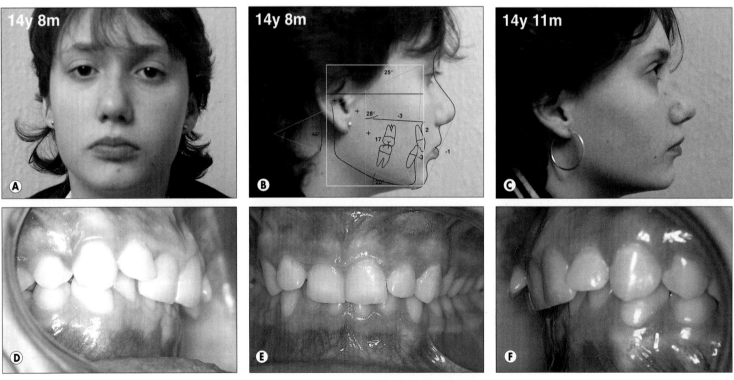

13.9 Treatment:
A, B Appearance before treatment at age 14 years 8 months.
C Profile change after 3 months treatment.
D–F Occlusion before treatment..
G Upper archform before treatment.
H Upper fixed appliance in phase 2.

J Upper archform after treatment.
K Lower archform before treatment.
L Wilson lingual arch in phase 2.
M Lower archform after treatment.
N, P, Q Occlusion after treatment at age 17 years 2 months.
R, S Facial appearance after treatment at age 16 years 32 months.

HK

HK

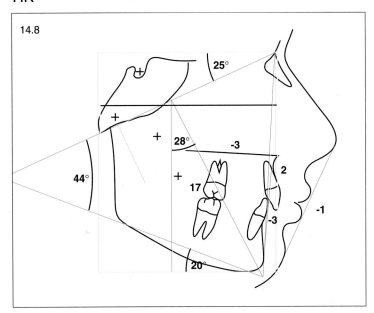

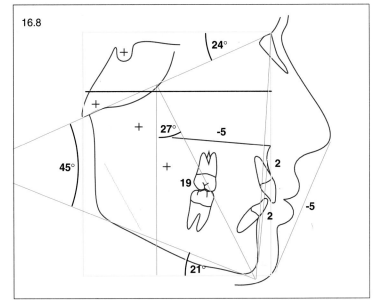

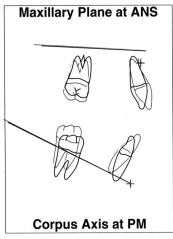

Maxillary Plane at ANS

Corpus Axis at PM

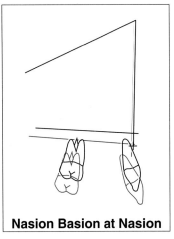

Nasion Basion at Nasion

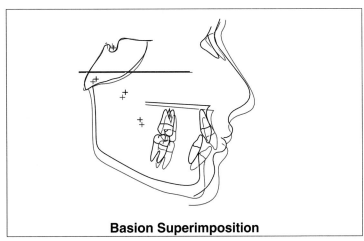

Basion Superimposition

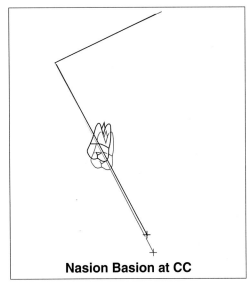

Nasion Basion at CC

H.K.-	Age 14.8	16.8 (Yr.Mon)
Cranial Base Angle	25	24
Facial Axis Angle	28	27
F/M Plane Angle	20	21
Craniomandibular Angle	44	45
Maxillary Plane	−3	−5
Convexity	2	2
U/Incisor to Vertical	12	22
L/Incisor to Vertical	21	43
Interincisal Angle	157	135
6 to Pterygoid Vertical	17	19
L/Incisor to A/Po	−3	2
L/Lip to Aesthetic Plane	−1	−5

Case report: S.Wa. aged 12 years 9 months

This girl is an example of treatment of a Class II division 2 malocclusion in the late mixed dentition with a combination of Twin Blocks and fixed appliances (**13.10 A–Q**).

Diagnosis, skeletal classification:
- Mild Class II.
- Facial type: severe brachyfacial.
- Maxilla: normal.
- Mild mandibular retrusion.

Diagnosis: dental classification:
- Class II division 2.
- 1|1 retroclined and 2|2 proclined.
- Lower incisors: mild retrusion.
- Good lower arch with no crowding.

Treatment plan:
- Orthopaedic phase to correct the distal occlusion and encourage vertical development to reduce the overbite.
- Orthodontic phase to detail the occlusion.

Appliances:
- Standard Twin Blocks with springs added to procline 1|1.
- Sectional fixed appliances and bioprogressive technique.

Bite registration. The intention of treatment in this Class II division 2 malocclusion is to limit forward translation of the mandible because the Class II skeletal discrepancy is mild. Therefore the bite is registered in an edge-to-edge incisor relationship and the upper incisors are advanced during the Twin Block stage to develop a positive overjet. Correction of the distal occlusion is achieved by encouraging vertical development of the lower molars that erupt forwards into a Class I occlusion with the upper molars.

The construction bite is registered with the blue exactobite and the handle is cut off to allow the incisors freedom to occlude edge-to-edge.

Clinical management. Twin Blocks were fitted and the springs were activated to advance 1|1. The upper Twin Block was trimmed occlusodistally to encourage lower molar eruption, to reduce the overbite and to increase facial height. After 2 months, brackets were added on 321|123 to correct anterior alignment in the upper arch at the same time as correcting the distal occlusion and reducing the overbite.

The distal occlusion was fully corrected with the molars in occlusion after 5 months, and the upper anterior alignment was corrected. The lower appliance was discarded and an anterior inclined plane used for 1 month only, to allow the buccal segments to settle, before fitting upper and lower sectional fixed appliances to complete the treatment.

Duration of treatment:
- Active phase: 5 months with Twin Blocks.
- Support phase: 1 month for the occlusion to settle.
- Orthodontic phase: 1 year 2 months.
- Retention: 1 year.

SWa

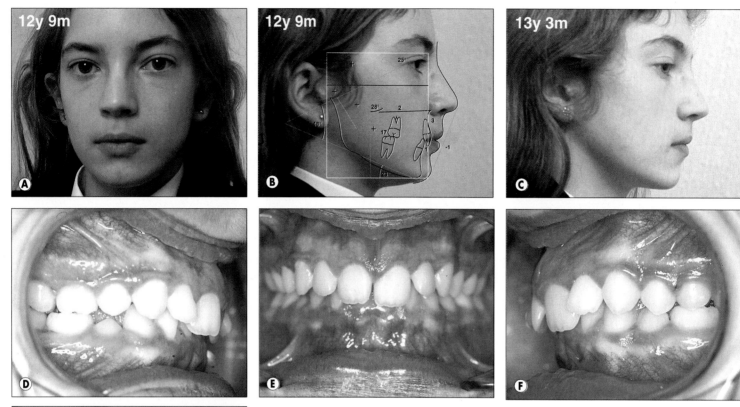

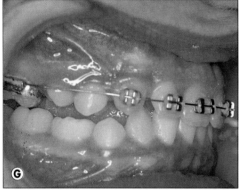

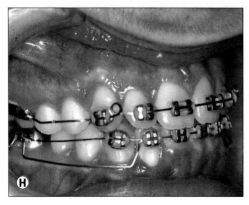

13.10 Treatment:
A, B Appearance before treatment at age 12 years 9 months.
C Profile change after 6 months with Twin Blocks.
D–F Occlusion before treatment.
G Orthodontic phase after 6 months of treatment.
H–K Fixed appliances to complete the treatment.

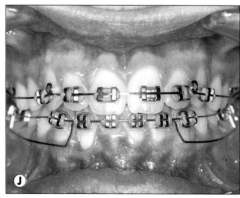

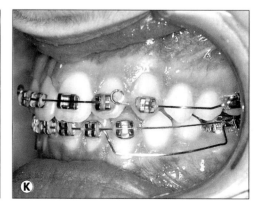

SWa

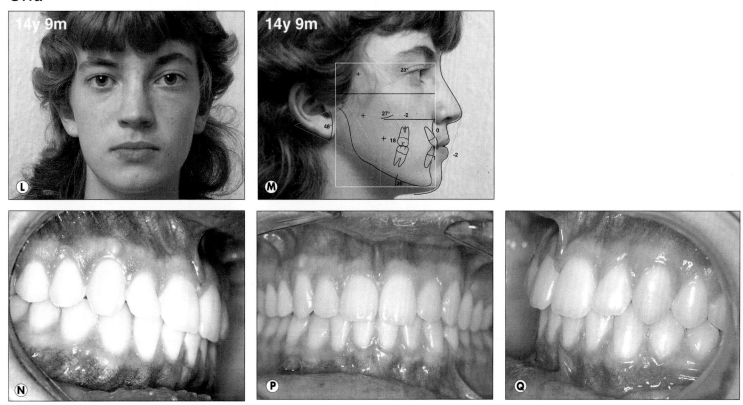

13.10 Treatment (cont.):
L, M Facial appearance after treatment at age 14 years 9 months.
N–Q Occlusion at age 17 years 3 months.

SWa

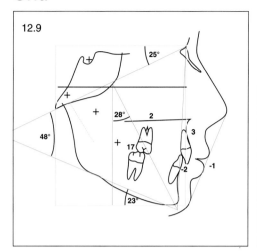

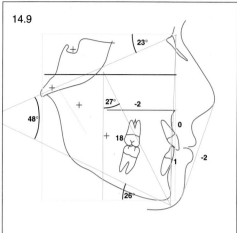

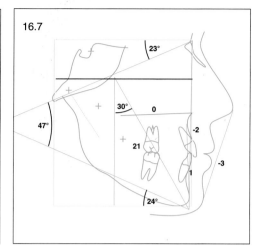

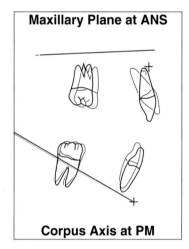

Maxillary Plane at ANS

Corpus Axis at PM

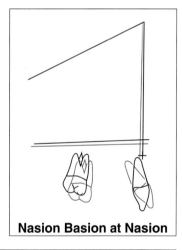

Nasion Basion at Nasion

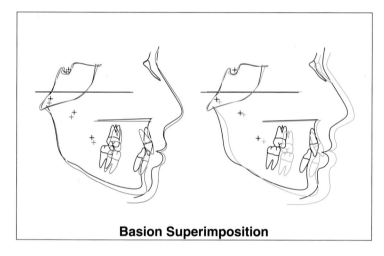

Basion Superimposition

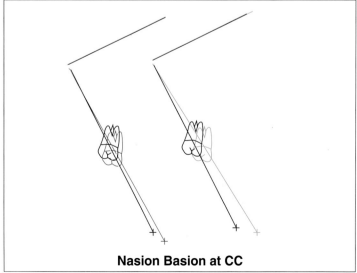

Nasion Basion at CC

S.Wa. -	Age	12.9	14.9	16.7	(Yr.Mon)
Cranial Base Angle		25	23	23	
Facial Axis Angle		28	27	30	
F/M Plane Angle		23	26	24	
Craniomandibular Angle		48	48	47	
Maxillary Plane		2	−2	0	
Convexity		3	0	−2	
U/Incisor to Vertical		8	27	29	
L/Incisor to Vertical		23	23	20	
Interincisal Angle		149	130	131	
6 to Pterygoid Vertical		17	18	21	
L/Incisor to A/Po		−2	1	1	
L/Lip to Aesthetic Plane		1	−2	−3	

SWn

THE CENTRAL SAGITTAL TWIN BLOCK

Combination therapy by Twin Blocks and fixed appliances

Case report: S.Wn. aged 12 years 6 months

This boy presented a Class II division 2 malocclusion in the permanent dentition. A central sagittal Twin Block was used to advance upper incisors, to reduce overbite and to correct distal occlusion. In the support phase, a three-way expansion screw combined lateral and anteroposterior expansion of the upper arch with a Wilson lower lingual arch, followed by a short period with fixed appliances to complete the treatment (**13.11**).

Failure to include lateral expansion during the first phase of sagittal correction resulted in the development of a lateral crossbite in the buccal segments. In this case, lateral expansion was carried out in the support phase, but it is normally better to combine transverse and sagittal expansion during the Twin Block phase.

Duration of treatment:
* Active phase: 12 months with Twin Blocks.
* Phase 2: 12 months for additional arch development.
* Orthodontic phase: 1 year 2 months.
* Retention: 1 year.

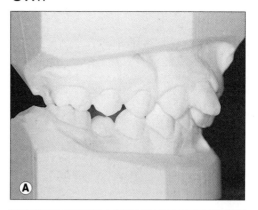
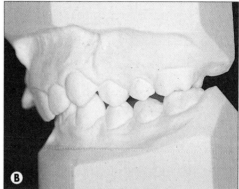
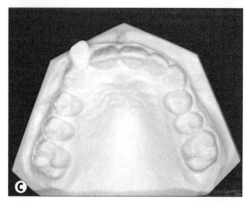
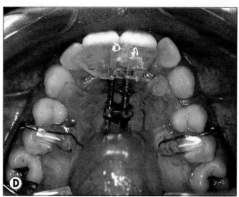

13.11 Treatment:
A–C Occlusion before treatment at age 12 years 6 months.
D Screw to advance the upper incisors.

SWn

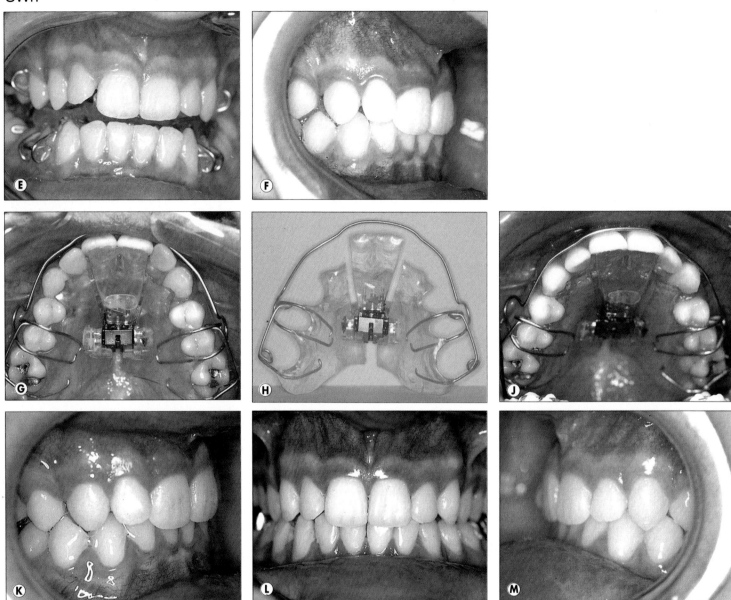

13.11 Treatment (cont.):
E Twin Block appliances.
F Occlusion after 1 year.
G–J Phase 2 appliance with a three-way expansion screw.
K–M Occlusion before fitting the fixed appliances at age 14 years 8 months.

SWn

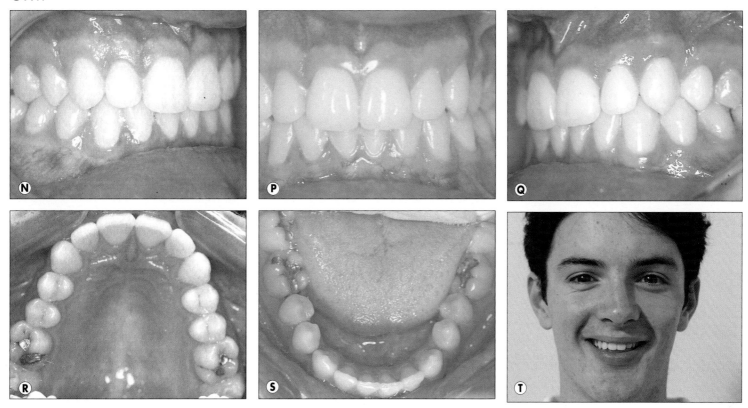

13.11 Treatment (cont.):
N–Q Occlusion at age 17 years 11 months.
R–T Occlusal views and facial appearance at age 17 years 11 months.

REFERENCES

Spahl, T.J. (1993). The Spahl split vertical eruption acceleration appliance system. *Functional Orthod.*, **10**(1): 10–24.

Witzig, J.W. & Spahl, T.J. (1987). The great second molar debate. In *The Clinical Management of Basic Maxillofacial Orthopedic Appliances, Vol. 1—Mechanics*, pp. 155–216.

CHAPTER
14

Treatment of Class III Malocclusion

REVERSE TWIN BLOCKS

Functional correction of Class III malocclusion is achieved in Twin Block technique by reversing the angulation of the inclined planes, harnessing occlusal forces as the functional mechanism to correct arch relationships by maxillary advancement, while using the lower arch as the means of anchorage. The position of the bite blocks is reversed compared to Twin Blocks for Class II treatment. The occlusal blocks are placed over the upper deciduous molars and the lower first molars.

Reverse Twin Blocks are designed to encourage maxillary development by the action of reverse occlusal inclined planes cut at a 70° angle to drive the upper teeth forwards by the forces of occlusion and, at the same time, to restrict forward mandibular development (**14.1**).

Prior to initiation of Class III Twin Block treatment it is important to ensure that the patient's condyles are not displaced superiorly and/or posteriorly in the glenoid fossae at full occlusion. In treatment with the reverse Twin Block, the occlusal force exerted on the mandible is directed downwards and backwards by the reverse inclined planes. No damaging force is exerted on the condyles because the bite is hinged open with the condyles down and forward in the fossae and the inclined planes are directed downwards and backwards on the mandibular teeth. The force vector in the mandible passes from the lower molar towards the gonial angle. This is the area of the mandible best able to absorb occlusal forces (**14.2**).

BITE REGISTRATION

It is not possible to build-in the same degree of activation in the construction bite for functional correction of a Class III malocclusion compared to a Class II correction, because there is less scope for distal displacement of the mandible.

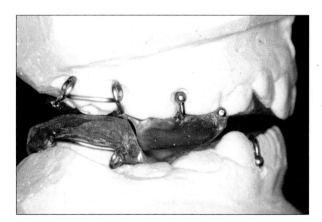

14.1 Reverse Twin Blocks.

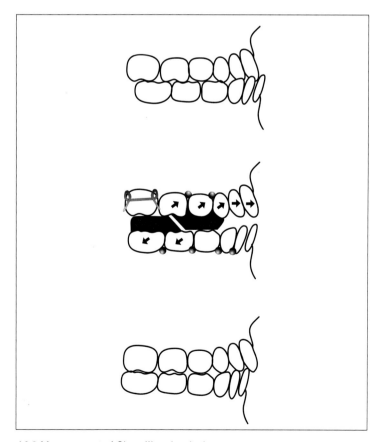

14.2 Management of Class III malocclusion.

The blue exactobite is used to register a construction bite with the teeth closed to the position of maximum retrusion, leaving sufficient clearance between the posterior teeth for the occlusal bite blocks. This is normally achieved by recording a construction bite with 2 mm inter-incisal clearance in the fully retruded position.

APPLIANCE DESIGN – REVERSE TWIN BLOCKS

The sagittal design is used to advance the upper incisors to correct the lingual occlusion in treatment of Class III malocclusion (**14.3**).

In many cases, the maxilla is contracted laterally in addition to occluding in a distal relationship to the mandible. This is an indication for combined sagittal and transverse expansion using a three-screw sagittal appliance which includes a midline screw to complement the action of the sagittal screws.

An alternative design uses a three-way expansion screw to combine transverse and sagittal expansion. This is also effective in expanding a contracted maxilla and in correcting lingual occlusion if used in combination with reverse inclined planes (**14.4 A,B**). Alternatively, a triple screw sagittal may be used for three way max-

illary development, as described for treatment of Class II division 2 malocclusion (see **13.4 A,B**).

Management of reverse Twin Blocks

With the sagittal appliance design, because of the curvature of the palate it is easier for the patient to operate the screws from the fitting surface of the appliance. The screws should be positioned so that both are opened by turning in the same direction. This is less confusing for a young patient. The lower appliance is retained with clasps on the lower molars and additional interdental clasps as required.

Opening the screws has the reciprocal effect of driving the upper molars distally and advancing the incisors. Distal movement of the upper molars is resisted by occlusion of the lower bite blocks on the reverse inclined planes. Therefore the net effect of opening the screws is a forward driving force on the upper dental arch. The position of the cut for the screws will influence their action on individual teeth. The cuts may be positioned distal to the lateral incisors to advance only the four upper incisors. Positioning the cuts mesial to the upper molars would increase the distalising component of force on the molars, but distal movement is resisted by occlusion with the lower

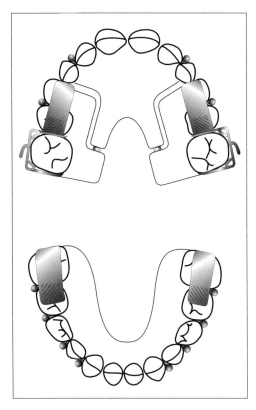

14.3 Detail of appliance design.

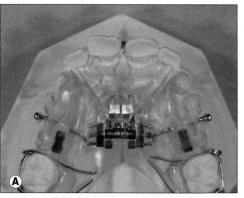
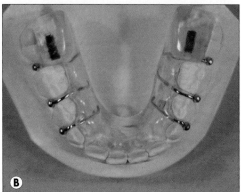

14.4 A, B Three-way screw appliance design.

bite blocks, and the reciprocal force acts to advance the entire upper arch mesial to the molars, using the lower arch as anchorage.

To enhance the forward movement of the upper labial segment, lip pads may be added to support the upper lip clear of the incisors with an action similar to that of the Frankel III. The lip pads need not be joined in the midline provided they are carried on heavy gauge wires that are self-supporting to hold the pads clear of the gingivae in order to avoid gingival irritation. It is important to attach the lip pads to the anterior segment of the appliance so that they advance as the screws are opened, otherwise the pads become compressed against the gingivae in the labial segment. In addition, they may be adjusted forwards clear of the gingivae as the incisors are advanced (**14.5 A,B**).

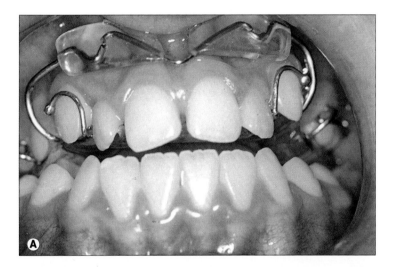

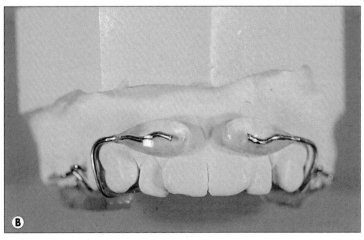

14.5 A, B Lip pads must be supported clear of the gingivae. The action is similar to the upper lip pads on the Frankel III.

TREATMENT OF CLASS III MALOCCLUSION WITH REVERSE TWIN BLOCKS

Case report: M.L. aged 7 years 5 months

This young girl presented an Angle's Class III malocclusion soon after eruption of the permanent incisors. There was lingual occlusion of the upper labial segment with no forward posture on closure and 2|2 were displaced lingual to 1|1 (**14.6 A–Q**).

Diagnosis, skeletal classification:
- Class III.
- Facial type: mesiofacial – dolichofacial tendency.
- Maxilla: moderate retrognathic.
- Mandible: normal.
- Convexity = –1 mm.

Diagnosis, dental classification:
- Class III.
- Lingual occlusion 21|12.
- Reverse overjet = 3 mm.
- Upper incisors: moderate retrusion.
- Lower incisors: mild protrusion.
- |2 blocked out of the arch lingual to |1.
- Cannot occlude edge-to-edge on upper incisors.
- No forward posture on closure.

Treatment plan. Advance the upper labial segment and apply a retrusive force downwards and backwards to the lower dental arch.

Appliances:
- Reverse Twin Blocks with sagittal design to advance the upper incisors. Additional springs to be added to advance 2|2.
- After correction of lingual occlusion Class III intermaxillary traction to be added to the lower labial segment to help increase the overbite and stabilise the occlusion.

Clinical management. A positive overjet was established after 6 weeks and light Class III traction was applied. Reverse Twin Blocks were worn for 5 months full time, and night-time wear for 3 months to correct the Class III occlusion.

Duration of treatment:
- Active phase: 5 months.
- Retention: 3 months.
- Total treatment time: 8 months. This short period of treatment was successful in reversing the Class III growth tendency, and in establishing a Class I occlusion that was maintained 6 years out of retention without further treatment.

ML

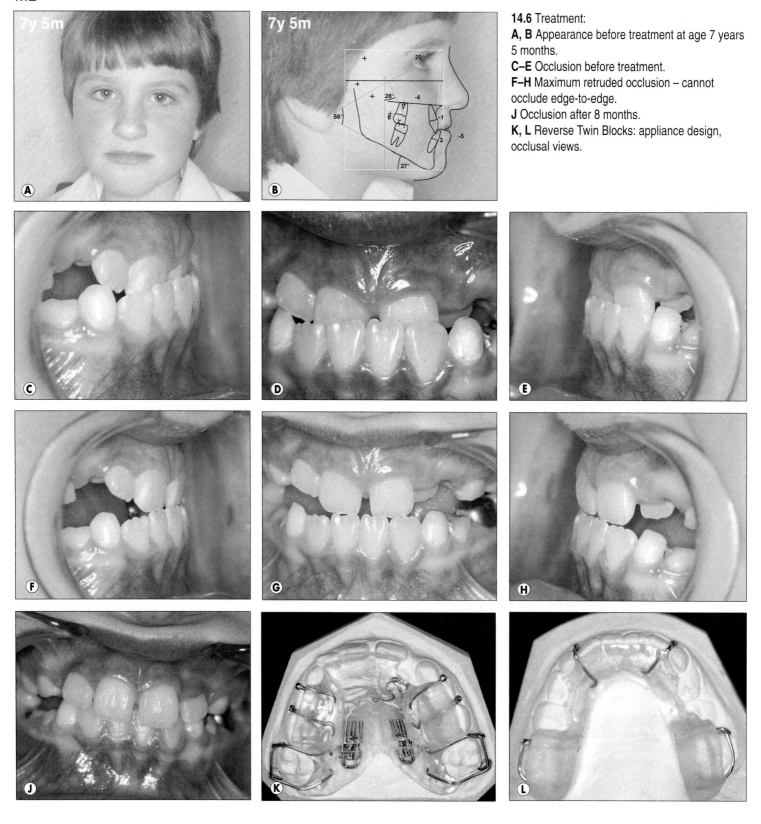

14.6 Treatment:

A, B Appearance before treatment at age 7 years 5 months.

C–E Occlusion before treatment.

F–H Maximum retruded occlusion – cannot occlude edge-to-edge.

J Occlusion after 8 months.

K, L Reverse Twin Blocks: appliance design, occlusal views.

ML

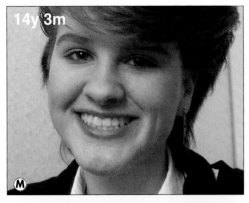

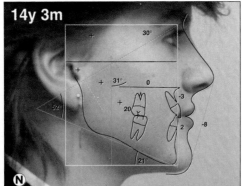

14.6 Treatment (cont.):
M, N Facial appearance at age 14 years 3 months.
P–R Occlusion 6 years out of retention at age 14 years 3 months.

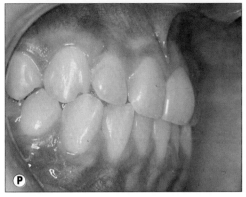

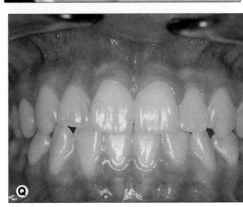

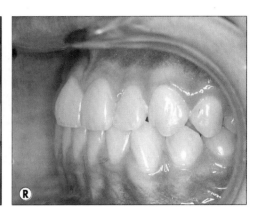

ML

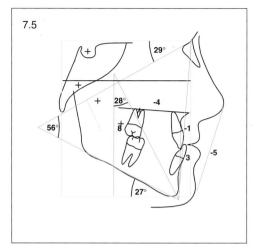

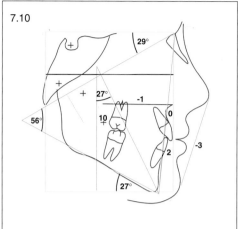

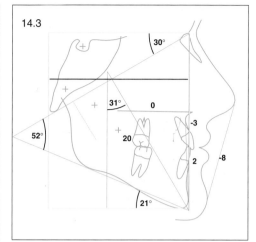

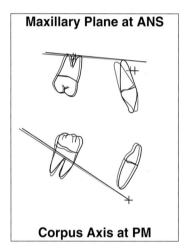

Maxillary Plane at ANS

Corpus Axis at PM

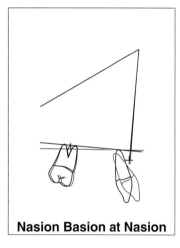

Nasion Basion at Nasion

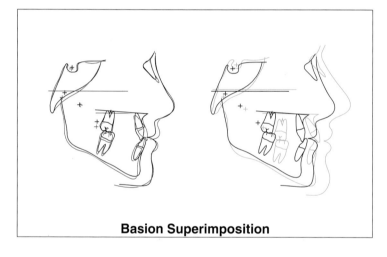

Basion Superimposition

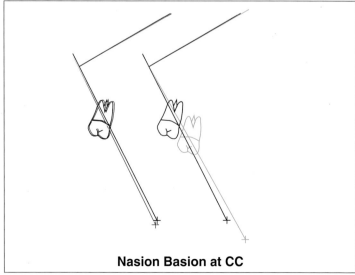

Nasion Basion at CC

M.L. -	Age	7.5	7.10	14.3	(Yr.Mon)
Cranial Base Angle		29	29	30	
Facial Axis Angle		28	27	31	
F/M Plane Angle		27	27	21	
Craniomandibular Angle		56	56	52	
Maxillary Plane		−4	−1	0	
Convexity		−1	0	−3	
U/Incisor to Vertical		11	29	30	
L/Incisor to Vertical		26	26	18	
Interincisal Angle		143	125	132	
6 to Pterygoid Vertical		8	10	20	
L/Incisor to A/Po		3	2	2	
L/Lip to Aesthetic Plane		−5	−3	−8	

REVERSE PULL FACIAL MASK

The reverse pull facial mask applies an additional component of orthopaedic force to advance the maxilla by elastic traction (Delaire, 1971, 1976; Delaire *et al.*, 1972; Petit, 1982, 1983, 1984, 1991; McNamara, 1987, 1993). This mechanism can be attached to the upper Twin Block to maximise the forward component of force on the maxilla, converting the technique to a functional orthopaedic system. The addition of three-way expansion in the appliance design enhances treatment of maxillary deficiency. Sagittal screws cut anterior to the upper molars have the effect of increasing the activation of the inclined planes to advance the premaxillary segment by driving the blocks distally against the resistance of the lower inclined planes (**14.7 A,B; 14.8**).

The elastic force applied should be increased gradually from the time the facial mask is fitted and as the patient adapts to the pressure. A starting pressure using bilateral 3/8 in (9.5 mm), 8 oz (227 g) elastics is recommended for the first two weeks. The force may then be increased by using 1/2 in (13 mm), 14 oz (397 g) elastics, and later to a maximum by 5/16 in (8 mm), 14 oz (397 g) elastics. If the patient experiences pain or soft-tissue irritation, the elastic force should be reduced to a more comfortable level.

The face mask is most effective if worn for a short period of 4–6 months using heavy forces. The additional functional forces make it unnecessary to wear the facial mask during the day and it can be applied as a night-time auxilliary force.

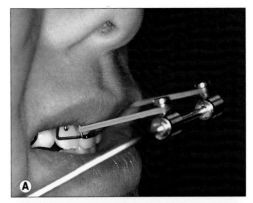

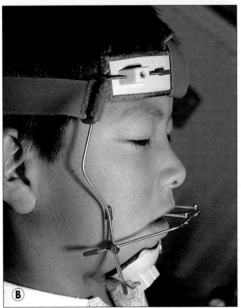

14. 7 A, B An example of a facial mask for maxillary advancement.

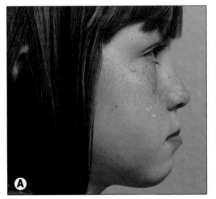
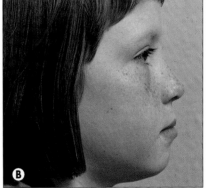

14. 8 A, B Facial change after 2 months treatment combining reverse magnetic Twin Blocks with reverse pull headgear.

REFERENCES

Delaire, J. (1971). Confection du masque orthopedique. *Rev. Stomat., Paris*, **72**: 579–84.

Delaire, J. (1976). L'articulation fronto-maxillaire. Bases theoretiques et principles generaux d'application le forces extra-orales postero-anterieures sur masque orthopedique. *Rev. Stomat., Paris*, **77**: 921–30.

Delaire, J., Verson, P., Lumineau, J.P., Gegha-Negrea, A., Talmont, J. & Boisson, M. (1972). Quelques resultats des tractions extra-orales à apput fronto-mentonnier dans de traitment orthopedique des malformations maxillo mandibulaires de Class III et des sequelles osseues des fente labio-maxillaires. *Rev. Stomat., Paris*, **73**: 633–42.

McNamara, J.A. (1987). An orthopedic approach to the treatment of class III malocclusion in young patients. *J. Clin. Orthod.*, **21**: 598–608.

McNamara, J.A. (1993). Orthopedic facial mask therapy. In *Orthodontic and Orthopedic Treatment in the Mixed Dentition*. pp. 283–95.

Petit, H. P. (1982). Syndromes prognathiques: schemas de traitement 'global' autour de masques facieux. *Rev. Orthop. Dent. Faciale*, **16**: 381–411.

Petit, H.P. (1983). Adaptation following accelerated facial mask therapy. In *Clinical Alteration of the Growing Face,* eds J.A. McNamara, Jr, J.A. Ribbens & R.P. Howe. Monograph No. 14, Craniofacial Growth Series. Ann Arbor, University of Michigan.

Petit, H.P. (1984). Orthopadie et/ou Orthodontie. *Orthod. Fr.*, **55**: 527–33.

Petit, H.P. (1991). Normalisation morphogenetique, apport de l'orthopadie, *Orthod. Fr.*, **62**: 549–57.

CHAPTER
15

Differential Diagnosis

EXTRACTION OR NON-EXTRACTION THERAPY

Since the turn of the century, the pendulum has swung back and forth between extraction and nonextraction therapy. At the beginning of the twentieth century, Angle believed unconditionally that all 32 teeth should be accommodated in every case, regardless of the growth pattern or the relationship of the size of the teeth to the basal bone. His philosophy insisted that if the teeth were moved into normal interdigitation, functional stimulation would result in compensatory basal bone growth to accommodate the teeth in their corrected position. It was heresy for a disciple of Angle even to think about extraction of teeth as a part of orthodontic therapy.

As a student of Angle, Tweed practised nonextraction therapy for 6 years and observed a high percentage of relapse by reappearance of crowding in cases with a tooth/supporting tissue discrepancy. In edgewise mechanics, correction of a Class II dental relationship in permanent dentition by intermaxillary traction was accompanied by forward movement of the lower dentition. He related lack of harmony in facial contour to the extent to which the denture was displaced mesially into protrusion and concluded that the orthodontist must find a means of accurately predetermining the anterior limits of stability of the denture in functional balance.

Tweed gained acceptance for premolar extraction therapy and established an entire orthodontic treatment philosophy based on the concept that facial balance and harmony are dependent on the mandibular incisors being upright over basal bone. He expressed a mean angulation of the lower incisor to the Frankfort plane of $65° \pm 5°$ as a position of balance.

Tweed differentiated facial growth trends into three basic types to account for patients who exhibited balanced growth, vertical growth and horizontal growth patterns . He believed that extractions were mandatory in vertical growth patterns for patients with high ANB angles, anticipating that point B would always drop down and back in treatment. He observed that lower incisors often had to be proclined in treating patients with vertical growth patterns to compensate for skeletal discrepancies, but as a rule these teeth then remained stable

and devoid of rotations after treatment. Conversely, in patients with horizontal growth patterns, the mandible grows forwards faster than the maxilla, resulting in lingual tipping of the lower incisors and development of crowding in the lower labial segments.

In developing the 'bioprogressive philosophy', Ricketts *et al.* (1979) moved away from a dogmatic approach to extraction therapy. They related treatment planning to facial aesthetics and the pattern of facial growth.

Studies of the long-term results of treatment were carried out by the bioprogressive group, assisted by Rocky Mountain Data Systems (Ricketts *et al.*, 1979). This resulted in improved methods of differential diagnosis for the selection of extraction or nonextraction therapy. These studies also provided a foundation for computerised growth prediction based on average increments of growth. Ricketts defined parameters in cephalometric analysis to assist more accurate treatment planning related to facial aesthetics.

The position of the lower incisor relative to the anterior limit of the skeletal base is crucial in facial aesthetics. The principle of relating lower incisor position to the skeletal apical base by means of linear measurements was originally described by Downs (1948) and elaborated by Ricketts (1960). The A–Po line joins point A and pogonion, the anterior points on the maxillary and mandibular skeletal bases, respectively. This line defines the anterior limit of the skeletal base.

In dental prosthetics we follow the principle of placing the lower incisors upright over the ridge to stabilise a lower denture. Positioning the incisors too far labially results in an unstable denture and placing them too far lingually encroaches on tongue space. The same principle applies in the natural dentition.

Lower incisor position is always reflected in the position of the lower lip and has a significant influence on the profile and, therefore, on facial aesthetics. Ricketts recommends positioning the tip of the lower incisor at +1 to +3 mm relative to the A–Po line for the best aesthetic result (**15.1**). This positions the lower incisor over basal bone close to the anterior limit of the skeletal base, and gives a pleasing contour to the lower lip- in profile-related to the nose and chin.

ARCH LENGTH DISCREPANCY

Arch length discrepancy defines the amount of crowding present in the dental arch by comparing the space available with the space required to accommodate all the teeth in the arch in correct alignment. The degree of crowding is determined by examining the models from the occlusal aspect, starting at the mesial contact point of the first permanent molar on one side and estimating the amount of crowding at each contact point, passing round the arch to the mesial contact point of the first molar on the opposite side. The summmation of crowding at each contact point gives the arch length discrepancy in mm. Allowance may also be made for potential crowding of second or third molars. The same calculation in the mixed dentition is referred to as a mixed dentition analysis and, if space is maintained by holding the position of the first molars after loss of second deciduous molars, provision should be made for an additional 4 mm of arch length during the transition to permanent dentition.

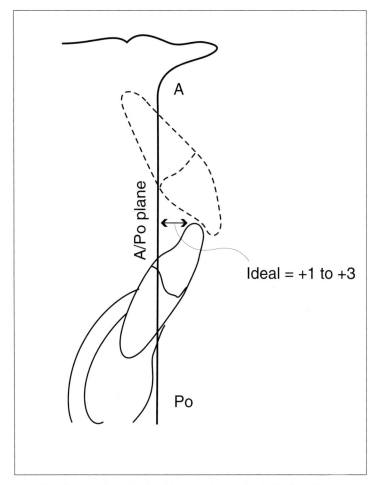

15.1 The distance from the tip of lower incisor to the A–Po line. For the best aesthetic result the range is +1 to +3 mm.

The 'Richter Scale'

It is helpful in treatment planning to classify the degree of difficulty of the malocclusion as mild, moderate or severe. In arch length discrepancy:

*   Mild crowding is in the range 1–3 mm.
*   Moderate crowding is classified as 4–5 mm.
*   Severe crowding is 6 mm or more.

This is a sliding scale (the author describes it as the 'Richter scale') expressing degree of difficulty for dental correction by nonextraction therapy. The higher the value, the more difficult it is to resolve crowding permanently without extractions.

Two factors improve the prognosis for non-extraction therapy in moderate or severely crowded dentitions:

*   First, early treatment by arch development to increase archwidth before permanent premolars and canines erupt.
*   Secondly, lingual positioning of the lower dentition relative to the skeletal base requires a nonextraction approach.

The 'Richter scale' can also be applied when the measure of convexity is used to determine the skeletal discrepancy:

*   A skeletal convexity of 1–3 mm is within the range of normal.
*   4 –5 mm convexity is a moderate Class II skeletal discrepancy.
*   6 mm or more is severe Class II.

The higher the convexity, the more likely that functional orthopedics is indicated to improve the skeletal relationship.

TREATMENT PLANNING IN CROWDED DENTITIONS

Ricketts' parameters for a lower incisor position relative to the A–Po line serve as a base line from which to plan the treatment of crowding. The degree of crowding in the lower arch is related to the labiolingual position of the lower incisor as a guide to determine a differential diagnosis for extraction or non-extraction therapy.

Assessing arch length discrepancy and lower incisor position determines whether the lower incisors can be advanced to a stable position relative to the skeletal base after treatment. This depends on the degree of protrusion or retrusion of the lower incisors related to the degree of crowding in the lower arch. Before moving the lower incisors it should be established that good bony support is available to accommodate the proposed movement.

If the lower incisors are retroclined and positioned lingual to the A–Po line, arch length can be increased by advancing the lower incisors. As a guide, proclination of the lower incisors by 1 mm increases arch length by 2 mm (equivalent to a gain of 1 mm on each side).

Conversely, if lower incisors are proclined and positioned too far labial to the A–Po line they should be retracted to improve facial aesthetics. Each 1 mm of retraction will reduce total arch length by 2 mm.

According to the position of the lower incisors before treatment, the space required to correct crowding can be calculated by repositioning the tip of the lower incisors within the range of +1 to +3 mm to the A–Po line. This is a reliable guideline to relate treatment to facial aesthetics in extraction and nonextraction therapy (**15.2**).

One other factor should be taken into account. Functional mandibular advancement carries pogonion forward and invariably results in a relative forward movement of the lower incisors as the A–Po line becomes more upright. The lower incisor position should therefore be reviewed after functional therapy when the occlusion has settled.

LIP CONTOUR

The fullness of the lips provides an additional aesthetic guideline for extraction or nonextraction therapy. The angulation of the upper lip is a crucial factor in facial aesthetics. Ideally the upper lip should be angled between 20 and 30° to the nasion vertical for the best aesthetic appearance. If the angle between the upper lip and the undersurface of the nose is more than 90°, the patient's appearance in profile is progressively less aesthetic as the naso-labial angle becomes more obtuse.

Extraction of premolars should be avoided at all costs if the lips are a thin red line and the lower lip lies well behind the aesthetic line (tangent to the nose and chin). The resulting loss of lip support would cause further damage to the facial appearance, and may compromise temporomandibular joint function.

When the lip contour is good before treatment it is important not to destroy good facial balance and premolar extractions should be avoided. In an ideal profile the lower lip lies fractionally behind the aesthetic line (2 mm in the child and 4 mm in the adult). The characteristic flattening of the profile that occurs in the late teens should be taken into account when we plan treatment for a young patient. If we produce a flat profile in a young child, the lips will become retrusive in the profile as the child grows into adulthood.

When the lips extend beyond the aesthetic line this reflects a labial position of the lower incisors. Crowding associated with bimaxillary protrusion is an indication for extraction of premolars.

NONEXTRACTION THERAPY

Non-extraction therapy has become a popular misnomer because it refers to nonextraction of premolars. Crowding may still be relieved by extraction of second or third molars after a period of nonextraction therapy. This approach lends itself to early intervention to combine arch development and functional therapy in a first phase of interceptive treatment, followed by an orthodontic phase for detailed finishing in the permanent dentition.

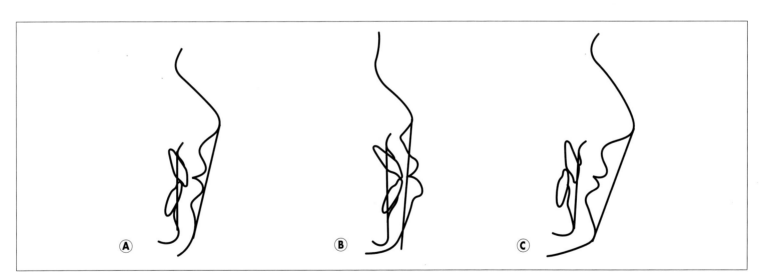

15.2 Diagram of three profiles to show the relationship of lip position to lower incisor position:
A The profile on the left shows good facial balance. Nonextraction treatment is preferred to maintain balance.
B The middle profile shows the lower incisor positioned significantly forward to the skeletal base (+7 mm to the A–Po line). Extraction therapy is indicated to improve the lip position.
C The profile on the right shows the lower incisor positioned significantly lingual to the skeletal base (–5 mm to the A–Po line). Extraction therapy is contraindicated and nonextraction therapy should aim to advance the upper and lower labial segments to improve the profile.

Extraction of second molars

Extraction of second molars has long been recognised as an effective alternative to premolar extraction in gaining arch length in the lower arch without the disadvantage of sacrificing lip support and damaging facial aesthetics (Wilson, 1964, 1966, 1971; Liddle, 1977; Witzig & Spahl, 1987). Reporting on 500 cases where second molars had been extracted, Wilson (1974) noted that 87% showed the third molars erupted in acceptable position. Richardson (Richardson & Burden, 1992; Richardson & Mills, 1990) followed the effects of extraction of second molars and found that extraction of second molars is effective in reducing the incidence of late lower arch crowding and third molar impaction.

Examining the effect of second molar extraction in the treatment of lower premolar crowding it was concluded that up to 4 or 5 mm of lower premolar crowding can be successfully treated by extraction of lower second premolars, with or without the use of simple orthodontic appliances. Early extraction of lower second molars, before second premolar eruption, seems to create the most favourable conditions for spontaneous premolar alignment.

Richardson & Richardson (1993), investigating lower third molar development subsequent to second molar extraction, found that 99% of third molars upright mesiodistally, but few became as upright as the second molars they replaced. Model analysis showed that 96% of the lower third molars erupted in good and acceptable positions.

REFERENCES

Liddle, D.W. (1977). Second molar extraction in orthodontic treatment. *Am. J. Orthod.*, **72**: 599–616.

Richardson, M.E. & Burden, D.J. (1992). Second molar extraction in the treatment of lower premolar crowding. *Brit. J. Orthod.*, **19**(4): 299–304.

Richardson, M.E. & Mills, K. (1990). Late lower arch crowding. The effect of second molar extraction. *Am. J. Orthod. Dentof. Orthop.*, **98**: 242–6.

Richardson, M.E. & Richardson, A. (1993). Lower third molar development subsequent to second molar extraction. *Am. J. Orthod. Dentof. Orthop.*, **104**: 566–74.

Ricketts, R.M. (1960). A foundation for cephalometric communication. *Am. J. Orthod.*, **46**, 330–57.

Ricketts, R.M. *et al.* (1979). *Bioprogressive Therapy*. Denver, Rocky Mountain Orthodontics.

Wilson, H.E. (1964). Extraction of second molars in treatment planning. *Orthod Fr.*, **25**: 61–7.

Wilson, H.E. (1966). The extraction of second molars as a therapeutic measure. *Eur. Orthod. Soc.*, 141–5.

Wilson, H.E. (1971). Extraction of second molars in orthodontic treatment. *Orthodontist*, **3**: 1–7.

Wilson, H.E. (1974). Long term observation on the extraction of second molars. *Eur.Orthod Soc.*, **50**: 215–21.

Witzig, J.W. & Spahl, T.J. (1987). The great second molar debate. In *The Clinical Management of Basic Maxillofacial Orthopedic Appliances, Vol. 1—Mechanics*, pp. 155–216.

16

Management of Crowding

NONEXTRACTION THERAPY

Interceptive treatment – arch development

Crowding and irregularity of the dental arches may necessitate an interceptive stage of treatment to align the arches and improve the archform as a preliminary to the correction of arch-to-arch relationships. Interceptive treatment should be initiated as early as possible in the mixed dentition to develop correct archform before permanent successors erupt.

Examination of the occlusion prior to treatment establishes the necessity for an interceptive phase of arch development. If significant crowding is present, the upper and lower archform does not match and, as a result, a preliminary stage of interceptive treatment becomes necessary.

A diagnostic guideline is observed by posturing the mandible forward to see if the teeth will fit in good occlusion when the mandible is advanced. This is confirmed by examining study models with the lower model advanced to reduce the overjet and correct the buccal segment relationships. If this produces a poor occlusion it may be necessary to correct the archform first before advancing the mandible by functional therapy.

Integration of Twin Blocks and Fixed Therapy

Combined orthopaedic and orthodontic treatment may be planned in two phases, depending on the age of the patient at the start of treatment and the degree of severity of the skeletal and dental problems. Arch development and functional therapy in the mixed dentition is frequently followed by a finishing phase of orthodontic treatment at a later stage of development.

In the permanent dentition fixed appliance treatment may precede Twin Block treatment to correct an irregular archform where the irregularity is moderate or severe. Alternatively, in less crowded cases fixed appliances may be integrated with Twin Blocks by the addition of brackets to correct anterior alignment. Further integration with fixed appliances can continue in the lower arch during the support phase, when the lower Twin Block is left out or, alternatively, a transition to full fixed appliances may be made on completion of functional correction. The treatment of patients presenting a combination of crowding, dental irregularity and skeletal discrepancy requires more time compared to the treatment of uncrowded cases with good archform.

ARCH DEVELOPMENT BEFORE FUNCTIONAL THERAPY

Combination fixed/functional therapy

Case report: K.C. aged 11 years 2 months

Diagnosis, skeletal classification:
- Moderate Class II.
- Facial type: severe brachyfacial retrognathic.
- Maxilla: normal.
- Mandible: mild retrognathic.
- Convexity: 7 mm.

Diagnosis, dental classification:
- Severe Class II division 1.
- Overjet = 13 mm.
- Overbite excessive with the lower incisors biting heavily into the soft tissues of the palate.
- Upper incisors: severe protrusion.
- Lower incisors: moderate retrusion (–4 mm to A–Po line).
- Crowding in both dental arches (ALD = 7 mm).
- Upper arch constricted with 2|2 displaced lingually.
- Lower arch: 3| blocked out of the arch.
- Lower centre line displaced to the right.
- Buccal segments: full unit distal occlusion.

The position of the lower incisors 4 mm lingual to the A–Po line compensates for the degree of crowding in the lower arch. The 7 mm of crowding can be resolved by advancing the lower incisors by 4 mm during arch development prior to functional therapy.

Treatment concept. The upper and lower archforms must be compatible to achieve a stable occlusion. This can be checked before treatment by sliding the lower model forwards to eliminate the overjet. If the archform does not match it is not possible to fit the models together correctly. It is necessary to correct the archform before mandibular translation, i.e. correct the archform prior to correcting arch-to-arch relationships (**16.1 A–U**).

Treatment plan:
- Orthodontic phase: to develop the archform and improve alignment.
- Orthopaedic phase: to translate the mandible downwards and forwards and improve the skeletal relationship.

Appliances:
- Upper arch: quad helix to expand the maxillary arch; bonded upper fixed appliance to correct alignment.
- Lower arch: bihelix to correct the archform.
- Twin Blocks for major correction of arch relationships.
- Anterior inclined plane to retain.

Stage 1: orthodontic phase. The archform was corrected using cross-arch anchorage to accommodate the blocked-out canine. The Curve of Spee improved during arch development. An overjet of 10 mm and a full unit distal occlusion remained after arch development.

Stage 2: orthopaedic phase.

Bite registration. A construction bite was registered with the blue exactobite to record an edge-to-edge occlusion with 2 mm interincisal clearance, and the centre lines correct.

Clinical management. The Twin Blocks required little adjustment apart from supervising the screw to match the arch width.The response to treatment was rapid and the overjet reduced from 10 mm to 3 mm after 5 months of treatment. The facial muscles responded quickly to the new functional environment and a dramatic change in facial balance was recorded on photographs after 8 weeks. The improvement in facial balance proved stable 18 months out of retention.

Duration of treatment:
- Orthodontic phase: 11 months to complete arch development.
- Orthopaedic phase: 7 months.
- Support and retention: 7 months to retain the corrected position as the buccal segments settled into occlusion.
- Total period of treatment: 25 months.

Final records. 18 months out of retention at age 14 years 9 months.

16.1 Treatment:
A Profile before treatment at age 11 years 2 months.
B Profile after 9 months of arch development at age 11 years 11 months.
C Rapid improvement after 8 weeks with Twin Blocks at age 12 years 2 months.
D–F Occlusion before treatment.
G, H Bihelix to improve the lower archform at age 11 years 2 months and 11 years 11 months.
J Upper fixed appliance to improve the upper archform.
K–M Twin Blocks in phase 2.

KC

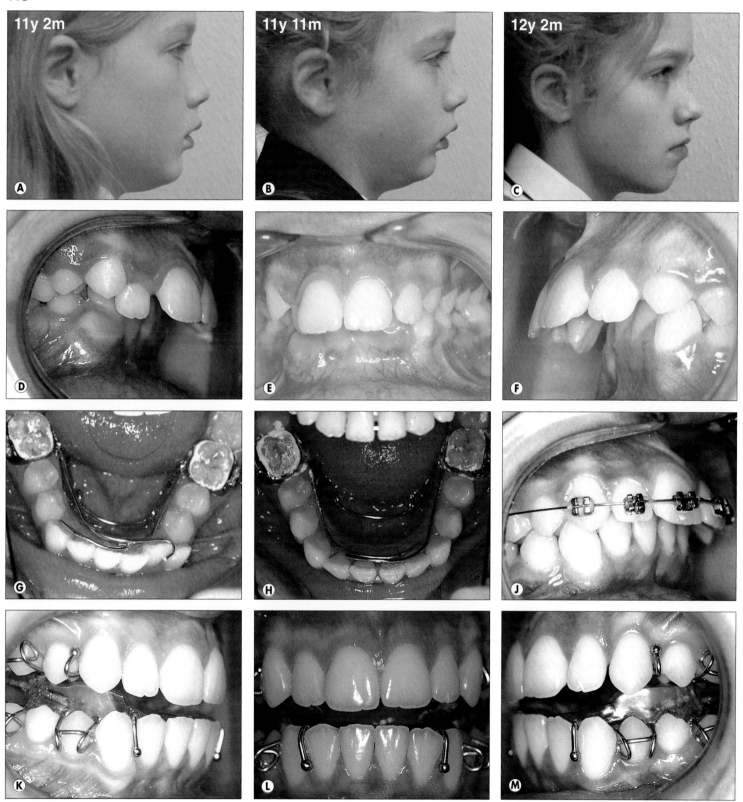

KC

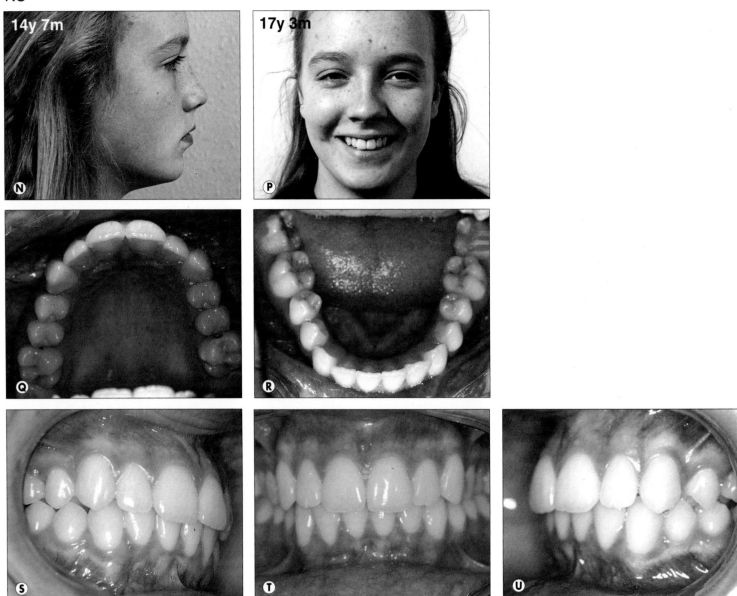

16.1 Treatment (cont.):
N Profile at age 14 years 7 months, 18 months out of retention.
P Facial appearance at age 17 years 3 months.
Q, R Upper and lower archform after treatment.
S–U Occlusion at age 14 years 7 months.

KC

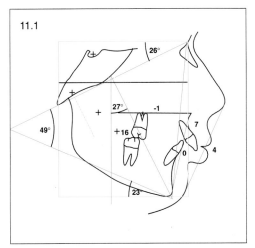

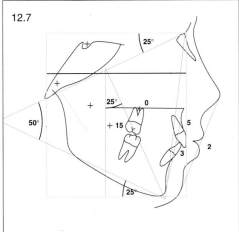

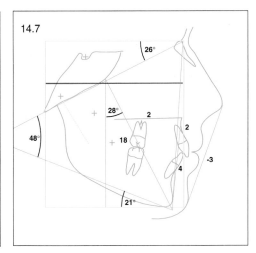

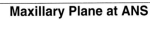

Maxillary Plane at ANS

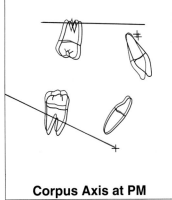

Corpus Axis at PM

Nasion Basion at Nasion

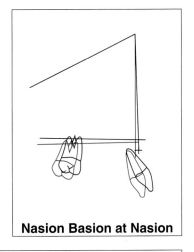

Basion Superimposition

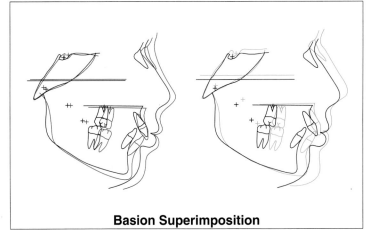

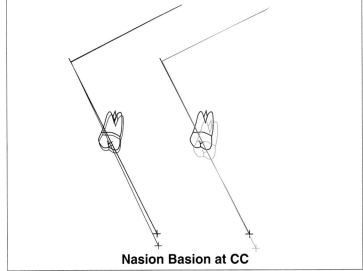

Nasion Basion at CC

K.C. -	Age	11.1	12.7	14.7 (Yr.Mon)
Cranial Base Angle		26	25	26
Facial Axis Angle		27	25	28
F/M Plane Angle		23	25	21
Craniomandibular Angle		49	50	48
Maxillary Plane		−1	0	2
Convexity		7	5	2
U/Incisor to Vertical		31	22	21
L/Incisor to Vertical		37	42	36
Interincisal Angle		112	116	123
6 to Pterygoid Vertical		16	15	18
L/Incisor to A/Po		0	3	4
L/Lip to Aesthetic Plane		4	2	−3

MANAGEMENT OF CROWDING – NONEXTRACTION THERAPY

Case report: N.K. aged 11 years 11 months

When a Class II division 1 malocclusion is associated with a severe lip trap the conspiring labial muscle imbalance can lead to collapse of the lower labial segment and crowding in the lower arch. The profile determines whether the patient should be treated by extraction or nonextraction therapy, taking into account the degree of crowding in the lower arch, the position of the lower incisors relative to the anterior limit of the skeletal base and the lip contour relative to the aesthetic line (**16.2 A–Z**).

Diagnosis, skeletal classification:
- Class I.
- Facial type: severe brachyfacial.
- Maxilla: normal.
- Mandible: normal.
- Convexity = 2 mm.

Diagnosis, dental classification:
- Severe Class II division 1.
- Upper incisors: severe protrusion.
- Lower incisors: moderate retrusion (–4 mm to A–Po line).
- Deep overbite and reduced lower facial height.
- Overjet =11 mm.
- Trapped lower lip.
- Strong mentalis activity and lower alveolar retrusion.
- Lower arch crowding (ALD = 9 mm).

Treatment plan. A nonextraction approach was selected because the skeletal growth pattern was severe brachyfacial, with a strong horizontal growth tendency in the mandible. In view of the retrusive lips, the profile favoured nonextraction therapy. Lower arch crowding of 9 mm could be resolved by advancing the lower incisors. They were positioned 4 mm behind the A–Po line before treatment and could be advanced to +1 mm to gain 10 mm of arch length. Tight lip musculature with the lower lip trapped in the overjet indicates that extraction of the premolars would damage the profile by loss of support for the lips. The extraction of the second molars was planned during the course of treatment to accommodate the third molars and to relieve the pressure from distal crowding in the lower arch.

Stage 1. Align the lower and expand the upper arch to develop the archform.

Stage 2. Functional mandibular advancement to improve the profile. Correct the distal occlusion and reduce the overjet and overbite. Attempt to improve lip posture with a lip training appliance.

Appliances:
- Upper arch: quad helix to expand.
- Lower arch: bihelix to develop the archform.
- Lower lip bumper to improve lip posture.
- A bonded lower fixed appliance to level and align the lower arch.
- Twin Blocks for functional correction.

Clinical management. An initial stage of treatment with a bihelix and a lower lip bumper was followed by a bonded lower fixed appliance over a period of 6 months to align the lower arch in preparation for functional correction. During this stage there was little change in the overjet or the profile.

Twin Blocks were fitted after correcting the lower archform. An immediate improvement in profile was observed and the profile improved dramatically in the early stages of treatment. Arch relationships were corrected in 6 months and an anterior inclined plane was fitted with a Wilson lower lingual arch to retain the position.

Duration of treatment:
- Orthodontic phase: 6 months for arch development.
- Orthopaedic phase: 6 months with Twin Blocks.
- Support phase: 5 months for the occlusion to settle.
- Retention: 9 months with the lower lingual arch.

16.2 Treatment:
A, B Appearance before treatment at age 11 years 11 months.
C–E Occlusion before treatment.
F Lower arch crowding before treatment (ALD = 9 mm).
G Phase 1 arch development – bihelix and lip bumper.
H Detailing with the fixed appliance.
J Occlusion after arch development.
K Profile change after arch development at age 12 years 4 months.
L Phase 2 – Twin Blocks.

NK

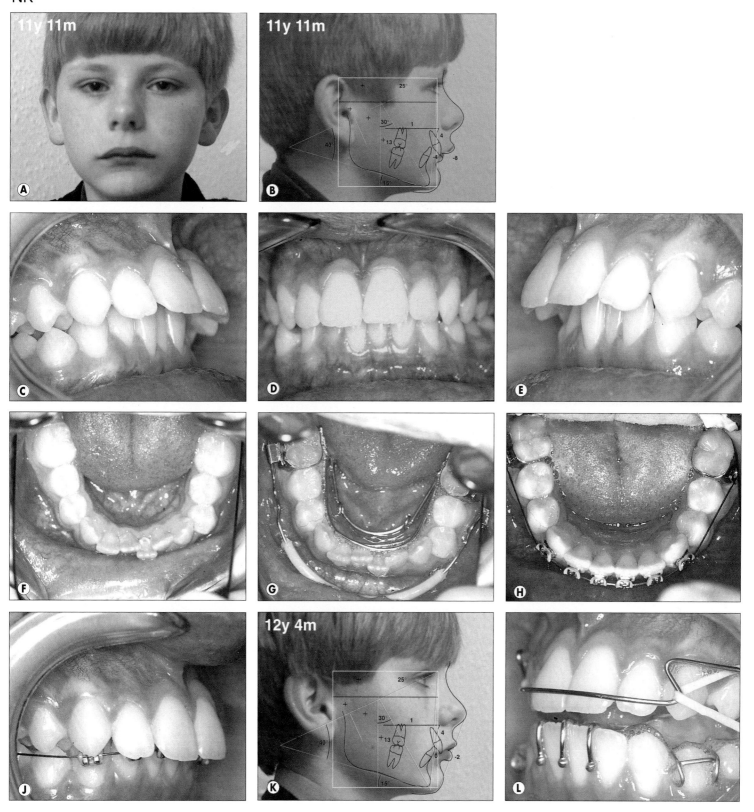

NK

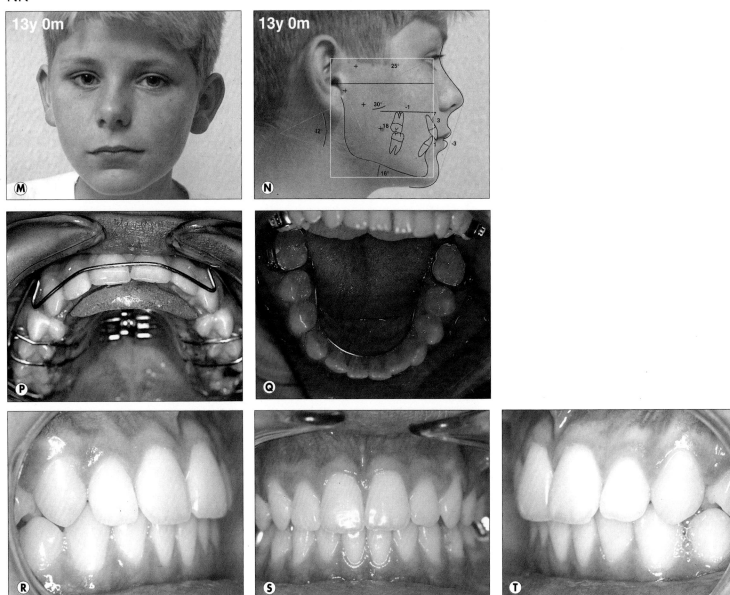

16.2 Treatment (cont.):

M, N Appearance after Twin Blocks at age 13 years.

P, Q Support phase appliances, anterior inclined plane and lingual arch.

R–T Occlusion after support phase at age 13 years 9 months.

NK

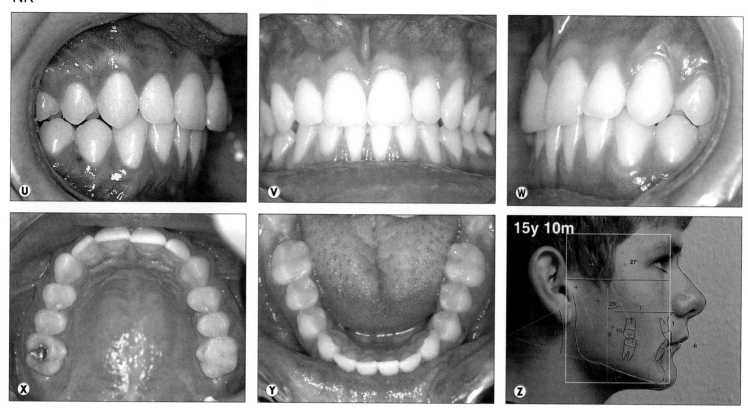

16.2 Treatment (cont.):
U–W Occlusion out of retention at age 15 years 10 months.
X–Z Upper and lower archforms and profile at age 15 years 10 months.

NK

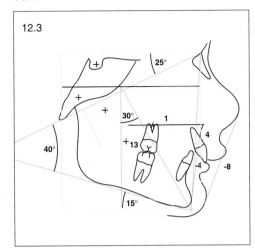

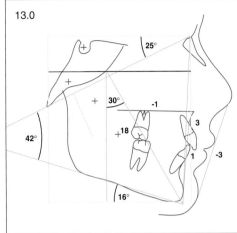

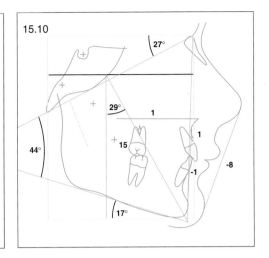

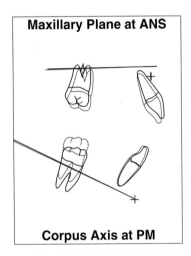

Maxillary Plane at ANS

Corpus Axis at PM

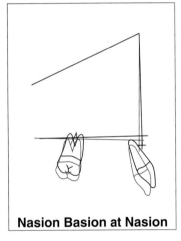

Nasion Basion at Nasion

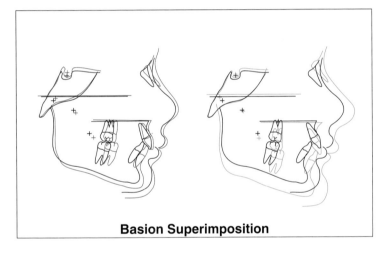

Basion Superimposition

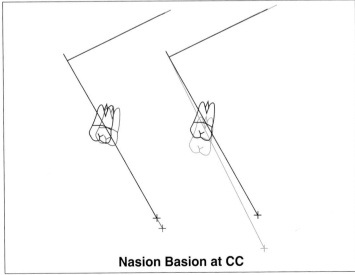

Nasion Basion at CC

N.K. -	Age	12.3	13.0	15.10 (Yr.Mon)
Cranial Base Angle		25	25	27
Facial Axis Angle		30	30	29
F/M Plane Angle		15	16	17
Craniomandibular Angle		40	42	44
Maxillary Plane		1	−1	1
Convexity		4	3	1
U/Incisor to Vertical		28	23	13
L/Incisor to Vertical		37	25	28
Interincisal Angle		115	132	139
6 to Pterygoid Vertical		13	18	15
L/Incisor to A/Po		0 - 4	1	−1
L/Lip to Aesthetic Plane		−8	−3	−8

Case report: J.S. at age 12 years 6 months

This boy presented a Class II division 1 malocclusion with mild lower labial crowding. The treatment first improved the archform, and was-followed by functional correction to the Class I occlusion and a final stage with fixed appliances to detail the occlusion. Severe retrusion of the lower incisors (9 mm lingual to the A–Po line before treatment) is an indication for arch development followed by functional mandibular advancement (**16.3 A–Z**).

Diagnosis, skeletal classification:
- Mild Class II.
- Facial type: severe brachyfacial.
- Maxilla: normal.
- Mandible: slight retrognathia.
- Convexity = 5 mm.

Diagnosis, dental classification:
- Class II division 1.
- Upper incisors proclined and vulnerable to breakage.
- L/ incisors severely retroclined and biting into the palate.
- Lower incisors to A–Po line = –9 mm.
- Overjet = 15 mm.
- Excessive overbite = 10 mm.
- Excessive curve of Spee – lower incisors overerupted.
- Mild lower labial crowding.

Treatment plan:
- Arch development to correct the archform.
- Orthopaedic phase to correct the distal occlusion.
- Support phase to allow the occlusion to settle.
- Orthodontic phase to detail the occlusion.

Appliances:
- Wilson quad helix and lower 3D lingual arch.
- Standard Twin Blocks.
- Full-bonded fixed appliances.

Clinical management:
- Arch development: This approach is popular with patients because the preformed Wilson lingual appliances are both comfortable and invisible behind the teeth. Gentle activation from the lingual aspect corrected the lower archform and expanded the upper arch, while at the same time correcting the mesiolingual rotation of upper molars.
- Orthopaedic phase: Because the overjet was in excess of 10 mm the bite was registered to reduce the overjet by 8 mm on the first activation. This correction was achieved in 4 months and the Twin Blocks were then reactivated to interincisal edge-to-edge. The occlusion was fully corrected after 9 months.
- Support phase: An anterior inclined plane was fitted and the Wilson lingual arch was used to maintain the lower archform. The occlusion at this stage was very near ideal, but it was decided to proceed with a finishing stage with fixed appliances.
- Orthodontic phase: First an upper utility arch was used in conjunction with the lower Wilson lingual arch and intermaxillary traction to reduce the overbite further. Bonded upper and lower appliances were fitted for 8 months to detail the occlusion.

Duration of treatment:
- Arch development: 3 months with lingual appliances.
- Orthopaedic phase: 9 months with Twin Blocks.
- Support phase: 10 months. The occlusion was good at this stage, but on review it was decided to proceed with an orthodontic phase.
- Orthodontic phase: 8 months with upper and lower fixed appliances to detail the occlusion.

JS

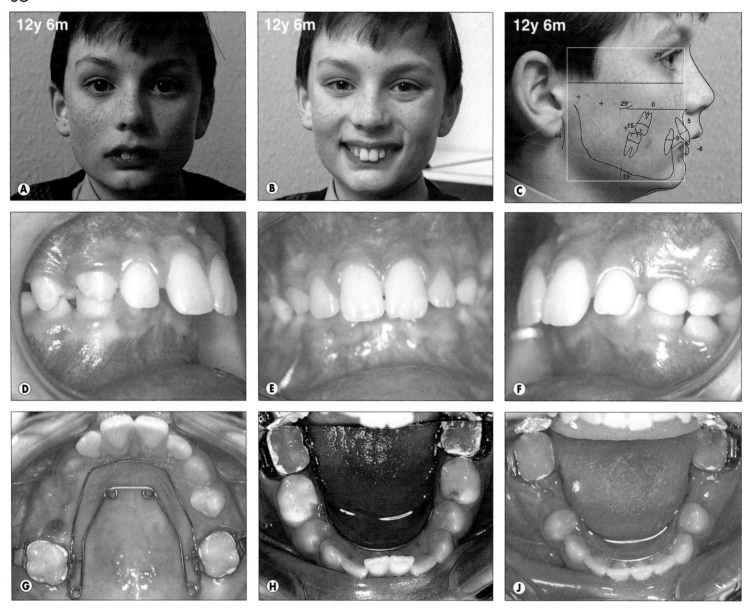

16.3 Treatment:

A–C Appearance before treatment at age 12 years 6 months.

D–F Occlusion before treatment.

G–J Phase 1 – arch development, Wilson quad helix and lingual arch.

JS

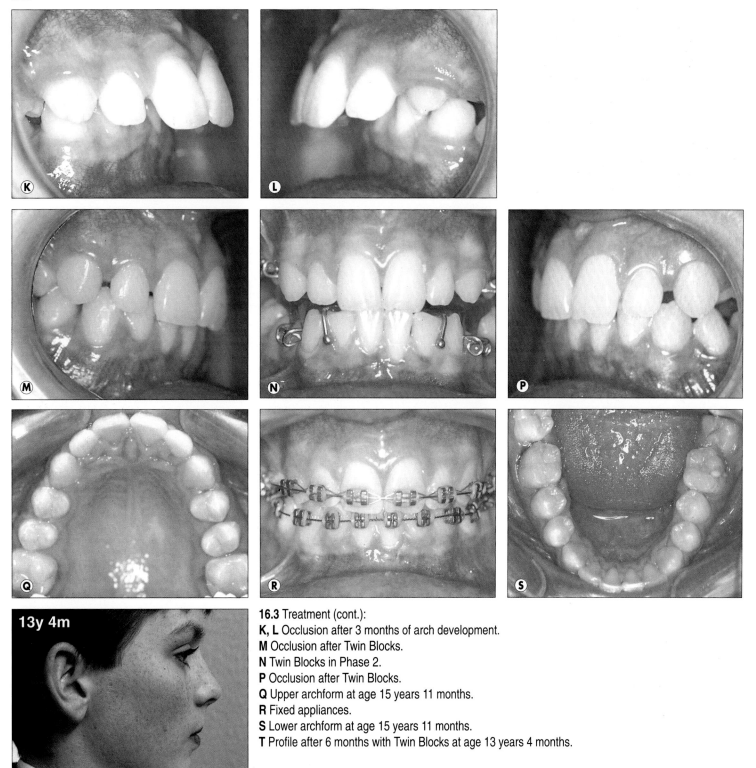

16.3 Treatment (cont.):
K, L Occlusion after 3 months of arch development.
M Occlusion after Twin Blocks.
N Twin Blocks in Phase 2.
P Occlusion after Twin Blocks.
Q Upper archform at age 15 years 11 months.
R Fixed appliances.
S Lower archform at age 15 years 11 months.
T Profile after 6 months with Twin Blocks at age 13 years 4 months.

JS

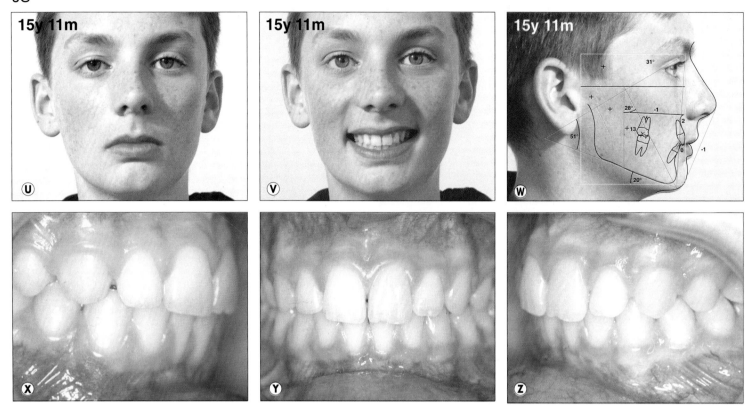

16.3 Treatment (cont.):
U–W Appearance at age 15 years 11 months.
X–Z Occlusion at age 15 years 11 months.

JS

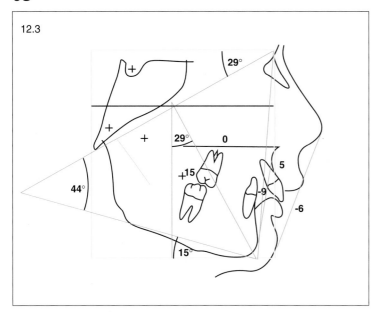

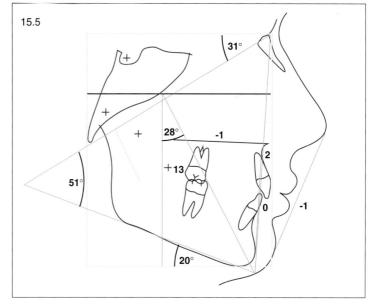

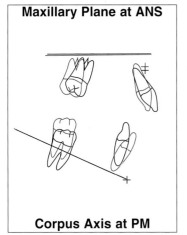

Maxillary Plane at ANS

Corpus Axis at PM

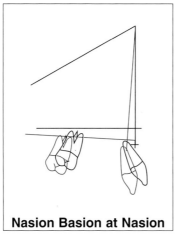

Nasion Basion at Nasion

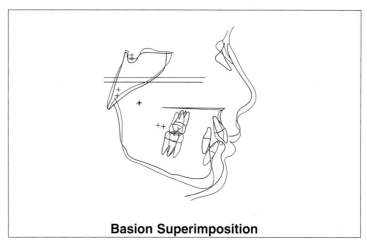

Basion Superimposition

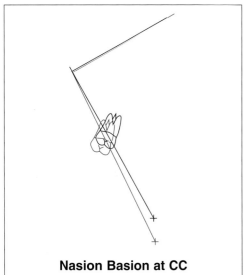

Nasion Basion at CC

J.S. -	Age	12.3	15.5	(Yr.Mon)
Cranial Base Angle		29	31	
Facial Axis Angle		29	28	
F/M Plane Angle		15	20	
Craniomandibular Angle		44	51	
Maxillary Plane		0	−1	
Convexity		5	2	
U/Incisor to Vertical		27	15	
L/Incisor to Vertical		12	33	
Interincisal Angle		141	132	
6 to Pterygoid Vertical		15	13	
L/Incisor to A/Po		−9	0	
L/Lip to Aesthetic Plane		−6	−1	

CLASS II DIVISION 1 MALOCCLUSION WITH CROWDED CANINES

Combination therapy by Twin Blocks and fixed appliances

Case report: T.S. aged 14 years 2 months

The Twin Block sagittal appliance can be used to treat upper labial segment crowding and, at the same time, will correct distal occlusion and reduce overjet (**16.4 A–T**).

Diagnosis, skeletal classification:
- Moderate Class II.
- Facial type: severe brachyfacial – horizontal growth.
- Maxilla: mild prognathic.
- Mandible: normal.
- Convexity = 5 mm.

Diagnosis, dental classification:
- Severe Class II division 1.
- Upper incisors: retroclined.
- Lower incisors: normal.
- Overjet = 3 mm.
- Mild upper labial crowding.
- Minimal lower arch crowding.

In view of the horizontal mandibular growth pattern, maxillary retraction is contraindicated. It is better to reposition the mandible to match the maxillary position. This diagnosis is confirmed as the profile improves when the mandible postures forwards.

Treatment plan:
- Orthopaedic phase: Advance retroclined incisors to resolve the upper arch crowding. Functional correction to improve the profile and correct the distal occlusion.
- Support phase: Allow the buccal segments to settle into Class I occlusion, and during this phase resolve the slight lower labial crowding.
- Orthodontic phase. Detail the occlusion with fixed appliances.

Appliances:
- Upper sagittal/ lower standard Twin Blocks.
- Upper sagittal with anterior inclined plane. Lower Wilson lingual arch.
- Straightwire technique with ceramic brackets.

Clinical management. The palatal screws in the sagittal Twin Block were turned two quarter turns per week to align the upper incisors. The appliance was trimmed clear of 1, which was positioned slightly labially, so that the activation of the screws advanced only the retroclined upper incisors. The palatal acrylic on the upper appliance was trimmed to relieve the pressure on the palatal gingivae lingual to 21|12 during treatment that is incidental to screw expansion. It is important to maintain appliance contact on the lingual surfaces of the teeth that are being advanced, and therefore no trimming was done where the appliance contacts these teeth.

The transition to fixed appliances was made after a short support phase when the buccal teeth settled into Class I occlusion, during which period a lower lingual arch corrected the lower archform. Subsequent detailing of the occlusion was simple after achieving the major correction during the Twin Block phase of treatment.

Duration of treatment:
- Orthopaedic phase: 8 months to correct to Class I occlusion.
- Support phase: 6 months for the occlusion to settle and to develop the lower archform.
- Orthodontic phase: 9 months to detail the occlusion.
- Retention: 1 year.
- Total treatment time: 3 years, including retention.

TS

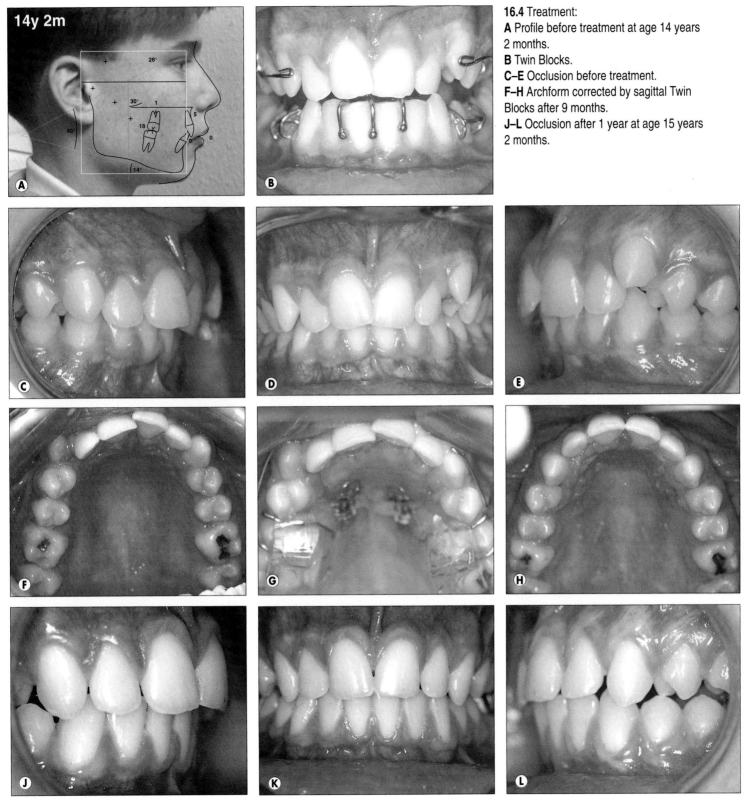

16.4 Treatment:
A Profile before treatment at age 14 years 2 months.
B Twin Blocks.
C–E Occlusion before treatment.
F–H Archform corrected by sagittal Twin Blocks after 9 months.
J–L Occlusion after 1 year at age 15 years 2 months.

TS

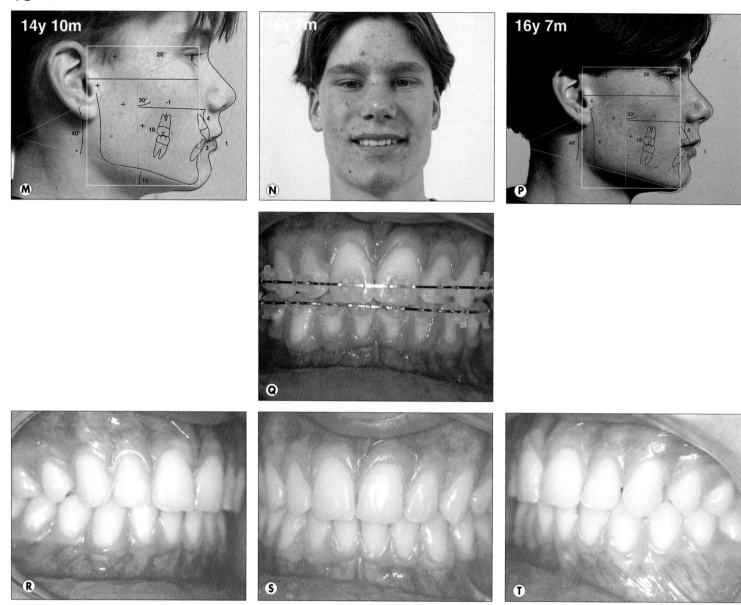

16.4 Treatment (cont.):
M Profile after 1 year.
N, P Appearance after treatment.
Q Fixed appliances.
R–T Occlusion 1 year out of retention at age 16 years 7 months.

TS

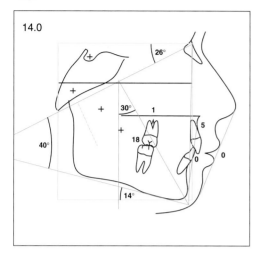

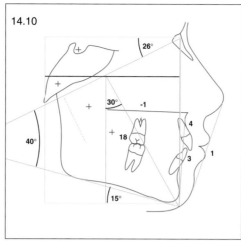

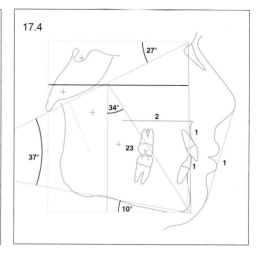

Maxillary Plane at ANS

Corpus Axis at PM

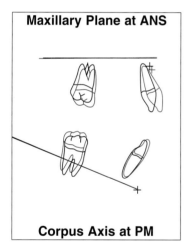

Nasion Basion at Nasion

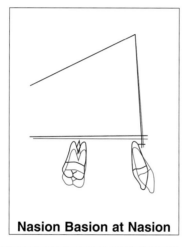

Basion Superimposition

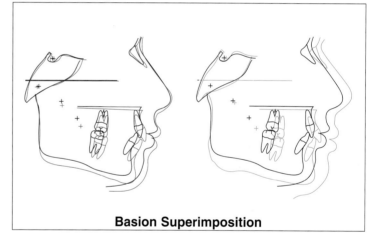

Nasion Basion at CC

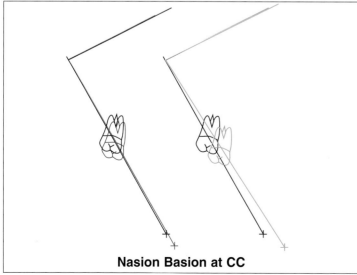

T.S. -	Age	14.0	14.10	17.4 (Yr.Mon)
Cranial Base Angle		26	26	27
Facial Axis Angle		30	30	34
F/M Plane Angle		14	15	10
Craniomandibular Angle		40	40	37
Maxillary Plane		1	−1	2
Convexity		5	4	1
U/Incisor to Vertical		11	22	26
L/Incisor to Vertical		33	33	23
Interincisal Angle		136	125	131
6 to Pterygoid Vertical		18	18	23
L/Incisor to A/Po		0	3	1
L/Lip to Aesthetic Plane		0	1	1

MANAGEMENT OF CROWDING WITH AN ANTERIOR OPEN BITE

Case report: R.G. aged 11 years 6 months

A girl with an anterior open bite and mild lower labial crowding is treated in two stages by a combination of orthopaedic and orthodontic treatment (**16.5 A–Y**).

Diagnosis, skeletal classification:
*   Severe Class II.
*   Facial type: severe brachyfacial – horizontal growth.
*   Maxilla: moderate prognathic.
*   Mandible: mild retrognathic.
*   Convexity = 10 mm.

Diagnosis, dental classification:
*   Severe Class II division 1.
*   Upper incisors: severe protrusion.
*   Lower incisors: mild retrusion (–1 mm to A–Po line).
*   Mild lower labial crowding (5 mm with $\overline{E|E}$ present)
*   Overjet = 9 mm.
*   Anterior open bite.
*   History of thumbsucking, now stopped.
*   Full unit distal occlusion.

Holding the lower molar position when the deciduous molars shed would gain 4 mm of arch length leaving a minimal space deficit in the lower arch, with the lower incisors positioned 1 mm behind the A–Po line before treatment.

Treatment plan:
*   Orthopaedic phase: functional mandibular advancement and expansion of both arches with Twin Blocks.
*   Support phase: an upper anterior inclined plane combined with a lower fixed appliance to correct alignment in the lower arch.
*   Orthodontic phase: upper and lower bonded fixed appliances to detail the occlusion.

Appliance design. Standard Twin Block design with a midline screw for expansion of both arches.

Bite registration. An edge-to-edge incisor occlusion was registered with the blue exactobite, giving 2 mm interincisal clearance.

Clinical management. Both screws were turned for the first 4 months of treatment. At that stage the molar relationship was corrected to Class I and the overjet reduced to 3 mm. Twin Blocks were worn for a further 5 months to overcorrect the incisors to edge-to-edge occlusion. A lower fixed appliance was fitted during the support phase to align the lower arch before making the transition to bonded fixed appliances to complete treatment.

Duration of treatment:
*   Orthopaedic phase: 9 months to correct arch relationships.
*   Support phase: 4 months to settle the occlusion and align the lower arch.
*   Orthodontic phase: 18 months to detail the occlusion.
*   Retention: 1 year.

RG

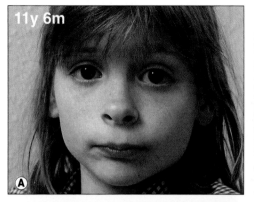

11y 6m

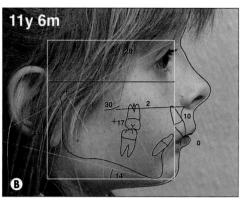

11y 6m

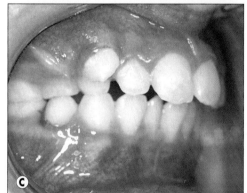

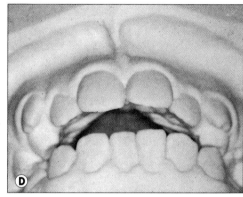

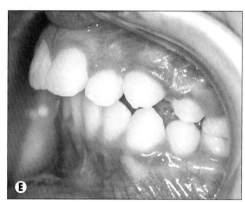

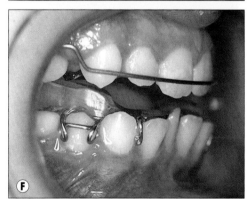

16.5 Treatment:

A, B Appearance before treatment at age 11 years 6 months.

C–E Occlusion before treatment.

F Twin Blocks.

G–J Correction after 8 weeks of treatment with the Twin Blocks.

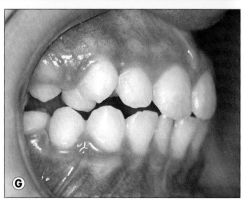

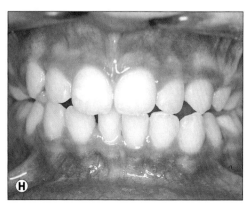

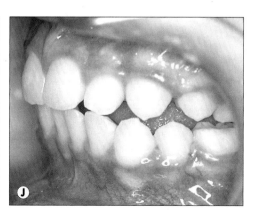

RG

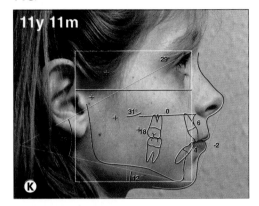

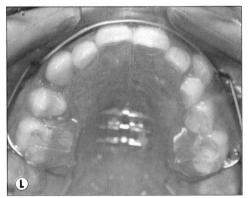

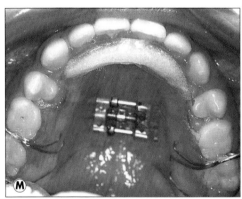

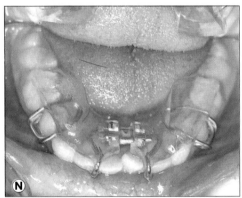

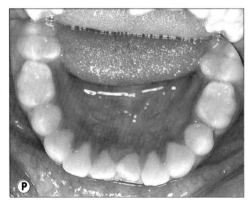

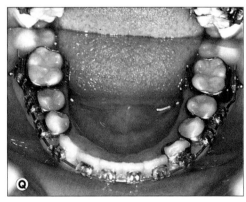

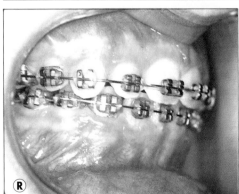

16.5 Treatment (cont.):
K Profile after 5 months treatment with Twin Blocks at age 11 years 11 months.
L, M Upper archform and appliances.
N, P Lower archform after expansion with Twin Blocks.
Q, R Fixed appliances.

RG

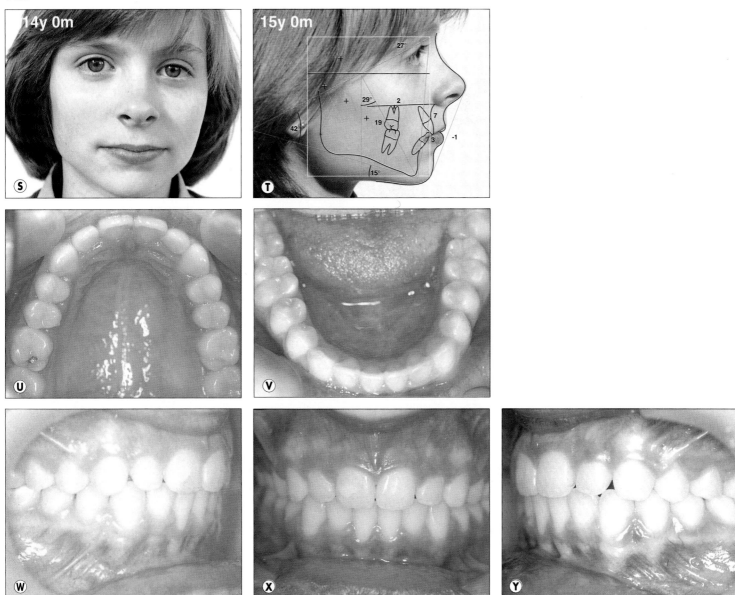

16.5 Treatment (cont.):
S Appearance after treatment at age 14 years.
T Profile at age 15 years.
U, V Upper and lower archforms at age 16 years.
W–Y Occlusion 1 year out of retention at age 16 years.

RG

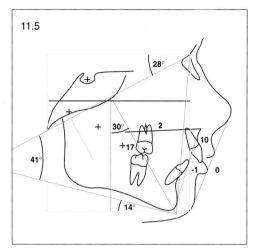

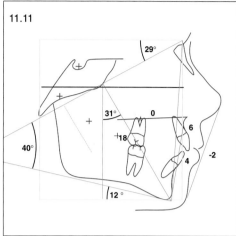

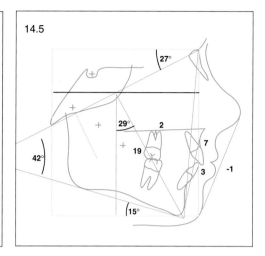

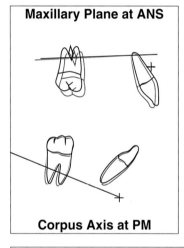

Maxillary Plane at ANS

Corpus Axis at PM

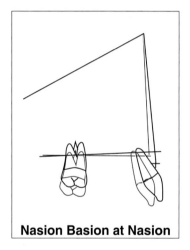

Nasion Basion at Nasion

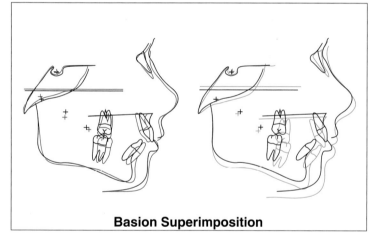

Basion Superimposition

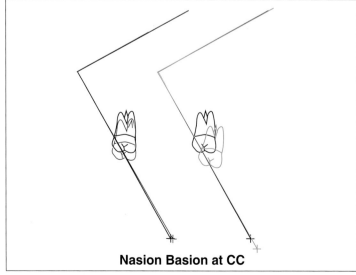

Nasion Basion at CC

R.G. -	Age	11.5	11.11	14.5 (Yr.Mon)
Cranial Base Angle		28	29	27
Facial Axis Angle		30	31	29
F/M Plane Angle		14	12	15
Craniomandibular Angle		41	40	42
Maxillary Plane		2	0	2
Convexity		10	6	7
U/Incisor to Vertical		26	19	30
L/Incisor to Vertical		47	40	40
Interincisal Angle		107	121	110
6 to Pterygoid Vertical		17	18	19
L/Incisor to A/Po		−1	4	3
L/Lip to Aesthetic Plane		0	−2	−1

TREATMENT OF CONTRACTED ARCHFORM

Case report: S.M. aged 12 years 5 months

This girl presented a severe Class II division 1 malocclusion with crowding and narrow archforms, and was treated by a combination of Twin Blocks with arch development and fixed appliances. In this case, functional correction was carried out first, followed by arch development (**16.6 A–Z**).

Diagnosis, skeletal classification:
- Moderate Class II.
- Facial type: mild retrognathic – vertical growth tendency.
- Maxilla: mild retrognathic.
- Mandible: mild retrognathic.
- Convexity = 6 mm.

Diagnosis, dental classification:
- Severe Class II division 1.
- Upper incisors: severe protrusion.
- Lower incisors: severe retrusion (–5 mm to A–Po line).
- Overjet = 13 mm.
- Excessive overbite with the upper incisors biting in the palate.
- Full unit distal occlusion.
- Narrow contracted archform.
- Crowding of the lower canines (ALD = 9 mm).
- Potential crowding of the third molars.

Treatment plan. The patient's age and stage of development favoured immediate functional correction of distal occlusion, especially as the upper incisors were vulnerable to damage due to their exposed position. The position of the lower incisors 5 mm lingual to the A–Po line before treatment was favourable for arch development and treatment of crowding in the second stage. This was followed by detailed finishing with fixed appliances in the final stage. In the course of treatment relief of crowding was planned by extraction of the second molars on eruption to accommodate the third molars.
- Orthopaedic phase: to correct the distal occlusion and reduce the overjet by functional mandibular advancement, accompanied by maxillary expansion.
- Support phase and arch development: to allow the buccal segments to settle into occlusion and to correct the archform in the lower arch and continue expansion in the upper arch.
- Orthodontic phase: detailed finishing with upper and lower fixed appliances.

Appliances:
- Standard Twin Blocks to correct the arch relationship.
- Upper anterior inclined plane with midline expansion. Lower Wilson lingual arch to correct archform and accommodate erupting canines.
- Upper and lower full bonded appliances to detail the occlusion.

Bite registration. The overjet was partly reduced on first activation using the blue exactobite to allow a 2 mm interincisal clearance, and selecting the appropriate groove to achieve an 8 mm activation.

Clinical management. The overjet reduced from 13 to 4 mm after 3 months of treatment, when the Twin Blocks were reactivated slightly to complete the correction. The overjet was fully reduced and the distal occlusion corrected after 5 months. In view of the vertical growth tendency, the bite blocks were trimmed only after the overjet had been reduced, in order to reduce the overbite partly by molar eruption and partly by incisor intrusion.

Maxillary expansion continued during the support stage, and a Wilson lower lingual arch was fitted. All second molars were extracted which allowed 6|6 to be distalised to accommodate the lower canines. There was a resting phase in treatment in this case due to delayed eruption of the canines. The mandibular position was maintained during this stage. The final orthodontic phase with fixed appliances progressed slowly to a successful conclusion.

Duration of treatment:
- Orthopaedic phase: 9 months with Twin Blocks.
- Support phase: 4 months for the occlusion to settle.
- Arch development: 6 months to make space for the canines.
- Resting phase: awaiting eruption for 14 months.
- Orthodontic phase: 2 years to completion.
- Retention: 1 year.

SM

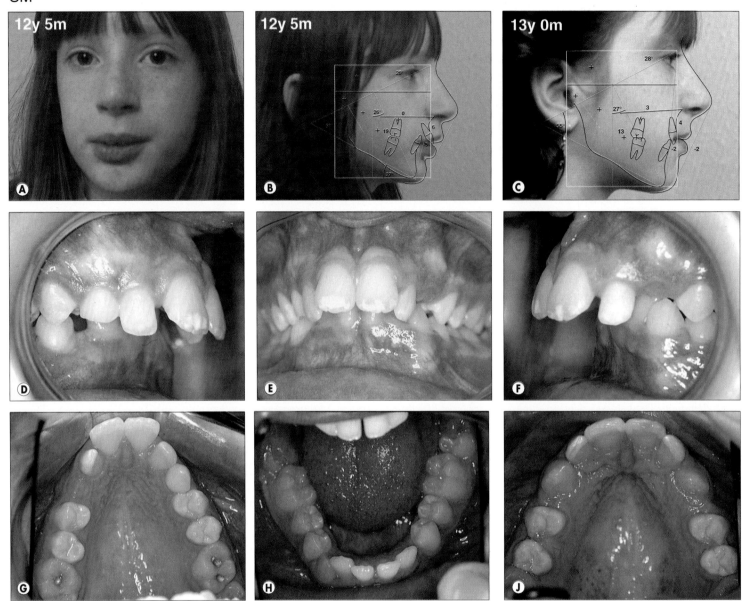

16.6 Treatment:

A, B Appearance before treatment at age 12 years 5 months.

C Profile after 7 months with Twin Blocks.

D–F Occlusion before treatment.

G, H Contracted upper and lower archform before treatment.

J Upper arch development after twin block phase.

SM

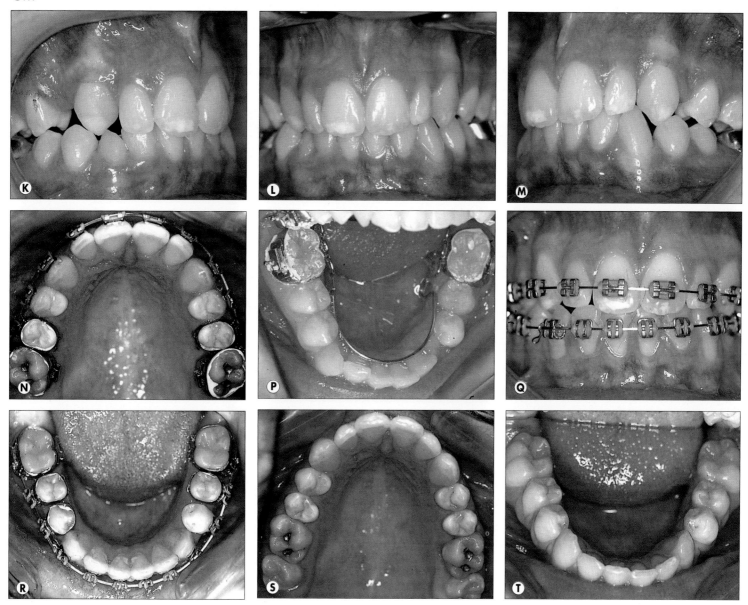

16.6 Treatment (cont.):

K–M Occlusion after arch development in the support phase at age 14 years.

N–P Arch development continues in fixed appliance treatment.

Q, R Fixed appliances to detail the occlusion.

S, T Corrected archform at age 19 years 9 months.

SM

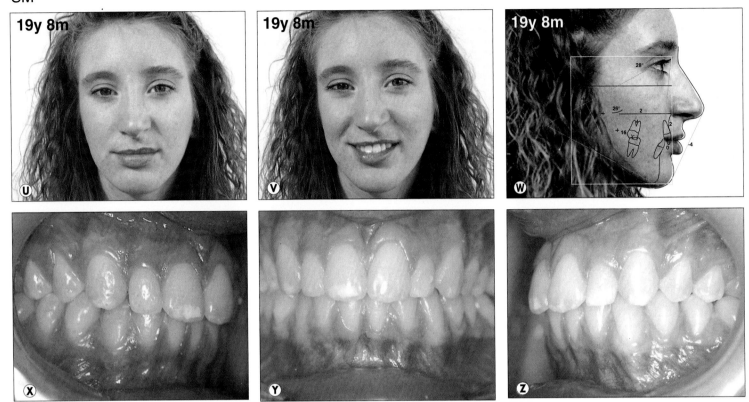

16.6 Treatment (cont.):

U–W Appearance at age 19 years 8 months.

X–Z Occlusion out of retention at age 19 years 8 months.

SM

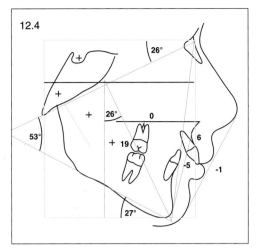

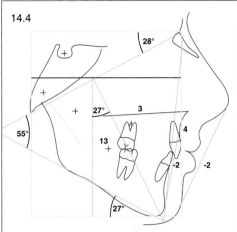

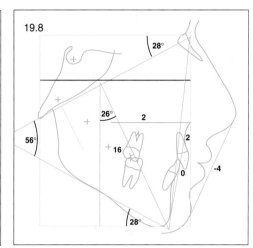

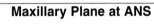

Maxillary Plane at ANS

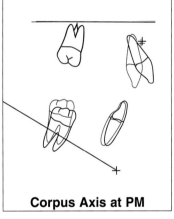

Corpus Axis at PM

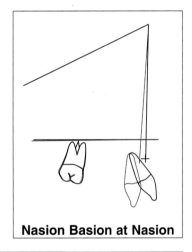

Nasion Basion at Nasion

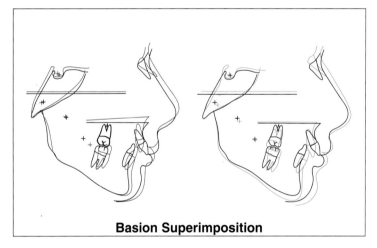

Basion Superimposition

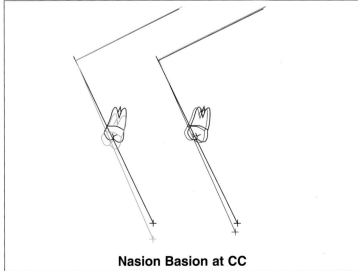

Nasion Basion at CC

S.M. -	Age	12.4	14.4	19.8 (Yr.Mon)
Cranial Base Angle		26	28	28
Facial Axis Angle		26	27	26
F/M Plane Angle		27	27	28
Craniomandibular Angle		53	55	56
Maxillary Plane		0	3	2
Convexity		6	4	2
U/Incisor to Vertical		28	6	21
L/Incisor to Vertical		28	29	28
Interincisal Angle		124	145	131
6 to Pterygoid Vertical		19	13	16
L/Incisor to A/Po		−5	−2	0
L/Lip to Aesthetic Plane		−1	−2	−4

Extraction Therapy

EXTRACTION THERAPY

It is unusual to combine extraction of premolars with functional therapy. With certain exceptions, premolar extraction therapy and functional appliance therapy are almost contradictory terms. In a minority of cases, the degree of crowding mesial to the first permanent molars may be so severe that premolar extractions are inevitable, although the patient may still benefit from functional correction. In other cases, the patient may present too late to control crowding by interceptive treatment and arch development, but may still require functional mandibular protrusion. In these circumstances, fixed and functional therapy is required to correct archform, close spaces and correct arch relationships.

Patients presenting withvertical growth patterns and a high mandibular plane angle cannot be expected to grow favourably during treatment. In such cases, when significant crowding is present in the lower arch, it may only be resolved by premolar extractions.

Examples of patients in these categories are illustrated to demonstrate the management of these problems, which are exceptional rather than typical in Twin Block therapy.

Case report: K.M. aged 11 years 9 months

This is an example of Twin Block treatment for a girl who presented a Class II division 1 malocclusion in the permanent dentition with severe crowding in the lower premolar region and $\overline{5|5}$ blocked out and impacted. Twin Blocks were used to correct the distal occlusion and reduce the overjet, followed by extraction of premolars to relieve crowding (**17.1 A–M**).

Diagnosis, skeletal classification:
- Moderate Class II.
- Facial type: moderate brachyfacial.
- Maxilla: normal.
- Mandible: mild retrognathic.
- Convexity = 6 mm.

Diagnosis, dental classification:
- Severe Class II division 1.
- Overjet =12 mm.
- Overbite: incomplete with tongue thrust and lip trap.
- Buccal crossbite $4|4$.
- Lower buccal crowding with $\overline{5|5}$ impacted.
- Crowding in lower arch (ALD = 12 mm).
- Lower incisor to A–Po =–4 mm.

Treatment plan. Functional correction to advance the mandible. Re-evaluate the crowding on completing this stage of treatment and plan the extraction of the premolars or second molars.

Registration bite. The initial construction bite reduced the overjet by 7 mm with 2 mm interincisal clearance using a blue exactobite.

Appliances:
- Standard Twin Blocks in the active phase.
- Anterior inclined plane in the support phase.
- Sectional upper fixed appliance to close the spaces.

Clinical management. Little expansion of the upper arch was necessary in view of the crossbite of $4|4$. After 3 months of treatment the overjet reduced to 5 mm and the inclined planes were reactivated to an interincisal edge-to-edge occlusion by adding acrylic to the anterior incline of the upper Twin Block. The overjet was fully reduced after 6 months and the position was retained first with Twin Blocks for 4 months before moving on to an anterior inclined plane. At this stage $5|5$ and $\overline{4|4}$ were extracted to relieve crowding, and $\underline{6|6}$ were moved mesially. Space was now available for $\overline{5|5}$ to erupt.

KM

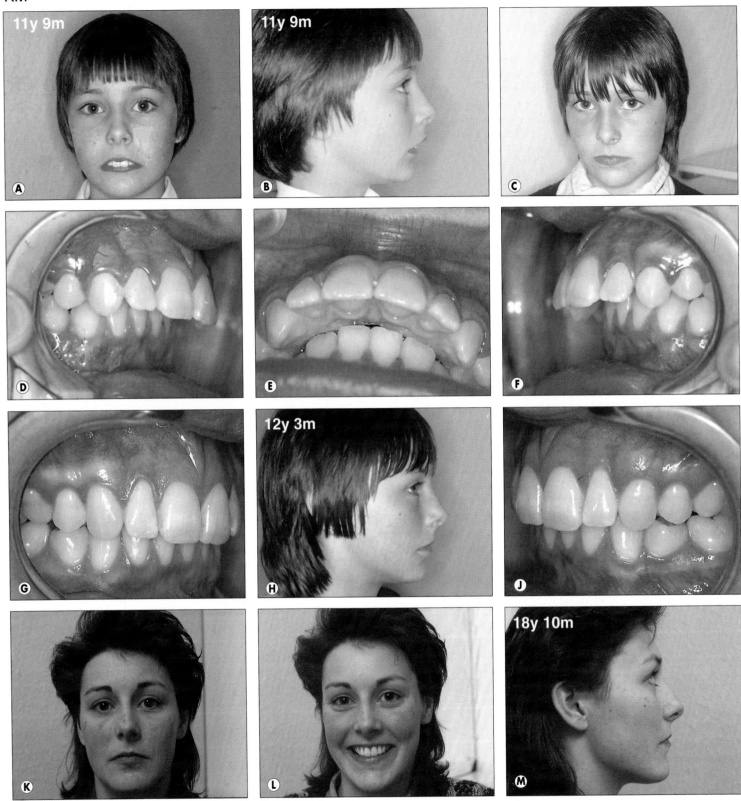

KM

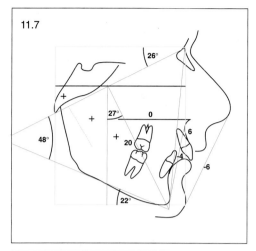

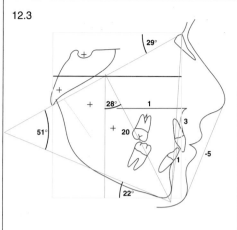

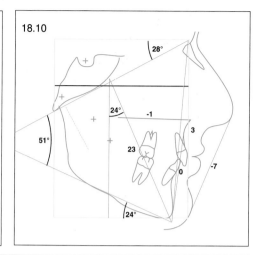

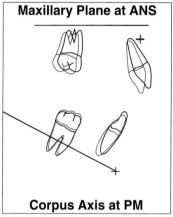

Maxillary Plane at ANS

Corpus Axis at PM

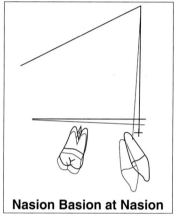

Nasion Basion at Nasion

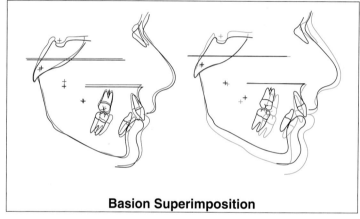

Basion Superimposition

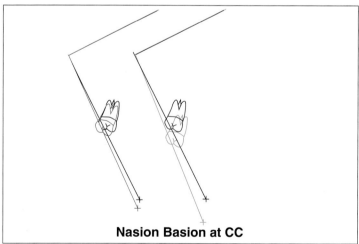

Nasion Basion at CC

17.1 Treatment:

A, B Appearance before treatment at 11 years 9 months.

C Appearance after 6 months treatment.

D–F Occlusion before treatment.

G, H, J Occlusion after treatment, and profile change after 6 months.

K–M Appearance at age 18 years 10 months.

K.M. -	Age	11.7	12.3	18.10 (Yr.Mon)
Cranial Base Angle		26	29	28
Facial Axis Angle		27	28	24
F/M Plane Angle		22	22	24
Craniomandibular Angle		48	51	51
Maxillary Plane		0	1	−1
Convexity		6	3	3
U/Incisor to Vertical		26	17	16
L/Incisor to Vertical		30	39	34
Interincisal Angle		124	124	130
6 to Pterygoid Vertical		20	20	23
L/Incisor to A/Po		−4	1	0
L/Lip to Aesthetic Plane		−6	−5	−7

Case report: G.McD. aged 12 years 1 month

This patient presents a difficult problem with a severe Class II skeletal relationship, mandibular retrusion, a vertical growth pattern and severe lower labial crowding and deep overbite. Because of the vertical growth pattern, the profile does not significantly improve when the mandible postures forwards. Extraction of the premolars is indicated to improve the profile (**18.2 A–M**).

The combination of a high mandibular plane angle and deep overbite is a warning sign that facial height will increase if the mandible is translated forwards. This is confirmed in the profile change observed when the patient postures forwards before treatment. In such cases, an alternative approach is to intrude the incisors with fixed appliances, for example, using utility arches, before the functional phase of treatment. The mandible may then be translated forwards without increasing the facial height.

The degree of crowding in the lower arch and the position of the lower dentition relative to the basal bone are the factors which determine whether or not extractions are required, and influence the choice of extraction. If the lower dentition is crowded and significantly protrusive beyond the anterior limit of basal bone, extraction therapy is indicated. The normal position of the tip of the lower incisor relative to the A–Po line is +1 to +3 mm.

Diagnosis, skeletal classification:
- Severe Class II.
- Facial type: moderate dolichofacial – vertical growth.
- Maxilla: prognathic.
- Mandible: severe retrusion.
- Convexity = 10 mm.

Diagnosis, dental classification:
- Severe Class II division 1.
- Overjet = 9 mm.
- Overbite: increased.
- Upper incisors: severe protrusion.
- Lower incisors: normal (1 to A–Po = +3 mm).
- Severe lower labial crowding.
- Mixed dentition analysis (ALD = 11 mm with $\overline{E|E}$ present).
- Lower canines displaced buccally.
- Class I molar relationship.

Treatment plan. In an effort to improve the profile it was decided to advance the mandible in the first stage of treatment, followed by the extraction of four premolars to relieve crowding and the use of bonded fixed appliances to close the spaces and reduce the prominence of the lips.

Clinical management. The overjet reduced from 8 to 2 mm in 4 months with Twin Blocks, but the profile did not improve due to a lengthening of the lower facial height. After the extraction of four premolars, a Wilson lower lingual arch was fitted to maintain arch length and align the lower labial segment. After closing buccal segment spaces and establishing a Class I occlusion, the upper and lower incisors were retracted by space closing mechanics, allowing the profile to improve as the lips were retracted.

Duration of treatment:
- Orthopaedic phase: 4 months.
- Orthodontic phase: 2 years.
- Retention: 1 year.

17.2 Treatment:

A Profile before treatment at age 12 years 4 months.

B Forward posture before treatment does not improve profile.

C Profile not improving after 10 months with Twin Blocks.

D, E, F, G Contracted upper to lower archform and occlusion before treatment.

H, J Upper and lower archform after extractions and space closure in phase 2.

K, L, M Occlusion and profile after treatment at age 15 years 2 months.

GMcD

GMcD

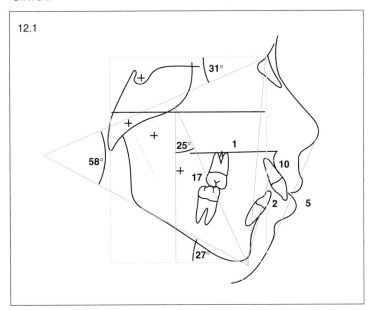

12.1

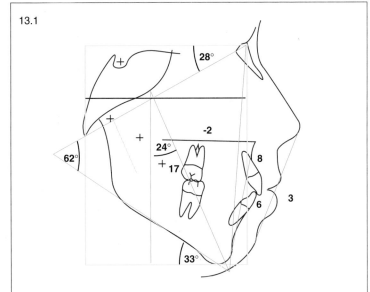

13.1

Maxillary Plane at ANS

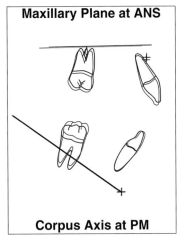

Corpus Axis at PM

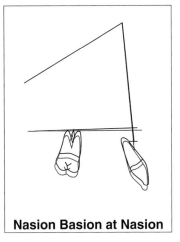

Nasion Basion at Nasion

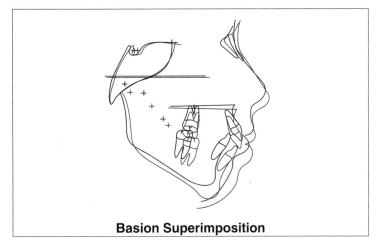

Basion Superimposition

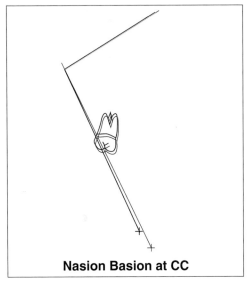

Nasion Basion at CC

G.McD. -	Age	12.1	13.1	(Yr.Mon)
Cranial Base Angle		31	28	
Facial Axis Angle		25	24	
F/M Plane Angle		27	33	
Craniomandibular Angle		58	62	
Maxillary Plane		1	–2	
Convexity		10	8	
U/Incisor to Vertical		28	22	
L/Incisor to Vertical		36	40	
Interincisal Angle		116	118	
6 to Pterygoid Vertical		17	17	
L/Incisor to A/Po		2	6	
L/Lip to Aesthetic Plane		5	3	

Case report: L.C. aged 10 years 9 months

This girl presented a severe Class II division 2 malocclusion with severe crowding in both arches, and was treated with extractions and a combination of Twin Blocks and fixed appliances. It is very unusual to extract premolars in Class II division 2 malocclusion; this case is an exception to the general rule, due to the severity of lower arch crowding (ALD = 19 mm) presenting in permanent dentition(**17.3 A–R**).

Diagnosis, skeletal classification:
- Severe Class II.
- Facial type: severe brachyfacial.
- Maxilla: mild prognathic.
- Mandible: mild retrognathic.
- Convexity = 10 mm.

Diagnosis, dental classification:
- Severe Class II division 2.
- Upper incisors severely retroclined.
- Overjet = 1 mm.
- Overbite: excessive (10.5 mm).
- Lower incisors severely retroclined (1 to A–Po = -7 mm).
- Interincisor angle = 175°.
- Low mandibular plane angle.
- Reduced lower facial height.
- Severe crowding in lower arch (ALD = 19 mm).

Treatment plan:
- Orthopaedic phase: procline the upper incisors to free the occlusion. Advance the mandible to improve the mandibular retrusion and correct to Class I occlusion. Relieve crowding by extraction of one unit in each quadrant, the choice of extractions to be confirmed after establishing the response to treatment.
- Support phase: to allow the occlusion to settle.
- Orthodontic phase: full bonded upper and lower fixed appliances to correct the angulation and torque and to detail the occlusion.

Bite registration. The construction bite was taken with a blue exactobite after cutting off the handle to register an edge-to-edge incisor occlusion. In view of the excessive overbite no additional interincisal clearance was necessary in this case.

Appliances. The upper Twin Block incorporated springs to advance the upper incisors and a midline screw to expand the upper arch. The lower appliance was simply designed to advance the lower arch.

Clinical management. Twin Blocks were worn for 6 months to advance the mandible, and, at the same time, procline the upper incisors and expand the upper arch before reactivating the inclined planes to an incisal edge-to-edge occlusion. Treatment continued for an additional 10 months to complete the mandibular advancement, and during this period $\frac{4|4}{2|4}$ were extracted to relieve crowding.

Towards the end of the Twin Block stage, brackets were fitted on the upper anterior teeth to improve alignment. An anterior inclined plane was worn for 2 months to allow the occlusion to settle before fitting the fixed appliances. The finishing stage was slow and extended over a period of 3 years.

Duration of treatment:
- Orthopaedic phase: 16 months with Twin Blocks.
- Support phase: 2 months with an anterior guide plane.
- Orthodontic phase: 3 years.
- Retention: 1 year.

LC

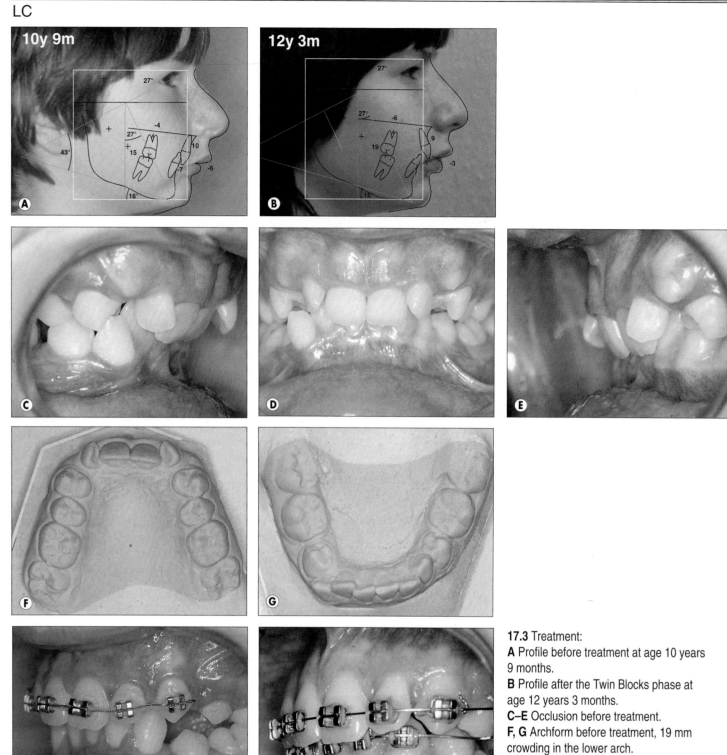

17.3 Treatment:
A Profile before treatment at age 10 years 9 months.
B Profile after the Twin Blocks phase at age 12 years 3 months.
C–E Occlusion before treatment.
F, G Archform before treatment, 19 mm crowding in the lower arch.
H Brackets on upper anterior teeth during the Twin Block phase.
J Phase 2 – fixed appliances.

LC

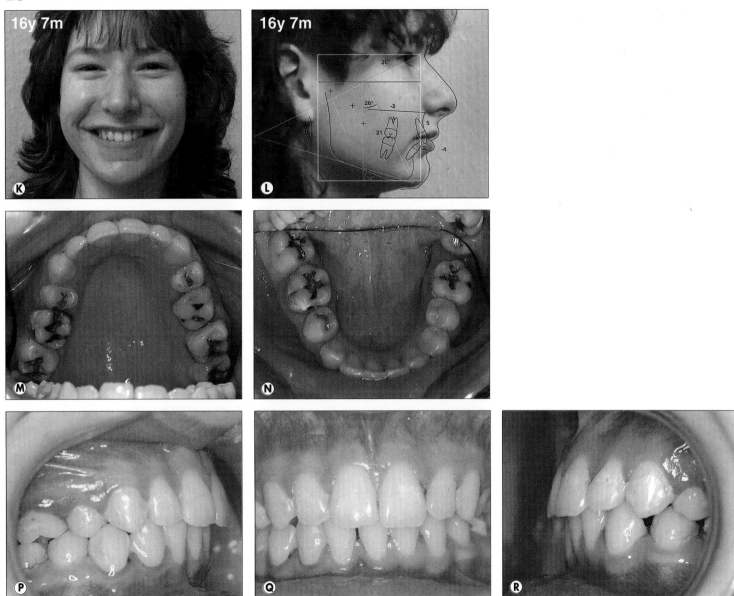

17.3 Treatment (cont.):
K, L Appearance after treatment at age 16 years 7 months.
M, N Archform at age 18 years 3 months.
P–R Occlusion at age 18 years 3 months.

LC

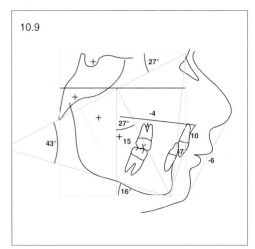

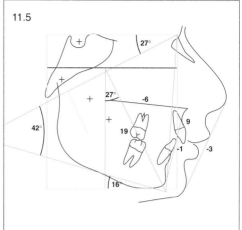

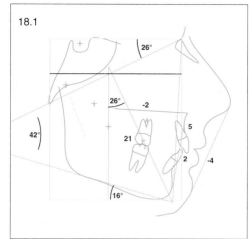

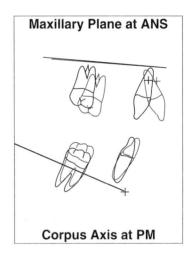

Maxillary Plane at ANS

Corpus Axis at PM

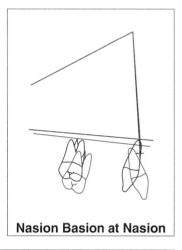

Nasion Basion at Nasion

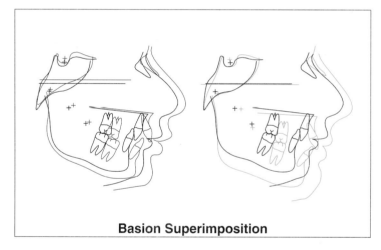

Basion Superimposition

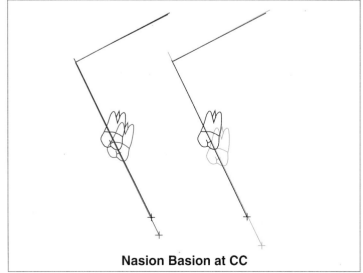

Nasion Basion at CC

L.C. -	Age	10.9	11.5	18.1 (Yr.Mon)
Cranial Base Angle		27	27	26
Facial Axis Angle		27	27	26
F/M Plane Angle		16	16	16
Craniomandibular Angle		43	42	42
Maxillary Plane		−4	−6	−2
Convexity		10	9	5
U/Incisor to Vertical		−17	16	21
L/Incisor to Vertical		22	35	40
Interincisal Angle		175	129	119
6 to Pterygoid Vertical		15	19	21
L/Incisor to A/Po		−7	−1	2
L/Lip to Aesthetic Plane		−6	−3	−4

CHAPTER
18
Treatment of Facial Asymmetry

The occlusal inclined plane is an ideal functional mechanism for unilateral activation, and Twin Blocks are extremely effective in the correction of facial and dental asymmetry. The sagittal Twin Block is the appliance of choice for correction of asymmetry because the sagittal design allows unilateral activation to restore symmetry in buccal and labial segments.

Case report: M.McK. aged 10 years 4 months
This girl presented facial and dental asymmetry with the lower centre line displaced to the right. In the anterior facial view the chin point was displaced to the right in open and closed position, confirming a true skeletal asymmetry. Orthopaedic treatment to improve the asymmetry was followed by an orthodontic phase of detailed finishing with fixed appliances.

Diagnosis, skeletal classification:
- Moderate Class II.
- Facial type: moderate brachyfacial.
- Dental and facial asymmetry.
- Maxilla: normal.
- Mandible: mild retrusion.

Diagnosis: dental classification:
- Asymmetrical Class II division 1.
- Upper incisors: mild protrusion.
- Lower incisors: moderate retrusion.
- Lower midline displaced to the right.
- Distal occlusion more marked on the right side.
- Asymmetrical overjet with 21|2 retroclined.
- Deep overbite.

- Lower archform good with minimal crowding.

Treatment:
- Orthopaedic phase: to improve facial asymmetry and, at the same time, correct the mandibular retrusion.
- Support phase: to allow the buccal teeth to settle into occlusion, and to initiate fixed appliance treatment.
- Orthodontic phase: to detail the occlusion

Appliances:
- Twin Blocks designed to improve the asymmetry.
- Anterior inclined plane to settle the occlusion. Initiate fixed appliance treatment with the lower fixed appliance and sectional upper fixed appliance.
- Full bonded fixed appliances to detail the occlusion.

Bite registration. Correction of asymmetry in the construction bite ensures that the occlusal forces activate the appliance to restore symmetry. The construction bite is registered with the incisors edge-to-edge with 2 mm vertical clearance, and the centre lines correct. This will improve the facial asymmetry and reduce the mandibular retrusion.

Appliance design. An upper Twin Block sagittal appliance with two palatal screws is designed to advance retroclined upper incisors and drive upper molars distally. The screw is turned more frequently on the side that requires more distal movement. The mechanical action of the palatal screws is reinforced by occlusal forces on the inclined planes, favouring the working side to correct the midline displacement (**18.1**).

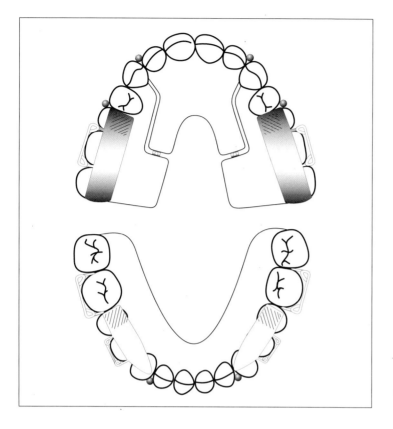

18.1 Sagittal Twin Blocks give better control for correction of dental or facial asymmetry. Good fixation is necessary in the lower arch.

Clinical management. The initial response to treatment resulted in rapid correction of the asymmetry and reduction of the overjet. After 7 weeks of treatment, at the second visit for adjustment, the centre lines were corrected and the overjet was fully reduced. A new muscle balance position was established whereby it was not possible for the patient to retract the mandible into its former retruded asymmetrical position. The rapid improvement in muscle balance is evident in the facial photographs at this stage and there is already a marked improvement in the facial asymmetry and profile.

At the start of treatment the upper bite block was trimmed occlusodistally to encourage lower molar eruption. At the second visit the inclined planes on the left side were trimmed out of contact in order to reinforce the corrective occlusal forces on the active right side.

At this stage the lateral open bite is increased on the right side. Asymmetry is normally associated with a vertical discrepancy, which can be identified when the centre lines are corrected in the construction bite. The vertical space between the posterior teeth is more marked on the side to which the mandible is displaced. The height of the occlusal blocks in the premolar region on the right side was slightly reduced over a period of 2 months to encourage vertical correction.

After 6 months of treatment the buccal segment occlusion was corrected to Class I with the overjet and overbite reduced. The centre lines were now correct, and the lateral open bite was closed sufficiently to proceed to the next stage.

The lower Twin Block was replaced by a lower fixed appliance to commence orthodontic correction in the lower arch. An upper appliance with an anterior inclined plane was fitted to support the corrected incisor relationship, leaving the posterior teeth free to erupt fully into occlusion.

Brackets were placed on the upper anterior teeth to improve alignment during the support phase. A full transition to fixed appliances was made after 10 months of treatment, when the distal occlusion and dental asymmetry corrected, and there was considerable improvement in the facial asymmetry. Treatment continued in an orthodontic phase with full-bonded fixed appliances, followed by retention (**18.2 A–Z**).

Duration of treatment:
- Orthopaedic phase: 6 months to correct occlusion to Class I.
- Support phase: 5 months to settle occlusion and begin orthodontic correction.
- Orthodontic phase: 12 months to complete treatment.
- Retention: 1 year.
- Total treatment time: 2 years 11 months including retention.

Final records. 1 year out of retention.

The rapid improvement in facial and dental asymmetry in this case was achieved by unilateral activation of the occlusal inclined planes. This improvement was maintained out of retention.

MMcK

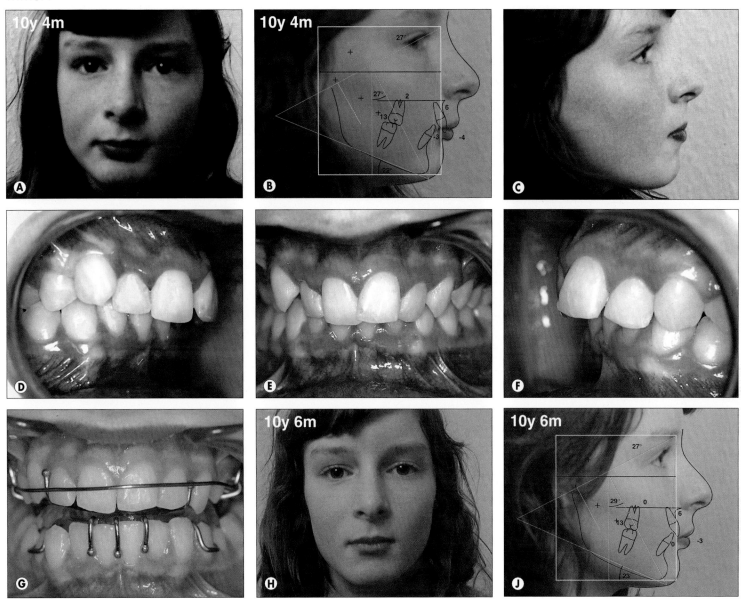

18.2 Treatment:

A, B Appearance before treatment at age 10 years 4 months.

C Improvement in profile on fitting the Twin Blocks.

D–F Asymmetrical occlusion before treatment.

G Construction bite corrects the asymmetry.

H, J Improvement in asymmetry and profile after 10 weeks at age 10 years 6 months.

MMcK

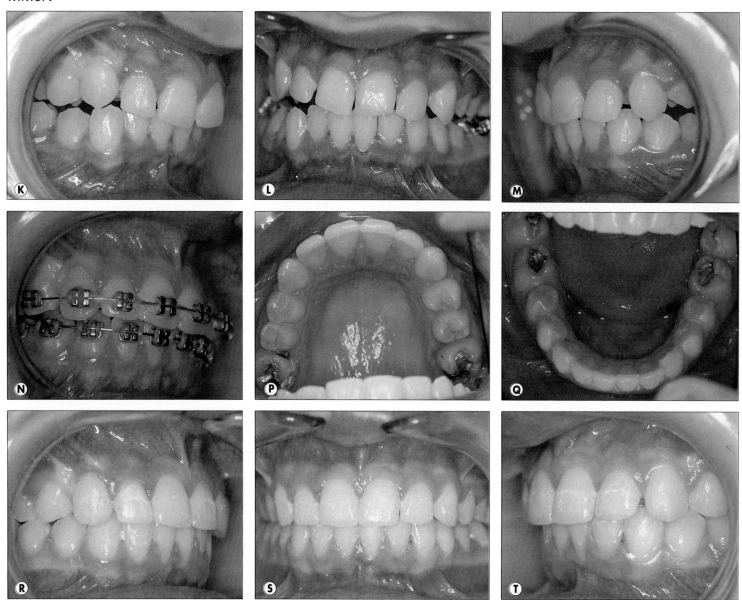

18.2 Treatment (cont.):

K–M Correction of occlusion at age 10 years 7 months.

N Fixed appliances to detail the occlusion.

P, Q Archform after treatment.

R–T Occlusion at the end of treatment.

MMcK

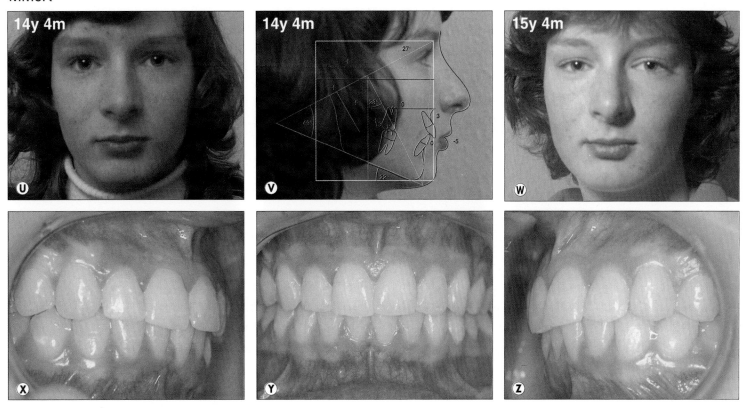

14y 4m 14y 4m 15y 4m

18.2 Treatment (cont.):

U, V Appearance after treatment.

W Correction of facial asymmetry is maintained at age 15 years 4 months, one year out of retention.

X–Z Occlusion 1 year out of retention at age 15 years 4 months.

Magnetic force in the correction of facial asymmetry

Inclined planes with attracting magnets provide an excellent training mechanism to improve facial balance by controlling muscle action. Magnetic Twin Blocks have the potential to accelerate the rate of correction achieved by conventional functional appliances (**18.3**).

The use of magnetic force will be discussed further in Chapter 19.

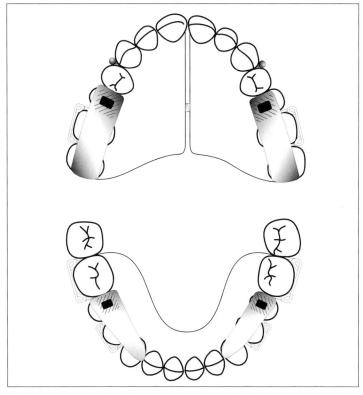

18.3 Magnetic Twin Blocks can accelerate the rate of correction.

MMcK

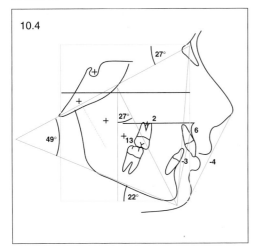

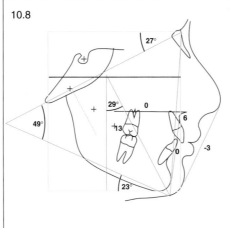

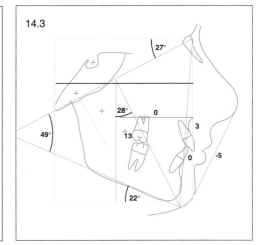

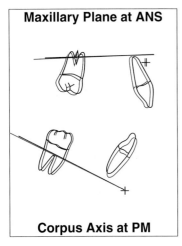

Maxillary Plane at ANS

Corpus Axis at PM

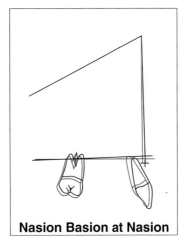

Nasion Basion at Nasion

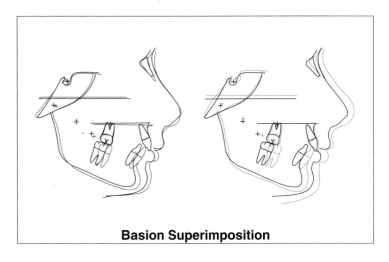

Basion Superimposition

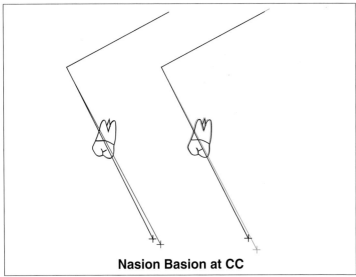

Nasion Basion at CC

M.McK -	Age	10.4	10.8	14.3 (Yr.Mon)
Cranial Base Angle		27	27	27
Facial Axis Angle		27	29	28
F/M Plane Angle		22	23	22
Craniomandibular Angle		49	49	49
Maxillary Plane		2	0	0
Convexity		6	6	3
U/Incisor to Vertical		19	22	27
L/Incisor to Vertical		24	36	35
Interincisal Angle		137	122	118
6 to Pterygoid Vertical		13	13	13
L/Incisor to A/Po		–3	0	0
L/Lip to Aesthetic Plane		–4	–3	–5

CHAPTER

19

Magnetic Twin Blocks

The role of magnets in Twin Block therapy is specifically to accelerate correction of arch relationships. The purpose of the magnets is to encourage increased occlusal contact on the bite blocks to maximise the favourable functional forces applied to correct the malocclusion.

Two types of rare earth magnet (samarium cobalt and neodynium boron) have been used to examine the response to attracting magnetic forces in Twin Block treatment. Both are effective, but neodynium boron delivers a greater force from a smaller magnet. At this stage no statistical comparison has been made by the author to evaluate the response to magnetic and nonmagnetic appliances, and the following observations are based on clinical evaluation.

Attracting magnets incorporated in occlusal inclined planes may be effective in maintaining forward mandibular posture when the patient is asleep. Patients who have magnets added to Twin Blocks during treatment report increased occlusal contact by day and observe also that the blocks are in contact on waking.

MAGNETIC FORCE

Magnetic force is a new factor under investigation as an activating mechanism in orthodontic and orthopaedic treatment. Animal experiments in mandibular advancement (Vardimon *et al.,* 1989, 1990) indicate an improved mandibular growth response to magnetic functional appliances compared to nonmagnetic appliances of similar design.

Similar experiments using a magnetic appliance with an adjustable screw for maxillary advancement showed midfacial protraction with horizontal maxillary displacement and anterosuperior premaxillary rotation (Vardimon *et al.,* 1989, 1990).

Clinical investigations are now proceeding to develop new appliance systems to utilise magnetic forces. The author has modified Twin Blocks by the addition of attracting magnets to occlusal inclined planes, using magnetic force as an activating mechanism to maximise the orthopaedic response to treatment. Darendeliler & Joho (1993) have described similar appliances which are based on the magnetic Twin Block.

ATTRACTING OR REPELLING MAGNETS

The first consideration on the use of magnets in inclined planes is whether the opposing poles should attract or repel. There are logical reasons to support the use of both systems. The advantages of both methods may be summarised as follows, with examples of current clinical research.

Attracting magnets

In favour of attracting magnets it may be said that increased activation can be built into the initial construction bite for the appliances. The attracting magnetic force pulls the appliances together and encourages the patient to occlude actively and consistently in a forward position. The functional mechanism of Twin Blocks stimulates a proprioceptive response by repeated contact on the occlusal inclined planes. Attracting magnets may accelerate progress by increasing the frequency and the force of contact on the inclined planes, thus enhancing the adaptive response to functional correction.

The author has used rare earth attracting magnets in five different clinical situations, described below.

Class II division 1 malocclusion with a large overjet
This resulted in more rapid correction of distal occlusion than would normally be expected without magnets. After 1 month's treatment, the overjet reduced from 10 mm to 6 mm, and after 2 months' treatment, a further reduction to 2 mm was observed (**19.1**).

Mild residual Class II buccal segment relationship
This was proving difficult to resolve and was mainly a unilateral problem. Magnetic inclined planes were used to accelerate correction of the buccal segment relationship to a 'super Class I' relationship, which was quickly achieved.

Mild Class II division 1 malocclusion with an overjet of 7 mm
The patient was failing to posture forwards consistently with conventional Twin Blocks and, as a result, was making slow progress. The addition of attracting magnets noticeably improved occlusal contact on the bite blocks, and progress improved in consequence. Patients with weak musculature fail to respond to functional therapy because they do not make the muscular effort required to engage the appliance actively by occluding on the inclined planes. It appears that

237

attracting magnets will benefit this type of patient by increasing the frequency of favourable occlusal contacts.

Unilateral Class II adult patient with temperomandibular joint pain
Magnets were fitted unilaterally to correct the mandibular displacement to the affected side. This was immediately effective in resolving the symptoms, and occlusal correction is proceeding to produce a long-term resolution of the problem.

Skeletal Class III malocclusion with persistent crossbite, failed to resolve with conventional mechanics
Class III magnetic Twin Blocks were used to apply orthopaedic forces to correct mandibular displacement and to advance the maxilla, with an additional sagittal expansion component. This was effective in resolving quickly the mandibular displacement. The initial response to Class III correction is excellent.

Treatment of facial asymmetry

Magnetic force may be used to counteract asymmetrical muscle action in the development of facial asymmetry. Mandibular displacement responds rapidly to correction with attracting magnets in the occlusal inclined planes on the working side. The nonactive side may be activated to a lesser degree to encourage centre line correction.

Repelling magnets

Repelling magnets may be used in Twin Blocks with less mechanical activation built into the occlusal inclined planes. The repelling magnetic force is intended to apply additional stimulus to forward posture as the patient closes into occlusion.

Moss & Shaw (1990) reported at the European Orthodontic Congress on a controlled study of 12 patients with repelling magnets placed in occlusal inclines of Twin Block appliances.The results indicated a 50% increase in the rate of correction of overjet compared to a similar group of patients where magnets were not used, although an improved growth response was not established.

The repelling magnets were intended to induce additional forward mandibular posture without reactivation of the blocks. A disadvantage of this method is that the amount of activation is not clear, and reactivation of the inclined planes would deactivate the magnets.

The appliances used in this study were not designed to allow vertical development in the buccal segments and, therefore, produced a large posterior open bite which subsequently had to be closed by fixed appliances. These appliances did not conform to the basic principles of Twin Block design for control of the vertical dimension.

After a short period of investigation it appears that magnetic Twin Blocks may help to resolve some of the problems encountered in the management of difficult cases. It is still to be established whether attracting or repelling magnets are more effective, although attracting magnets would appear to have an advantage by increasing contact on the inclined planes.

Magnets should be used only where speed of treatment is an important consideration, or where the response to nonmagnetic appliances is limited.

Case report: F.H. aged 14 years 11 months

This boy attended for treatment in his mid-teens and presented labial segment crowding and irregularity in both arches, requiring three stages of treatment. An initial stage of arch development was followed by functional correction and a finishing stage with fixed appliances. Magnetic Twin Blocks with attracting magnets were used to accelerate the orthopaedic stage of treatment (**19.1 A–Z**).

Diagnosis, skeletal classification:
- Moderate Class II.
- Facial type: severe brachyfacial.
- Maxilla: mild protrusion.
- Mandible: normal.
- Convexity = 5 mm.

Diagnosis, dental classification:
- Severe Class II division 1.
- Buccal segments: full unit distal occlusion.
- Overjet = 10 mm.
- Deep traumatic overbite = 7 mm.
- Labial displacement $\overline{1}$ with gingival recession.
- Upper and lower labial segment crowding.

Clinical diagnosis confirmed that functional therapy was indicated, as the profile improved significantly when the patient postured the mandible forwards to reduce the overjet and correct the distal occlusion. This simple clinical guide takes precedence over cephalometric evaluation in assessing suitability for functional therapy.

Treatment plan:
- Arch development: to correct the archform and improve alignment.
- Orthopaedic phase: to correct the distal occlusion.
- Orthodontic phase: detailed finishing.

Appliances:
- Quad helix and a lower lingual arch to develop the archform.
- Magnetic Twin Blocks to correct to Class I occlusion.
- Full-bonded fixed appliance to detail the occlusion.

Clinical management:
- Arch development: a Wilson quad helix and lower lingual arch were fitted first with brackets on the upper anterior teeth to improve the upper and lower archform. This objective was achieved after 6 months of treatment.
- Orthopaedic phase: attracting magnets were incorporated in the inclined planes in the Twin Blocks to accelerate functional correction.This resulted in rapid progress as the overjet reduced from 10 to 2 mm in 2 months. The Twin Blocks were worn for a further 3 months to stabilise the corrected occlusion before discarding the lower appliance and fitting an upper appliance with an anterior inclined plane. There was a short period of passive retention at this stage, during which the lower labial fraenum was resected to improve the gingival recession on $\overline{1}$.
- Orthodontic phase: detailing of the occlusion was carried out with bonded fixed appliances. Lingual root torque was applied to $\overline{1}$ to position the root in the alveolar bone in order to stabilise the incisor relationship and improve the gingival attachment of this tooth.

FH

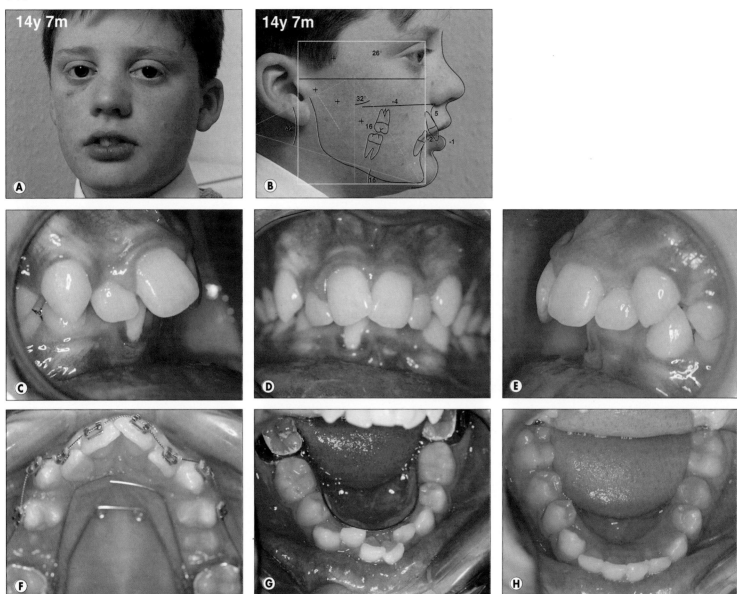

19.1 Treatment:

A, B Appearance before treatment at age 14 years 7 months.

C–E Occlusion before treatment – note the gingival recession of 1̄.

F, G Phase 1 – arch development (quad helix and Wilson lingual arch).

H Improved lower archform after arch development.

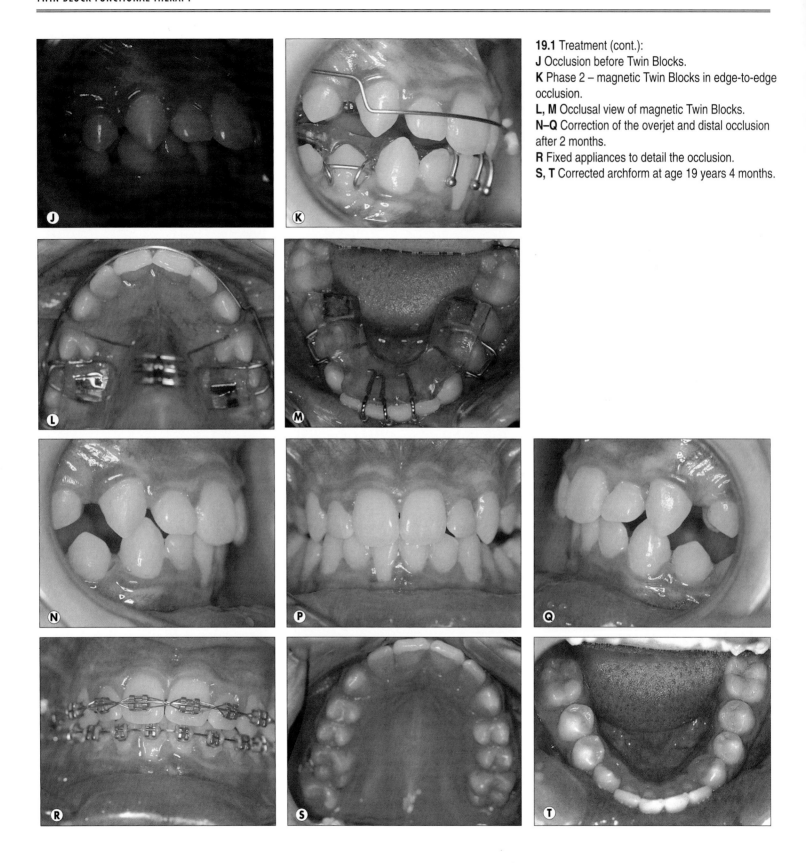

19.1 Treatment (cont.):
J Occlusion before Twin Blocks.
K Phase 2 – magnetic Twin Blocks in edge-to-edge occlusion.
L, M Occlusal view of magnetic Twin Blocks.
N–Q Correction of the overjet and distal occlusion after 2 months.
R Fixed appliances to detail the occlusion.
S, T Corrected archform at age 19 years 4 months.

FH

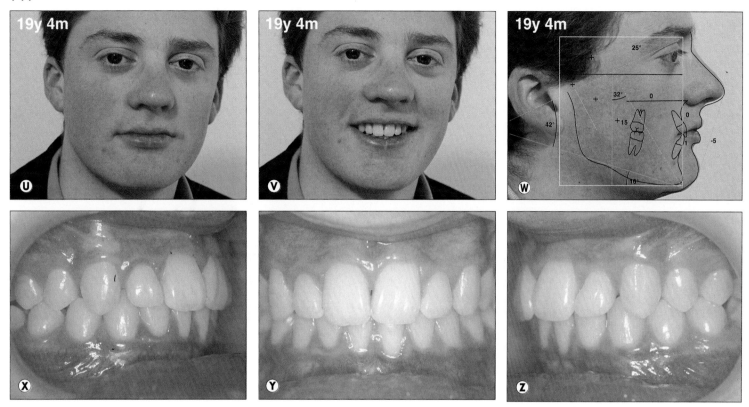

19.1 Treatment (cont.):
U–W Appearance at age 19 years 4 months.
X–Z Occlusion 1 year out of retention at age 19 years 4 months.

Duration of treatment:
- Arch development: 6 months.
- Orthopaedic phase: 5 months.
- Orthodontic phase: 20 months.
- Retention: 1 year.

Discussion. This case illustrates the management of a crowded dentition in three phases of arch development, functional correction and orthodontic finishing. The addition of attracting magnets in the inclined planes was successful in accelerating correction of the distal occlusion. This was followed by orthodontic correction with fixed appliances to detail the occlusion and overcorrect the labially displaced lower incisor.

REFERENCES

Darendeliler, M.A. & Joho, J.P. (1993). Magnetic activator device II (MAD) for correction of Class II Division I malocclusions. *Am. J. Orthod. Dentofac. Orthop.,* **103:** 223–39.

Moss, J. & Shaw (1990). European Orthodontic Congress, Copenhagen.

Vardimon, A.D., Graber, T.M., Voss, L.R. & Muller, T.M. (1990). Functional Orthopedic Magnetic Appliance (FOMA) III—modus operandi. *Am. J. Orthod. Dentofac. Orthop.,* **97:** 135–48.

Vardimon, A.D., Stutzmann, J.J., Graber, T.M., Voss, L.R. & Petrovic, A.G. (1989). Functional Orthopedic Magnetic Appliance (FOMA) II—modus operandi. *Am. J. Orthod. Dentofac. Orthop.,* **95:** 371–87.

FH

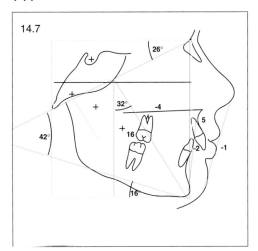

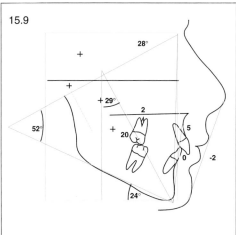

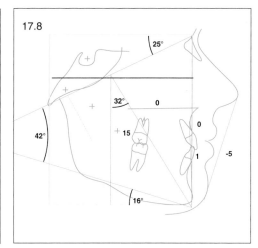

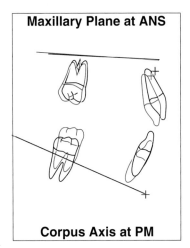

Maxillary Plane at ANS

Corpus Axis at PM

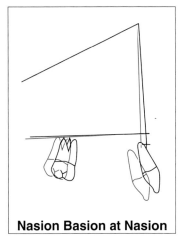

Nasion Basion at Nasion

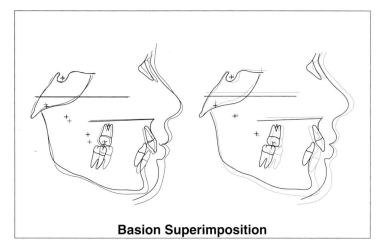

Basion Superimposition

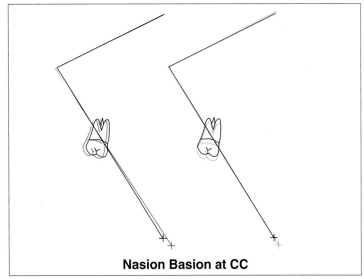

Nasion Basion at CC

F.H. -	Age	14.7	15.9	17.8 (Yr.Mon)
Cranial Base Angle		26	28	25
Facial Axis Angle		32	29	32
F/M Plane Angle		16	24	16
Craniomandibular Angle		42	52	43 42
Maxillary Plane		−4	2	0
Convexity		5	5	0
U/Incisor to Vertical		21	21	27
L/Incisor to Vertical		24	31	29
Interincisal Angle		135	128	126
6 to Pterygoid Vertical		16	20	15
L/Incisor to A/Po		−2	0	1
L/Lip to Aesthetic Plane		−1	−1	−5

CHAPTER

20

Adult Treatment

Tooth movements are slower in older patients, and the skeletal response diminishes with the patient's age. In adult orthodontic treatment we should anticipate a dentoalveolar response with limited skeletal adaptation. This still leaves scope for significant facial change, but only when the skeletal discrepancy is not severe. Surgical correction should be considered for cases of severe skeletal discrepancies in adults.

TREATMENT OF A YOUNG ADULT

Case report: P.W. aged 17 years 4 months

Treatment in late teens by Twin Blocks after the pubertal growth spurt (**20.1 A–F**).

Diagnosis, skeletal classification:
- Class I.
- Facial type: severe brachyfacial.
- Maxilla: normal.
- Mandible: normal.
- Pronounced chin eminence.
- Convexity = -2 mm.

Diagnosis, dental classification:
- Severe Class II division 1.
- Overjet = 10 mm.
- Traumatic deep overbite lingual to the upper incisors.
- Upper incisors proclined.
- Lower incisors to A–Po = –2 mm.
- Molar relationship: full unit distal occlusion.

Treatment plan. In the orthopaedic phase, in view of the patient's age, it was decided to reinforce the action of the inclined planes by a light traction force, to retract the maxillary dentition, using the Concorde facebow.

Duration of treatment:
- Orthopaedic phase: 9 months with Twin Blocks.
- Support phase: 3 months with anterior inclined plane.
- Retention: 6 months.

Discussion. There was a rapid response to treatment in this case as the overjet reduced from 10 to 6 mm within the first 6 weeks, and to 4 mm after 4 months of treatment. The patient declined a final stage of treatment to detail the occlusion with fixed appliances. The result proved to be stable although no significant growth changes are recorded at this age.

PW

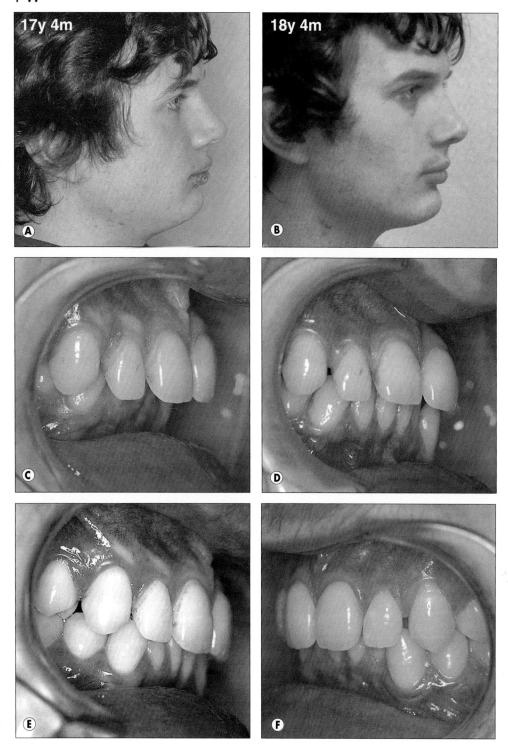

20.1 Treatment:
A, Profile before treatment at age 17 years 4 months.
B Profile after treatment at age 18 years 4 months.
C Occlusion before treatment
D Occlusion after 6 weeks of treatment.
E Occlusion after 18 months of treatment.
F Occlusion after 3 years, at age 20 years 4 months, 18 months out of retention.

PW

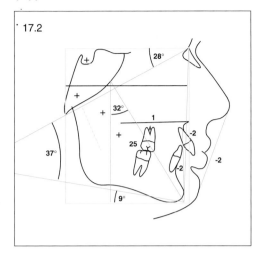

17.2

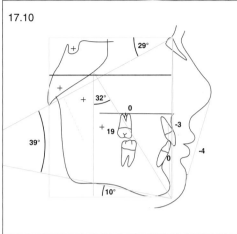

17.10

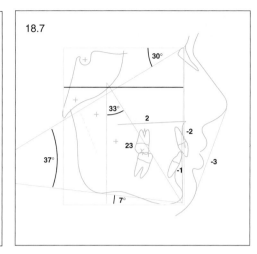

18.7

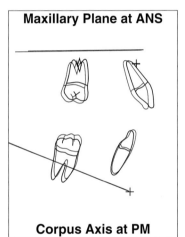

Maxillary Plane at ANS

Corpus Axis at PM

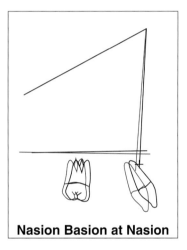

Nasion Basion at Nasion

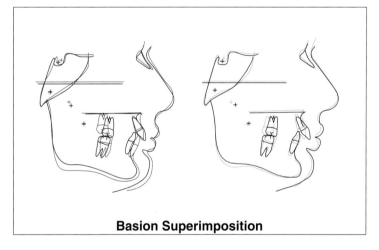

Basion Superimposition

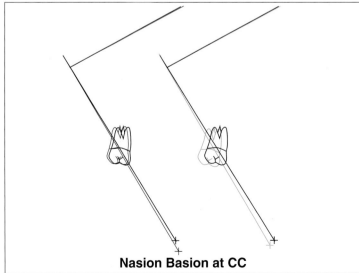

Nasion Basion at CC

P.W. -	Age	17.2	17.10	18.7 (Yr.Mon)
Cranial Base Angle		28	29	30
Facial Axis Angle		32	32	33
F/M Plane Angle		9	10	7
Craniomandibular Angle		37	39	37
Maxillary Plane		1	0	2
Convexity		–2	–3	–2
U/Incisor to Vertical		31	25	20
L/Incisor to Vertical		23	24	26
Interincisal Angle		126	131	134
6 to Pterygoid Vertical		25	19	23
L/Incisor to A/Po		–2	0	–1
L/Lip to Aesthetic Plane		–2	–4	–3

Case report: H.C. aged 42 years 8 months

This patient attended for treatment at the age of 42 because her upper incisors were migrating labially due to loss of bony support. This case shows a typical dentoalveolar response in adult treatment where periodontally compromised teeth are the weakest link in the biological chain of reaction due to lack of bony support. Combined extraoral and intermaxillary traction were applied at night during the orthopaedic phase of treatment, using the Concorde facebow to accelerate tooth movements. This was followed by an orthodontic phase with fixed appliances (**20.2 A–P**).

Diagnosis, skeletal classification:
- Class I.
- Facial type: mild brachyfacial.
- Maxilla: mild retrognathic.
- Mandible: mild retrognathic.
- Convexity = 2 mm.

Diagnosis, dental classification:
- Severe Class II division 1.
- Overjet = 11 mm.
- Traumatic deep overbite lingual to the upper incisors.
- Upper incisors proclined with central diastema.
- Lower incisors: normal.

Treatment plan:
- Orthopaedic phase: correct the dental relationship to Class I. Reinforce the anchorage with extraoral and intermaxillary traction to accelerate tooth movements using the Concorde facebow. Anticipate the minimal orthopaedic response in viewof the patient's age.
- Support phase.
- Orthodontic phase: finish with fixed appliances.

Appliances:
- An example of the early design of Twin Blocks.
- Anterior guide plane.
- Simple fixed appliances.

Clinical management. The early design of Twin Blocks shows the type of clasp used before the delta clasp was developed. The upper appliance had provision for the attachment of a facebow to a coiled tube incorporated in an Adams clasp. The Concorde facebow was worn at night to apply combined intermaxillary and extraoral traction.

The response to treatment was rapid and the overjet reduced from 10 to 4 mm in 4 months. The posterior teeth were still out of occlusion and an anterior inclined plane was worn for 3 months as the occlusion settled before making the transition to fixed appliances. Simple fixed appliances were worn for 8 months. Finally, upper and lower Rochette splints were fitted as fixed lingual retainers. These served the dual purpose of orthodontic retainer and splint to stabilise the anterior teeth for periodontal support.

Duration of treatment:
- Orthopaedic phase: 4 months with Twin Blocks.
- Support phase: 3 months with an anterior inclined plane.
- Orthodontic phase: 8 months with fixed appliances.
- Retention: permanent fixed lingual retainers.

Assessment of result. Superimposed x-rays confirm that the correction was due to dentoalveolar compensation, with no skeletal change. The upper dentition was retracted and the lower dentition moved mesially. Growth changes should not be anticipated in the treatment of adults who are beyond the growth stage and have loss of periodontal support.

HC

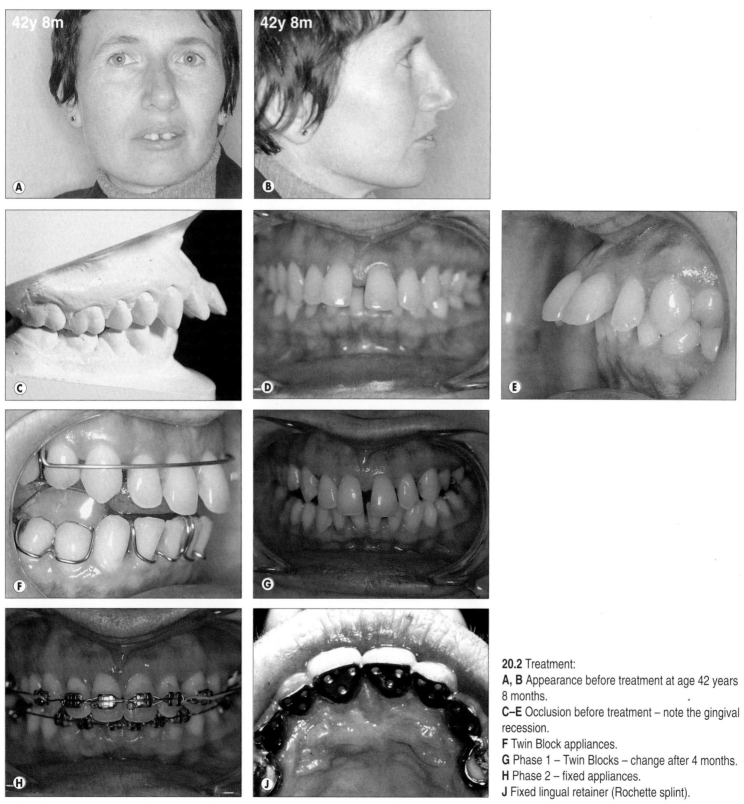

20.2 Treatment:
A, B Appearance before treatment at age 42 years 8 months.
C–E Occlusion before treatment – note the gingival recession.
F Twin Block appliances.
G Phase 1 – Twin Blocks – change after 4 months.
H Phase 2 – fixed appliances.
J Fixed lingual retainer (Rochette splint).

HC

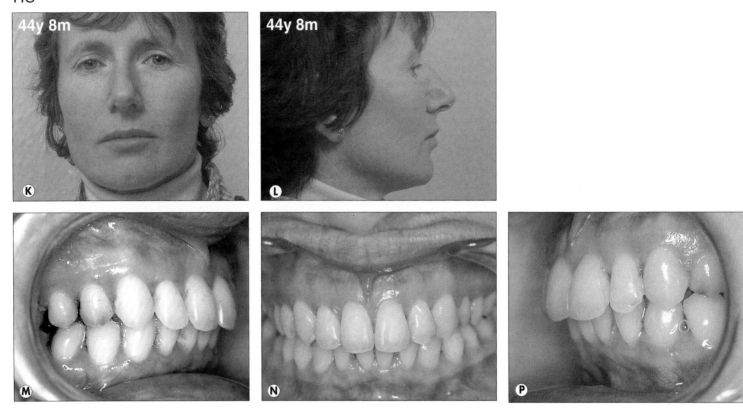

20.2 Treatment (cont.):

K, L Appearance after treatment.

M–P Occlusion after treatment at age 44 years 8 months.

HC

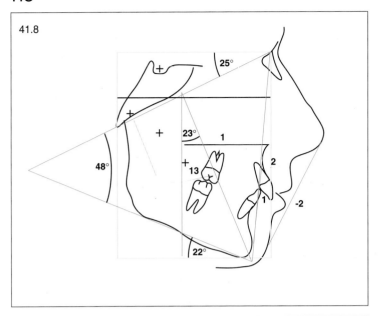

41.8

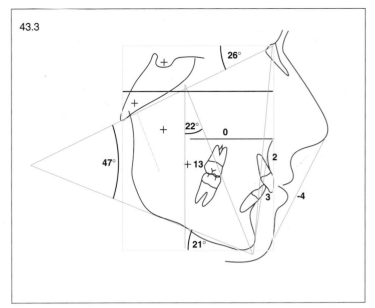

43.3

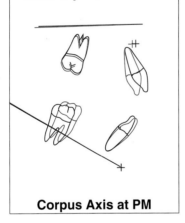

Maxillary Plane at ANS

Corpus Axis at PM

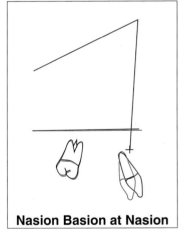

Nasion Basion at Nasion

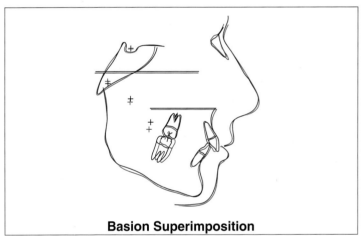

Basion Superimposition

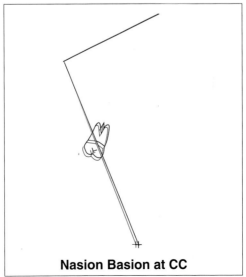

Nasion Basion at CC

H.C. -	Age	41.8	43.3	(Yr.Mon)
Cranial Base Angle		25	26	
Facial Axis Angle		23	22	
F/M Plane Angle		22	21	
Craniomandibular Angle		48	47	
Maxillary Plane		1	0	
Convexity		2	2	
U/Incisor to Vertical		26	21	
L/Incisor to Vertical		39	45	
Interincisal Angle		115	114	
6 to Pterygoid Vertical		13	13	
L/Incisor to A/Po		1	3	
L/Lip to Aesthetic Plane		−2	−4	

GJ

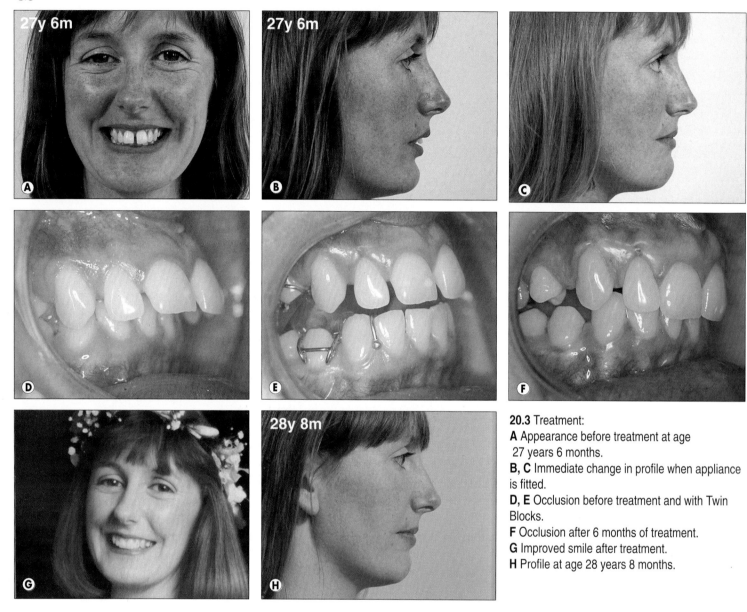

20.3 Treatment:
A Appearance before treatment at age 27 years 6 months.
B, C Immediate change in profile when appliance is fitted.
D, E Occlusion before treatment and with Twin Blocks.
F Occlusion after 6 months of treatment.
G Improved smile after treatment.
H Profile at age 28 years 8 months.

Case report: G.J. aged 27 years 6 months

When this patient attended for examination she asked if treatment to improve her smile could be completed before her wedding in 7 months time. Twin Blocks were fitted and sufficient progress was made to meet her request (20.3 A–H).

Diagnosis, skeletal classification:
- Class I.
- Facial type: mild retrognathic.
- Maxilla: mild retrognathic.
- Mandible: mild retrognathic.
- Convexity = 2 mm.

Diagnosis, dental classification:
- Severe Class II division 1.
- Overjet = 10 mm.
- Traumatic deep overbite lingual to the upper incisors.
- Upper incisors: protrusive.
- Lower incisors to A–Po line = –3 mm.
- Full unit Class II molar relationship.
- First premolars extracted previously.

Duration of treatment:
- Orthopaedic phase: 9 months with Twin Blocks.
- Support phase: 5 months with anterior inclined plane.
- Retention: continuing.

CHAPTER
21

Twin Blocks in
Temporomandibular Joint Therapy

TEMPOROMANDIBULAR JOINT PAIN AND DYSFUNCTION SYNDROME

Occlusion is inevitably related to the health and function of the temporomandibular (TM) joint. No dental condition is more distressing for a patient than chronic TM joint pain. A rationale of treatment is therefore important in dental and orthodontic practice. This is a litigious area of dental practice and second opinions should be sought before embarking on any treatment which may worsen an already established pathological condition.

The dental profession is increasingly aware of a multidisciplinary approach, recognising the role of chiropractors and craniosacral osteopaths in the diagnosis and resolution of TM joint dysfunction. Muscle spasm and joint pathology cannot be considered in isolation from a holistic examination of other possible causes in body posture and alignment of the vertebral column. Cooperation should be encouraged in interdisciplinary programmes of diagnosis and management.

Case history and diagnosis

Excellent record taking is an essential part of clinical management and treatment. A full case history is necessary to establish any cause-and-effect relationship of occlusal disharmony and mandibular displacement to pain and restriction of mandibular movement. This includes an assessment of any injury, headache, neck and back pain, neuromuscular tension, and tenderness to palpation.

Clinical and radiographic examinations of the TM joint are used to identify the position of the condyle in the glenoid fossae in the closed position, at rest and in the open position. Any radiographic evidence of flattening or irregularity in the shape of the condyle is a sign of pathological change, and patients with signs of osteoarthritic change in the joint should be referred for comprehensive investigation, and expert advice and treatment.

Some of the major signs and clinical symptoms of TM joint dysfunction of a functionally induced nature are diagnosed as pain, muscle tension, joint sounds, and limitation of movement. A displaced disc is often associated with clicks and limited opening. In unilateral disc displacement there is displacement of the mandible to the affected side, and limited transverse movement. It is sometimes possible to manipulate the mandible downwards and fowards to recapture the disc. If successful, this would have the immediate response of increased opening. However, manipulation to recapture the disc does not eliminate the cause of disc displacement, which may then recur. Limited opening is also a sign of disc displacement.

Freedom of mandibular movement

It is essential to diagnose any limitation of movement relative to the normal range of movement:

*   Normal opening is 48 mm (the three finger test).
*   Transverse movement is 12 mm to each side, measuring the lower midline displacement in maximum lateral movement.

The reciprocal click

A clicking joint is symptomatic of displacement of the articular disc off the head of the condyle. A reciprocal click describes the condition where a click is heard when the disc is recaptured by the head of the condyle on forward translation, and a reciprocal click is heard when the condyle is again displaced off the articular disc on closing. The opening click is louder than the closing click. Although the clicking joint may be otherwise asymptomatic, it is nevertheless already compromised internally and liable to present pathology at a later date due to the chronic displacement of the articular disc.

The timing of a click on opening is significant in the prognosis for resolution:

*   Early opening clicks: up to 22 mm opening are usually easy to resolve.
*   Midopening clicks: 22–35 mm opening are moderate to resolve.
*   Late opening clicks: over 35 mm opening are difficult to resolve.

Case selection for anterior repositioning of the mandible to relieve TM joint dysfunction is based on the severity of symptoms and condylar position at full occlusion. The prognosis is better for recapturing the disc for an early opening click. It becomes progressively more difficult for the mid- and late opening click, when pathological osteoarthritic change is likely to have occurred in the joint.

Spahl (1993) stresses that, neverthelss, disc recapture is not the main goal of treatment for patients with functionally induced TM joint pain dysfunction problems. The true goal is reduction of symptoms via condylar decompression procedures involving muscular advancement of the mandible followed by reconstruction of the occlusion in some manner to support the mandible/condyle in that advanced position.

THE CLOSED LOCK

Limitation of movement on opening is diagnostic of a disc which is displaced, usually anteromedially to the condyle, and is not recaptured on opening. In the initial stages, the patient may be pain free and may complain only of restriction of movement. This may be an episodic experience, where the disc is displaced from time to time and the patient may be able to periodically recapture the disc until the displacement becomes more severe. If not detected and treated, the disc may gradually become folded forwards and not recapturable, leading eventually to painful function and restricted opening due to osteoarthritis. A 'closed lock' should be diagnosed early from restricted movement and should be treated by anterior or vertical repositioning to recapture the disc. Treatment should then be effected to create vertical space in the joint by positioning the condyles downwards and forwards in the glenoid fossae, and to establish balanced occlusal support.

Internal derangement
The three stages of TM internal derangement are:

- Stage 1: painless clicking caused when an anteriorly displaced disc is recaptured on the condyle during opening translation.
- Stage 2: locking – persistent displacement of the disc which arrests condyle motion at midopening.
- Stage 3: disc displacement through all phases of jaw function. The anteromedially displaced disc becomes distorted and folded on opening, with chronic pain and signs of osteoarthritis. The disc remains permanently unrecapturable.

Stages 1 and 2 respond to splint therapy and anterior repositioning to recapture the disc, subject to correct case selection (Solberg, 1989) (**21.1 A–C**).

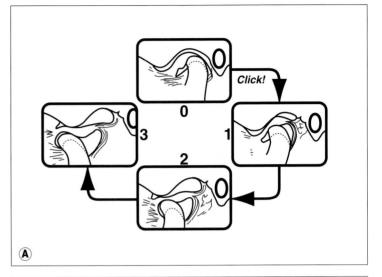

(A)

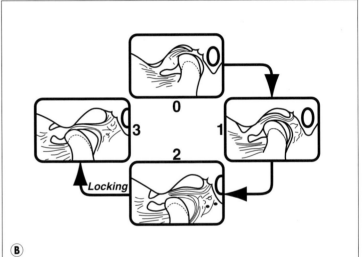

(B)

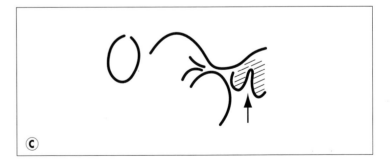

(C)

21.1 A A clicking joint: the sequence of opening and closing.
21.1 B, C The closed lock with a folded articular disc.
Reproduced from *Temporomandibular Disorders*, William K. Solberg, 1986, pp. 91, 92 and 93. Courtesy of the *British Dental Journal*, London.

Treatment rationale

Hawthorn & Flatau (1990) summarise the approach to joint dysfunction as follows:

> Conservative clinical treatment of joint dysfunction is based on the concept of the need to reduce loading within the joint itself in order to achieve satisfactory long term results, and to maintain the relationship of the meniscus to the condylar head.
>
> Conservative management of joint conditions ranging from arthritic degeneration to internal joint derangement is directed towards:
> 1. The reduction of functional loads exerted on the TM joint by restoration of interarch support.
> 2. The correction of the closing pathway as determined by tooth contacts. The constraints imposed on jaw movement in a sagittal plane by tooth contacts have a major effect on the movement of both the condyle and the meniscus during mandibular closure.

TM joint pain and dysfunction are frequently related to occlusal disharmony with premature occlusal contact, causing posterior or lateral shift of the mandible from centric relation and distal displacement of the condyles in the joint. Distal displacement of the condyle in occlusion is associated with anterior displacement of the articular disc.

The management of treatment in the past has been in three phases:

1. Sagittal expansion to advance the upper incisors, with occlusal cover to take the mandible out of occlusion and relieve pain.
2. Functional therapy to advance the mandible with a one piece functional appliance.
3. Vertical development of the posterior teeth using vertical elastic forces provided by appliances such as the Spahl vertical corrector or the biofinisher (Lynn, 1985), with occlusal reconstruction if required to increase the vertical dimension and to stabilise and balance the occlusion.

Temporomandibular joint therapy

Our efforts in treatment must not move the mandible back, or restrict the joint space. If occlusal imbalance is present, the muscles are the prime movers in causing mandibular displacement to avoid unfavourable premature occlusal contacts. Disc displacement and muscle spasm are secondary features of chronic occlusal imbalance, which causes the condyle to be displaced distally.

The goals of therapy are:
- Relieve the pain caused by distal displacement of the condyle.
- Retrain the muscles to a healthy pattern.
- Recapture the disc when possible by advancing the displaced condyle.
- Move the teeth that are causing occlusal imbalance and mandibular misguidance.
- Increase the vertical dimension to reduce deep overbite.

TWIN BLOCKS IN TEMPOROMANDIBULAR JOINT THERAPY

Case selection

A full diagnosis and case history is essential before proceeding to corrective treatment in TM joint therapy. If any signs of joint pathology are detected, expert advice should be sought. If in doubt, a diagnostic splint should first be supplied to resolve the pain and rest the joint before proceeding to more active therapy.

Twin Blocks are most likely to be indicated to resolve an early click when the condyle is displaced distal to the disc and the disc is recaptured at an early stage in the opening movement. Twin Blocks then achieve the following objectives in the first phase of treatment:

- Pain is relieved immediately when Twin Blocks are fitted or, in more difficult cases, within 4 days.
- The muscles are retrained automatically to a healthy pattern. A consistent feature of Twin Block therapy is the rapid improvement in facial balance. Muscle spasm is relieved when Twin Blocks are fitted, by changing the pattern of muscle activity to achieve a new position of equilibrium in muscle balance.
- The disc is recaptured by posturing the mandible downwards and forwards to advance the condyles.
- Rather than act as a passive splint, Twin Blocks are designed to move the teeth that are causing occlusal imbalance.
- The upper block may be trimmed selectively over the lower first molars only, using molar bands with vertical elastics to accelerate eruption of the first molars. To continue to rest the joint, a posterior occlusal stop is maintained by occlusal contact of the blocks with the second or third molars to support the vertical dimension.

The Twin Block sagittal appliance is usually appropriate to achieve all these objectives (**21.2**). In bite registration the exactobite is used to guide the mandible downwards and forwards to a comfortable position. It is important to recognise that if pain is not relieved by forward posture, and the disc does not appear to be recaptured, there may be internal derangement, or folding of the disc, which will not respond to Twin Block therapy.

A common cause of unilateral condylar displacement is occlusal interference causing a mandibular displacement and sideways shift, with the condyle displaced distally on the affected side, often associated with a unilateral distal occlusion. Unilateral sagittal activation to drive upper molars distally and advance the mandible simultaneously to correct the centre line and restore symmetry may help to resolve this type of occlusal imbalance.

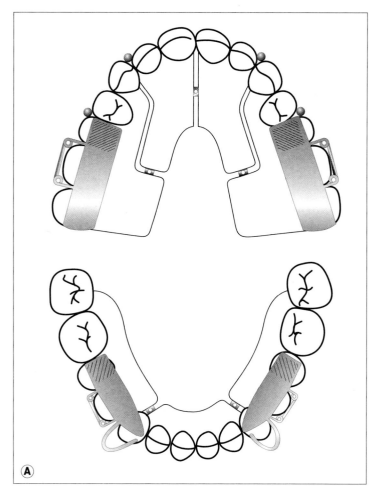
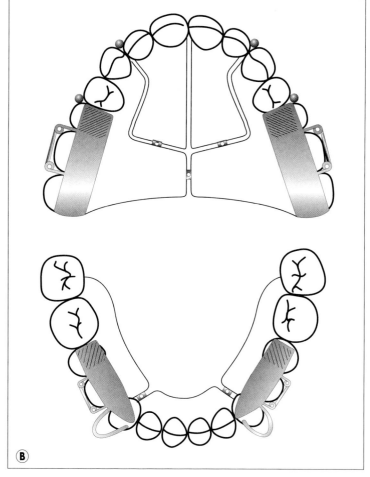

21.2 A, B The three-screw sagittal Twin Block to develop archform.

APPLIANCE DESIGN

The sagittal Twin Block is used to relieve compression on the joint by posturing the mandible downwards and forwards and advancing retroclined upper incisors. In sagittal appliance design, the further forwards the screws, the more anterior the movement; the further back the screws, the more posterior the movement.

Clinical management

In the management of deep overbite, the occlusal cover is trimmed progressively over the first molars only to allow the eruption of posterior teeth, without creating enough vertical clearance to allow the tongue to spread laterally between the teeth. Only after the first molars have erupted fully into occlusion may the blocks be trimmed selectively to encourage eruption of premolars or second or third molars as required.

It is especially important in the treatment of TM joint dysfunction to maintain posterior occlusal support at all times in order to relieve compression in the joint. A transition may be made to an anterior inclined plane to support the corrected occlusion after good posterior occlusal support is restored. This approach can be usefully combined with the Spahl vertical corrector in the support phase to accelerate correction of the vertical dimension.

Traction to open the bite

Vertical elastics may be used to accelerate the bite opening by stretching elastics from the upper appliance to hooks bonded to the lower posterior teeth, having first relieved occlusal acrylic to encourage selective eruption. This is not generally required in the treatment of the growing child, where eruption occurs naturally to close a posterior open bite. The addition of elastics is especially useful in adult treatment to accelerate eruption in patients who are no longer actively growing. Vertical traction assumes an increasingly important role as an effective method of increasing the vertical dimension in the treatment of patients who have TM joint dysfunction due to overclosure.

Stages of treatment

Treatment may be divided into into three separate objectives of sagittal development, functional repositioning and vertical development. Sagittal Twin Blocks are designed to allow all three corrective phases to proceed simultaneously to relieve a distally displaced condyle. Progressive trimming to encourage vertical development is crucial to the success of the treatment.

Detailed finishing of the occlusion to achieve a functional balance is necessary for long-term stability of joint symptoms. A finishing stage of treatment with bonded fixed appliances is frequently required to achieve this objective. When this is not possible, the alternative of occlusal rehabilitation by restorative means may be preferred if the occlusion is compromised by loss of teeth.

Round tripping

In the care of injured joints it is never effective to wear crutches part time and sometimes discard them – this results in relapse. This principle applies equally in TM joint therapy, whether a splint or a more active appliance is being used to rest the joint. Intermittent appliance wear only relieves the pain temporarily, and under certain circumstances may worsen it!

Pain is relieved when the appliance is worn and the condyle is positioned downwards and forwards in the joint. If the patient takes the appliance out for eating, or for any other reason, the condyle is again displaced up and back in the glenoid fossa and the pain returns.

It is important not to introduce splint dependency, but to endeavour to resolve the occlusal imbalance related to TM disorders. Successsful TM joint treatment requires a full-time commitment from the patient to see the treatment through until the occlusion is reconstructed with the condyles positioned correctly in the glenoid fossae. Depending on the aetiology of the condition this may involve orthopaedic repositioning, orthodontic balancing of the occlusion, occlusal reconstruction or a combination of these disciplines.

Case report: R.D. aged 36 years

This patient presented a severe Class II division 2 malocclusion and a history of chronic headaches 3 or 4 times a week for as long as he could remember. He had come to accept this as part of normal life until he learned that the headaches might be related to his dental occlusion, at which stage he presented for treatment.

The aim of the treatment was to relieve the compression in the TM joint by releasing the mandible from its trapped position in distal occlusion. This required upper anterior arch development followed by functional correction to advance the mandible. The objective was then to build the vertical dimension and position the condyles downwards and forwards in the glenoid fossae. A final restorative stage of

treatment is anticipated to increase the width of the upper incisors to correct the Bolton relationship after correcting the canines to a Class I occlusion (**21.3**).

Diagnosis, skeletal classification:
*   Class II.
*   Facial type: severe brachyfacial.
*   Maxilla: normal.
*   Mandible: mild retrusion.
*   Convexity = 5 mm.

Diagnosis, dental classification:
*   Severe Class II division 2.
*   Overjet = 3 mm.
*   Traumatic deep overbite lingual to the upper incisors.
*   Upper incisors: severe retrusion.
*   Lower incisors: severe retrusion.
*   1 to A/Po = –10 mm.
*   Interincisal angle = 180°.
*   Full unit Class II molar relationship.

Treatment plan:
*   Stage 1: arch development. An upper sagittal appliance to advance the upper incisors was the first step in releasing the mandible. This appliance includes occlusal cover over the upper posterior teeth to help relieve compression of the tissue behind the condyles in the TM joint.
*   Stage 2: orthopaedic phase. Sagittal Twin Blocks to continue to advance the upper incisors and simultaneously to posture the mandible downwards and forwards to initiate correction of the distal occlusion. This stage also built up the vertical dimension by adjustment and vertical traction to encourage eruption of the lower posterior teeth.
*   Stage 3: support phase. To maintain the corrected occlusion and support the vertical dimension.
*   Stage 4: orthodontic phase. Upper and lower fixed appliances to level and align the arches and detail the occlusion.
*   Stage 5: restorative phase. To restore the width of the upper anterior teeth to the correct Bolton relationship with the lower anterior teeth and maintain the intercanine width to stabilise the corrected occlusion.

Clinical management. The patient quickly experienced a remission of headaches during the first stage of treatment as the upper incisors advanced. The improvement continued throughout the treatment and the headaches did not return. After 9 months of treatment with the sagittal appliance, the patient occluded only on the upper and lower anterior teeth and a posterior open bite was present and showed no sign of resolving.

Twin Blocks were fitted to an edge-to-edge incisor occlusion with two sagittal screws in the upper appliance to continue to advance the upper incisors.

Separators were placed between the lower molars to free the contacts to facilitate the eruption of these teeth. The upper bite block was

RD

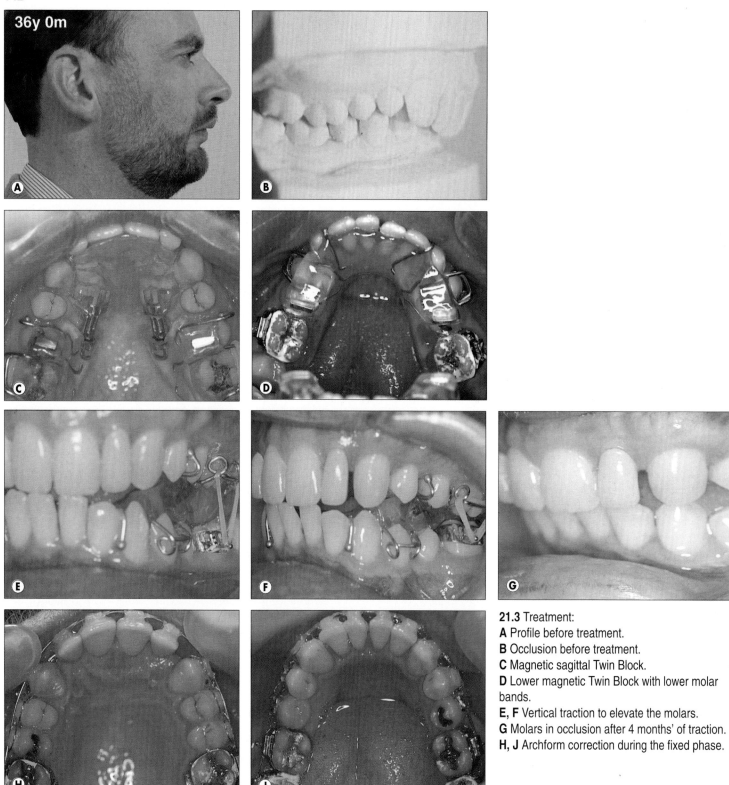

21.3 Treatment:
A Profile before treatment.
B Occlusion before treatment.
C Magnetic sagittal Twin Block.
D Lower magnetic Twin Block with lower molar bands.
E, F Vertical traction to elevate the molars.
G Molars in occlusion after 4 months' of traction.
H, J Archform correction during the fixed phase.

RD

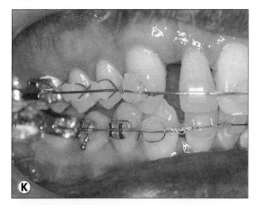

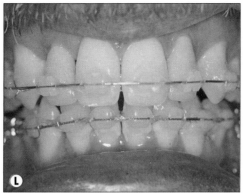

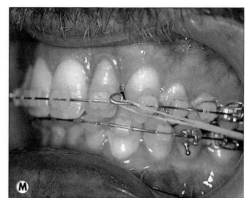

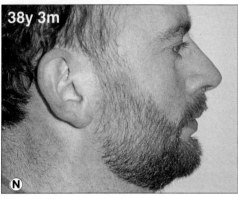

21.3 Treatment (cont.):
K–M Phase 2 – fixed appliances.
N Profile at age 38 years 3 months.

trimmed over the lower molars. Bands were fitted on the lower first molars a week later and vertical elastics were passed from the delta clasps on the upper molars to buccal hooks on the lower molar bands to accelerate eruption. The lingual flange of the lower Twin Block should extend distally to the molar region to prevent lingual tipping of the lower molars when a vertical elastic is applied.

Within 4 months of applying vertical elastics the lower molars erupted fully into occlusion with the upper and lower incisors in edge-to-edge occlusion. The intergingival distance increased from 7 to 20 mm with the molars in occlusion.

Adjustment of the screws continued to advance the upper incisors and to correct to a Class I molar relationship. After 9 months an anterior inclined plane was fitted with an occlusal stop to maintain the vertical correction, and vertical elastics were now applied to accelerate the eruption of the second lower premolars.

Four months later upper and lower fixed appliances were fitted to level and align the arches and detail the occlusion.

TM joint radiographs confirmed that the condyles were positioned downwards and forwards in the glenoid fossa after treatment and that the degree of movement is good. Progress TM joint images confirm that the condyles were displaced from the glenoid fossae when Twin Blocks were fitted but are observed in good position in the fossae 10 months later.

Duration of treatment:
- Arch development: 9 months with the upper sagittal appliance.
- Orthopaedic phase: 9 months with Twin Blocks.
- Support phase: 4 months with an anterior inclined plane.
- Orthodontic phase:
- Retention: continuing.

RD

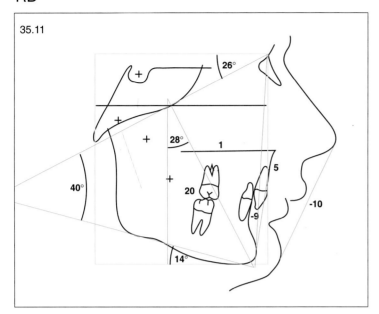

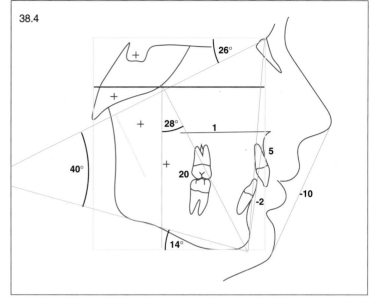

Maxillary Plane at ANS

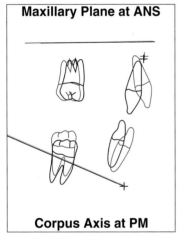

Corpus Axis at PM

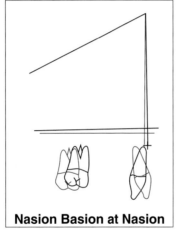

Nasion Basion at Nasion

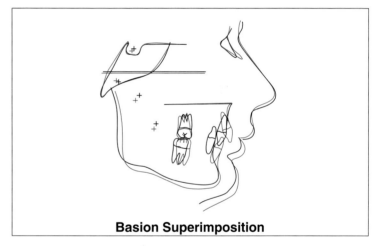

Basion Superimposition

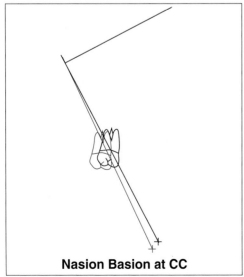

Nasion Basion at CC

R.D. -	Age 35.11	38.4	(Yr.Mon)
Cranial Base Angle	26	26	
Facial Axis Angle	28	28	
F/M Plane Angle	14	14	
Craniomandibular Angle	40	40	
Maxillary Plane	1	1	
Convexity	5	5	
U/Incisor to Vertical	−11	14	
L/Incisor to Vertical	14	28	
Interincisal Angle	177	138	
6 to Pterygoid Vertical	20	16	
L/Incisor to A/Po	−5 ~9	−2	
L/Lip to Aesthetic Plane	−10	−10	

THE TWIN BLOCK BIOFINISHER

The Twin Block biofinisher attachment is an alternative method of extruding lower molars by vertical traction in order to increase the vetical dimension to stabilise the temporomandibular joint. The biofinisher attachment has a hook for an elastic that extends above the upper molar in the vestibule. The objective is to achieve a longer elastic span for extrusion of lower molars. The attachment is inserted in horizontal tubes over the interdental embrasures in the molar region. The biofinisher attachment is removable, and may be worn at night and removed during the day. Alternatively, elastics may be attached directly to the delta clasps to be worn full time (**21.4 A,B**).

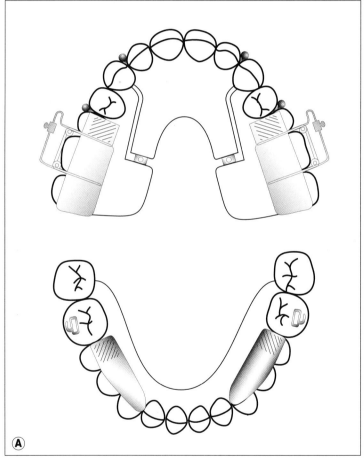

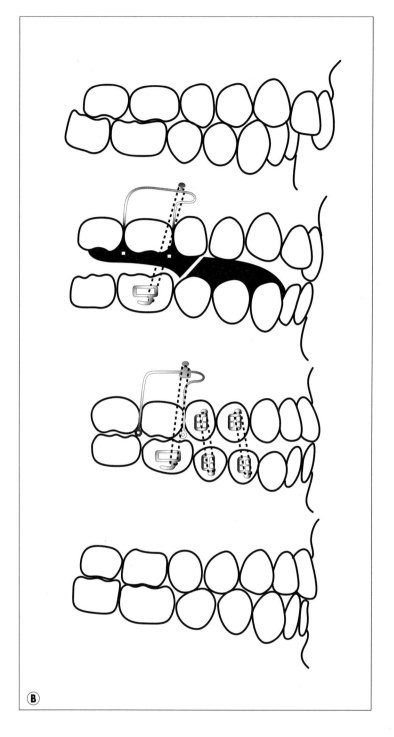

21.4 A, B Twin Block biofinisher. **A** Occlusal view. **B** Side view.

REFERENCES

Hawthorn, R. & Flatau, A. (1990). In *A Textbook And Colour Atlas of the Temporomandibular Joint Diseases, Disorders, Surgery*, eds J.E.deB Norman & Sir P. Bramley. London, Wolfe Medical Publications.

Llynn, J.M. (1985). "Biofinisher", *The Functional Orthodontist*, **2**(2): 36–41.

Solberg, W.K. (1989). *Temporomandibular Disorders*, 2nd edn. London, British Dental Journal, pp. 91, 92.

Spahl, T.J. (1993). The Spahl split vertical eruption acceleration appliance system. *Functional Orthod.*, **10**(1): 10–24

Fixed Twin Blocks

Any orthodontic or orthopaedic appliance system requires sufficient versatility to treat a wide range of malocclusions, and the facility to adapt to meet differing clinical requirements.

The advantage of fixed appliances compared to removable appliances is the increased control by the operator, which does not rely on the compliance of the patient. This is an essential feature of treatment planning when patient motivation does not ensure full-time wear. The patient's cooperation is assured if the appliance is either fixed permanently to the teeth, or is removable only by the operator as a fixed/removable component.

AESTHETIC APPLIANCE DESIGN

A major factor which improves patient cooperation and motivation is aesthetic appliance design. The aesthetic principle has been applied to fixed and fixed/removable Twin Block appliances with no visible anterior wires.

Integration with Wilson lingual appliances

The integration of the Twin Block with Wilson 3D modular appliances results in a fixed functional appliance system that is adaptable to the requirements of combined orthopaedic and orthodontic technique.

The Wilson 3D modular system is suitable for early intervention and arch development. The use of the Wilson 3D lingual tube as a retentive element on molar bands provides a means of attachment for occlusal Twin Block components, which may be fixed or fixed/removable, under the direct control of the operator. The facility to combine orthopaedic and orthodontic components by using a common retentive element extends the capabilities of both appliance systems.

Three distinct phases of treatment can be defined as follows:

- First phase: interceptive treatment and arch development by the Wilson modular appliance system.
- Second phase: orthopaedic treatment by the fixed/functional Twin Block system.
- Third phase: detailed orthodontic correction by bonded fixed appliances.

FIXED TWIN BLOCKS – FUNCTIONAL COMPONENTS

The Twin Block transpalatal arch

This component consists of a transpalatal arch with occlusal inclined planes over the posterior teeth that can be cemented in place. The inclined planes are secured by occlusal wire tags that are an extension of the transpalatal wire. The entire assembly is secured in Wilson lingual tubes on upper molar bands by the standard Wilson plug-in attachment.

The Twin Block lingual arch

The occlusal inclined plane component in the lower arch is combined with the Wilson 3D lingual arch, and extends over the occlusal surfaces of the lower deciduous molars, or premolars, depending on the stage of development. The appliance may be used in mixed dentition, when functional correction can be combined with interceptive treatment for arch development by the lingual arch. The Omega loop should be omitted to provide a more rigid attachment (**22.1**).

The Twin Block Hyrax appliance

The Hyrax screw is commonly used with fixed appliances for rapid maxillary expansion. Transverse development can be combined simultaneously with mandibular advancement by adding Twin Blocks to a rapid maxillary expansion appliance. The lower appliance may be anchored on lower second deciduous molars and may incorporate a lower lingual arch (**22.2**).

Occlusal inclined planes

The occlusal inclined planes are designed to occlude at a 70° angle mesial to the occlusion with the lower molar. The position of the inclined planes is critical in establishing vertical molar control in cases with deep overbite, where it is important to free the lower molar to erupt to control the vertical dimension.

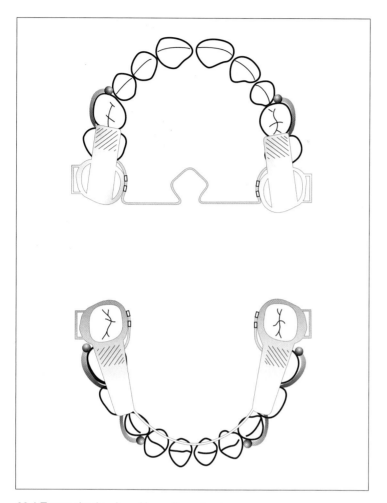

22.1 Transpalatal arch and lower lingual arch.

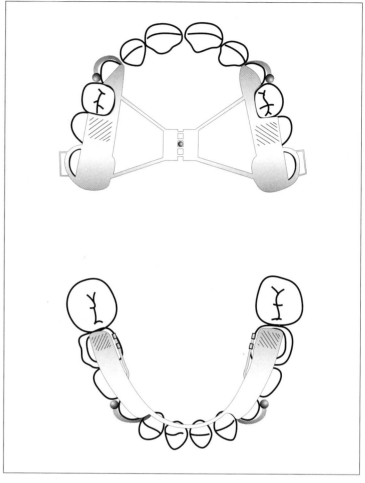

22.2 Hyrax design with lower lingual arch on second deciduous molars.

FITTING FIXED TWIN BLOCKS

It is recommended that the correct archform is established in both dental arches as a preliminary to fitting fixed Twin Blocks for functional orthopaedic correction. This ensures that the arches will occlude together correctly when the mandible is translated to a forward position. When this has been achieved, the lingual arches are removed and impressions are taken over molar bands to construct the fixed Twin Block appliances in the laboratory.

The occlusal components of Twin Blocks are designed to be removable from the lingual tubes on molar bands together with the Wilson lingual component. This allows the molar bands to be tried in

the mouth independently of the Twin Blocks, to check the fit of the bands. The next step is to assemble the Twin Block appliances and molar bands in one piece and to try it in the mouth as a unit. If the appliance is easily inserted in this way it may be cemented as a unit. Alternatively, the bands may be cemented first, before attaching the occlusal and lingual components. The same material may be used to attach the occlusal blocks or, alternatively, they may be bonded. Light cured composite offers the additional advantage of adequate working time to ensure that the blocks are fully engaged on the occlusal surfaces before the composite is activated to set.

As a precaution against occlusal caries it is essential to apply fissure sealant prior to fitting the occlusal blocks (**22.3**).

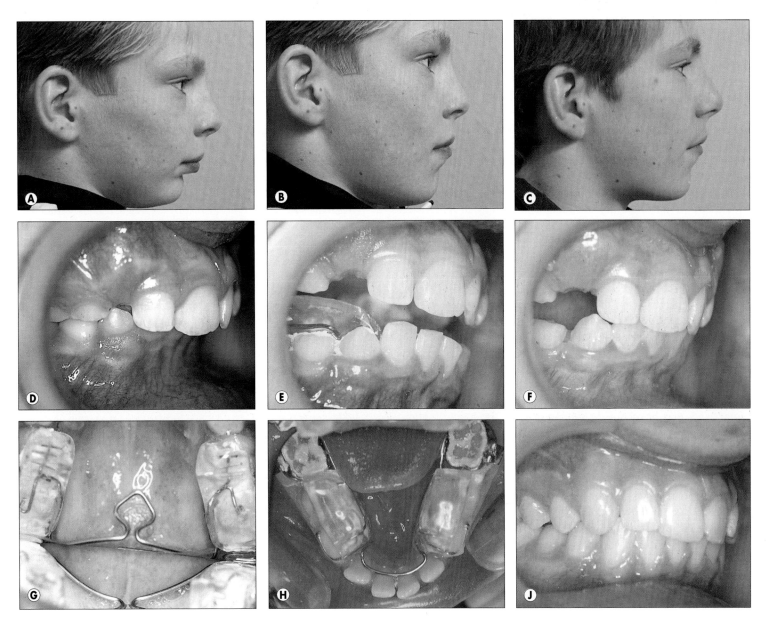

22.3
A, B Change in profile when fixed Twin Block was fitted.
C Profile at age 13 years 6 months.
D Occlusion before treatment at age 11 years 7 months.
F Change in occlusion after 8 months with Twin Blocks.
E, G, H Fixed Twin Blocks in position.
J Occlusion at age 15 years 7 months.
Treatment was completed with fixed appliances after eruption of
permanent teeth.

CLINICAL MANAGEMENT

The management of fixed Twin Blocks is very similar to the steps described in the management of removable Twin Blocks, except that fixed Twin Blocks are only removable by the operator for adjustment.

When the appliances are tried in the mouth, it is advisable to check that the blocks occlude correctly and are shaped correctly to allow the objectives of treatment to be achieved. This relates particularly to the patient being able to achieve a comfortable occlusion in a forward mandibular posture.

As described with removable Twin Blocks, the patient and parents should first be shown the dramatic improvement in facial appearance, from the anterior view and in profile, before cementing the appliance. This is a strong motivating factor, as it demonstrates an immediate improvement in facial balance.

Next, check the effect of the occlusal bite blocks on vertical dental development. The same provisions apply as for removable Twin Blocks.

To correct deep overbite the upper bite blocks are trimmed occluso-distally before fitting the appliance to allow eruption of lower molars to reduce overbite. Normally, vertical development of the molars can be delayed in the mixed dentition stage until the lower arch has been translated to a forward position. This allows the first permanent molars to be used as a means of fixation for the Twin Block lingual arch component. Vertical elastics to lingual and buccal hooks on opposing molar bands may be used in the support phase to accelerate eruption.

Appliance maintenance

In the early stages of treatment it is necessary to establish that the appliance settles in comfortably and that the patient is consistently occluding the mandible forwards in the desired position. Failure to do so would be indicated by an increased posterior open bite, which could be detected within a week of fitting the fixed Twin Blocks.

If the correct forward posture is not being achieved, there are two alternatives. First, the forward activation of the inclined planes may be reduced by removing the lower appliance and trimming the posterior inclines of the bite blocks, removing 1 mm at a time to reduce the activation, before checking the occlusion in the mouth to ensure that the patient can comfortably posture to the new position. If necessary, repeat the trimming until the patient occludes comfortably with forward guidance on the blocks.

Alternatively, an upper fixed appliance may be fitted, with provision for Class II intermaxillary elastics, to guide the mandible forwards.

When the patient has settled comfortably with fixed Twin Blocks and is posturing forwards correctly, maintenance should be routine at 3–4 week intervals. It is advisable to make more frequent checks than with removable appliances, and patients should be advised to contact the office immediately if anything breaks or comes loose. If the bite blocks become loose they may be removed with the Wilson lingual or transpalatal arch and reattached without necessarily removing the molar bands.

When the sagittal relationship is fully corrected, usually within 4–6 months, the lower molars may be freed from the Wilson attachment to allow them to erupt, with the help of vertical elastics if required.

Support phase: fixed anterior inclined plane

The anterior inclined plane is constructed from two Wilson 3D sectional appliances joined anteriorly by an inclined plane, which extends far enough around the upper arch to engage the six lower anterior teeth. For additional strength, the sectional wires may be replaced by a heavy-gauge lingual bar attachment soldered to Wilson lingual posts. This may be combined with a standard Wilson lower lingual arch to maintain the arch length and archform in the lower arch as the buccal segments erupt into occlusion.

In the support stage of treatment a full-bonded fixed appliance may be fitted to level the occlusal plane and detail correction in the lower arch.

Detailed orthodontic correction

Depending on the timing of treatment, orthodontic correction may be a separate phase of treatment after the permanent teeth have erupted, or may be a consecutive stage after the active treatment phase.

In the author's experience the management of fixed Twin Blocks is more difficult than the removable version. The blocks can become detached from the teeth, involving an immediate visit for repair. In addition, adjustment for control of the vertical dimension is limited after the appliance is fitted. If the lower molars are used for fixation of the appliance it is not possible for them to erupt for correction of deep overbite. Taking these disadvantages into account, removable Twin Blocks are preferred.

23

Growth Response to Twin Block Treatment

This study was designed to investigate the changes occurring in a group of 74 consecutively treated patients with Class II division 1 malocclusion, treated by the Twin Block traction technique. This study was of an early series of patients treated with a combination of Twin Blocks, with extraoral traction and intermaxillary traction, worn at night using the Concorde facebow., The sample consisted of 43 girls and 31 boys aged before treatment from 9 years 6 months to 14 years. The method of examination was by serial cephalometric analysis before and during treatment, at the end of retention, and on average 18 months out of retention. Where possible, patients were followed through to check the long-term results several years out of retention.

Tracings recorded 19 angular and 18 linear measurements to assess a range of craniofacial and dental changes for comparison with control values that relate age to growth changes. Allowance was made for sexual dimorphism in comparison with controls of untreated patients.

CONTROL GROUPS

Two sets of published cephalometric standards were selected as an appropriate basis for comparison as control values.

Control group 1
An Atlas of Craniofacial Growth, Riolo *et al.* (1979).
This study was based on examination of 83 individuals, 47 males and 36 females, with continuous attendance at the University School from their sixth to sixteenth birthdays, who were x-rayed on their birthday at yearly intervals.

Magnification
The distance from the x-ray target to the midsagittal plane of the subject was 5 feet (152.25 cm). The distance from the midsagittal plane of the head to the film surface was 7.625 in (17.84 cm). This geometry produces a 12.7% enlargement in all linear measurements reported in this control study.

Data for control group 2 was calculated at source to arrive at the same enlargement factor as the Michigan data, to allow direct comparisons to be made.

Control group 2
A Mixed Longitudinal Interdisciplinary Study of Growth and Development, Prahl Anderson *et al.* (1979).
This control sample examined a group of untreated patients biased towards a Class II dental relationship. This was, therefore, a more appropriate control sample to use for comparison with a series of patients with Class II malocclusion who received treatment.

MATERIAL AND METHOD

Cephalometric analysis
Serial cephalometric x-rays were taken at the following intervals:

* Before treatment commenced.
* When the overjet was reduced.
* On completion of stage 1 – the active Twin Block phase.
* On completion of stage 2 – the support phase.
* On completion of stage 3 – retention.
* Post-retention examination, on average 18 months out of retention.

In 57 cases the first x-ray was taken on average 6 weeks before treatment commenced. During that period normal growth occurred. No correction was made for this, and the calculation and summation of growth changes during treatment for statistical analysis includes this short period of normal growth before treatment commenced.

The average time between the first and second x-ray was 7.3 months, which included the 6 weeks pretreatment period in 57 cases. This was equivalent to an average active stage of treatment of 6 months with Twin Blocks in addition to the pretreatment period of 6 weeks.

The control values are based on annual growth increments and, in order to allow a direct comparison to be made, radiographs were selected as near as possible to a year after the initial cephalograms. A correction was made to annualise the changes in comparison to the control. On average this includes a period of 7.3 months from the initial cephalogram to the end of the Twin Block phase, followed by 4.7 months of passive support with an anterior inclined plane following the Twin Block stage.

STATISTICAL ANALYSIS COMPARED TO UNTREATED CONTROL SAMPLES

The results of analysis were subjected to Student's 't' test, and changes were assessed as follows:

$p < 0.001$ = highly significant (***)
$p < 0.01$ = significant (**)
$p < 0.01$ = probably significant (*)

Michigan series controls

A comparison with the Riola control values (Riolo *et al.*, 1979) revealed the following significant changes:

- Reduction of maxillary protrusion by retraction of the A-point (*/***).
- Reduction of anteroposterior skeletal discrepancy by a combination of maxillary retraction and, to a lesser degree, mandibular advancement (***).
- Retraction of the upper incisors (**/***).
- Increase in the interincisal angle (**/***).
- Reduction of convexity by retraction of the A-point relative to the facial plane (*/***).
- Advancement of the lower incisor tip relative to A–Pg (**/***).
- Retraction of the upper molars, measured to the pterygoid vertical (**/***).
- Increase in mandibular length, except in the age group 13–13.11 (**/***).
- Increase in ramus height, except in the age groups 11–11.11 and 14–14.11 (*/***).
- Increase in facial height, nasion–menton (**/***).

Nijmagen series controls

Significant changes were noted in the factors compared to controls in the Prahl Anderson series (Prahl Anderson *et al.*, 1979) as follows:

- Reduction of maxillary protrusion by retraction of the A-point (**/***).
- Reduction of anteroposterior skeletal discrepancy by a combination of maxillary retraction and, to a lesser degree, of mandibular advancement (***).
- Retraction of the upper incisors and reduction of the overjet (***).
- Increase in mandibular length in the age group 10–12.5 (articulare–gnathion) (***).
- Increase in facial height (nasion–menton) (*/***).
- Increase in the gonial angle, but not throughout the age range (*/**).

EVALUATION OF MEAN GROWTH CHANGES

Mandibular growth change in boys

This was asssessed by recording the dimension Ar–Gn as follows:

1 Period of treatment
For direct comparison with control values the changes were examined in 31 boys during the first year of treatment (mean age before treatment = 11 years 9 months). This represented on average 7.3 months of treatment from the initial cephalogram to the end of the Twin Block stage, followed by 4.76 months of passive support. The mean period examined was 12.06 months, and a slight conversion was made to record the annual change.

- Mean before treatment = 109.63 mm.
- Mean after treatment = 114.79 mm.
- Mean increase in Ar–Gn = 5.16 mm per annum.
- Mean annual growth rate of control for this age group = 2.71 mm.
- Increased growth compared with control = 2.45 mm.

2 Post-treatment observation period = 27.54 months
- Mean at end of treatment = 114.79 mm.
- Mean at end of observation = 121.02 mm.
- Mean increase in Ar–Gn = 2.71 mm per annum in the period of observation, exactly equivalent to the annual growth rate of the control sample.

Growth in facial height

Period of treatment (boys):
- Mean facial height before treatment = 116.90 mm.
- Mean facial height after treatment = 123.19 mm.
- Increase in facial height during treatment = 6.29 mm.
- Mean annual growth rate of control group for this age group = 2.58 mm.
- Increased vertical growth in treatment compared with control = 3.71mm.

Mandibular growth change in girls

A similar calculation was done for 43 girls, mean age before treatment = 11.6 years.
1 Period of treatment
- Mean before treatment = 106.81 mm.
- Mean after treatment = 110.84 mm.
- Mean annual increase in Ar–Gn = 4.0 mm.
- Mean annual growth rate of control for this age group = 1.83 mm.
- Increased growth compared with control = 2.17 mm.

2 Post-treatment observation period = 23.53 months
- Mean after treatment =110.84 mm.
- Mean after observation = 114.41 mm.
- Mean annual increase during observation = 1.89 mm.
- Mean annual growth rate for control group for this age group = 1.83 mm.

Growth during the observation period after treatment was exactly equivalent to the mean growth rate of the control sample.

Period of treatment (girls):
- Mean facial height before treatment = 117.40 mm.
- Mean facial height after treatment = 122.33 mm.
- Increase in facial height during treatment = 4.93 mm.
- Mean increase in control for this age group = 1.16 mm.
- Increased vertical growth in treatment compared to control = 3.77 mm.

A comprehensive account of the statistical analysis of growth changes in Twin Block functional therapy has been presented in a thesis submitted to the University of Dundee (Clark, 1995).

Discussion

It should not be expected that all patients who undergo functional therapy will show increased mandibular growth compared to the norm for their age. Some patients grow at a rate less than the norm while others exceed the normal rate of growth, with or without functional therapy. A lack of growth response may be related to the level of endocrine activity that prevails at the time of treatment. If treatment occurs during a resting phase of growth, the potential for increased mandibular growth is more limited.

As stated in Newton's third law of motion: 'To every action there is an equal and opposite reaction'. Functional appliances, therefore, exert equal and opposite forces in the opposing dental arch and have the reciprocal effect of restricting the forward component of maxillary growth. If a patient grows slowly during treatment, functional mandibular protrusion is more likely to retract the maxilla than advance the mandible.

On the question of the timing of treatment, Enlow (1983) stresses that 'the utilization of the pubertal growth spurt is coming rather late'. This observation applies especially to the treatment of Class II division 1 malocclusion where prominent upper incisors are vulnerable to trauma, and early treatment is indicated after eruption of permanent incisors. Class III malocclusion also responds to early intervention in the deciduous or mixed dentition, when the addition of forward pull traction to a facemask may be considered to increase the potential for maxillary advancement.

It is especially important to treat girls early because growth slows considerably after menstruation commences. There is more leeway in boys, who mature later and still show useful growth in their middle and late teens. As a general principle the response to treatment is related directly to the patient's rate of growth. Therefore, for patients beyond the middle teens,the older the patient the less growth we should expect and we should not presume growth changes in adults. But this does not preclude muscular advancement of retruded mandibles in adults with functional appliances, which may be indicated if the condyles are displaced posteriorly or superiorly in the glenoid fossae.

CONCLUSION

In the pursuit of ideals in orthodontics, facial balance and harmony are of equal importance to dental and occlusal perfection. We cannot afford to ignore the importance of orthopaedic techniques in achieving these goals by growth guidance during the formative years of facial and dental development.

As a new century approaches, the integration of orthodontic and orthopaedic techniques offers a new iniative in restoring facial balance for patients who present skeletal growth discrepancies

To catch dame Fortune's golden smile
Assiduous wait upon her,
And gather gear for ev'ry wile,
That's justified by honour.

Epistle to a Young Friend
Robert Burns, 1759–1796

REFERENCES

Clark, W.J. (1995). *Aspects of Twin Block Functional Therapy in Orthodontics and Dentofacial Orthodontics*. DDSc thesis submitted to the University of Dundee.

Enlow, D. (1983). On craniofacial growth. *ICI Interviews*, **17**: 669–79.

Prahl Anderson, B., Kowalski, C.J. & Heydendael, P.H.J.M. (1979). *A Mixed Longitudinal Interdisciplinary Study of Growth and Development*, University of Nijmagen, San Francisco Academic Press.

Riolo, M.L., Moyers, R.E., McNamara, J.A. Jr., Stuart Hunter, W. (1979).*Cephalometric Standards from the University School Growth Study*. Monograph No. 2. Craniofacial Growth Series, Center for Human Growth and Development, The University of Michigan.